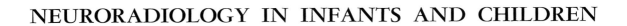
NEURORADIOLOGY IN INFANTS AND CHILDREN

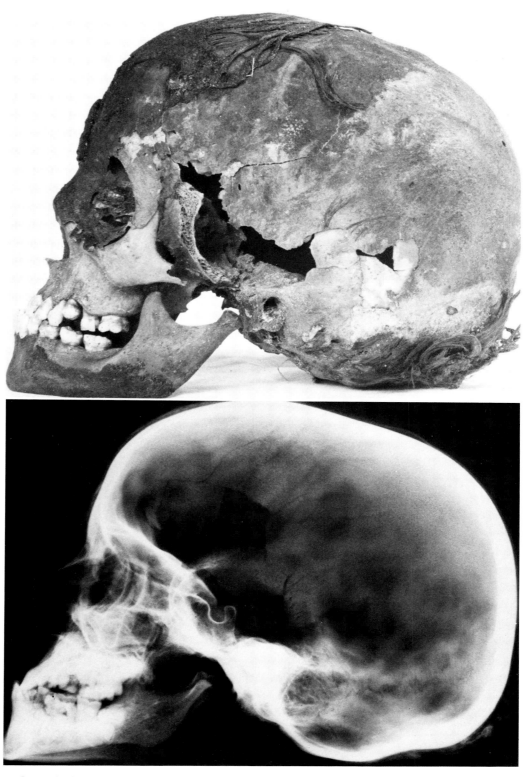

A lateral photograph and a lateral skull radiograph are of an 8-year-old female mummy from the Fayum area outside Cairo. The date of the burial is estimated to be 2,400 years ago. We believe she died of a severe comminuted skull fracture of the frontoparietal region, presumably due to a direct blow. The brain contents were removed prior to mummification via this defect rather than via a trocar-formed approach through the nose and sphenoid bone. A small glistening scarab beetle is seen in the left upper eyelid. (Mummy courtesy P. Lewin, M.D., Toronto.)

VOLUME THREE

NEURORADIOLOGY IN INFANTS AND CHILDREN

DEREK C. HARWOOD-NASH, M.B., Ch.B., F.R.C.P.(C)

Head, Division of Paediatric Neuroradiology,
The Hospital for Sick Children;
Professor of Radiology, University of Toronto,
Toronto, Ontario, Canada

with the assistance of

CHARLES R. FITZ, M.D.

Paediatric Neuroradiologist,
Department of Radiology, The Hospital for Sick Children;
Assistant Professor of Radiology, University of Toronto,
Toronto, Ontario, Canada

with 3931 *illustrations*

THE C. V. MOSBY COMPANY

Saint Louis   1976

Printed in the United States of America

Distributed in Great Britain by Henry Kimpton, London

Library of Congress Cataloging in Publication Data

Harwood-Nash, Derek C
  Neuroradiology in infants and children.

  Bibliography: p.
  Includes index.
  1. Pediatric neurology. 2. Nervous system—
Radiography. 3. Pediatric radiology. I. Fitz,
Charles R., joint author. II. Title. [DNLM:
1. Neuroradiography—In infancy and childhood.
WL141 H343n]
RJ488.H37   618.9′28′047572   76-27253
ISBN 0-8016-2086-4

CB/CB/B 9 8 7 6 5 4 3 2 1

CONTRIBUTORS

ROBERT E. CREIGHTON, M.D., F.R.C.P.(C)

Anesthetist, Department of Anesthesia, The Hospital for Sick Children;
Associate Professor of Anesthesiology, University of Toronto,
Toronto, Ontario, Canada

DAVID L. GILDAY, B.Eng., M.D., F.R.C.P.(C)

Head, Division of Nuclear Medicine, Department of Radiology,
The Hospital for Sick Children; Associate Professor of Radiology,
University of Toronto, Toronto, Ontario, Canada

BERNARD J. REILLY, M.B., Ch.B., M.A., F.R.C.P.(C)

Radiologist-in-Chief, Department of Radiology,
The Hospital for Sick Children; Professor of Radiology,
University of Toronto, Toronto, Ontario, Canada

**The generosity of the Physicians and Surgeons Foundation,
Incorporated, Toronto, is gratefully acknowledged.**

FOREWORD

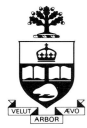

The motto on the coat of arms of the University of Toronto is well fulfilled by the publication of this pioneer work. "Growing like a tree through the ages" describes well the appearance and development of neuroradiology at this university medical center. Immediately after the conclusion of World War II, the development of clinical neurological sciences required that there be included on the team a radiologist devoted to the new discipline, neuroradiology. Thus was planted the seed from which sprang and grew a tree with three major branches—service, education, and research. The seed, planted at the Toronto General Hospital, grew through the 1950s and 1960s to a residency and fellowship program in neuroradiology. Its graduates became in turn the seed for new growths in other facilities of this university medical center and beyond.

Derek Harwood-Nash, a product of Rhodesia, obtained his early medical training at the University of Capetown, where his interest in surgery was awakened. Coming to the University of Toronto to commence training in that specialty, he was exposed, while in neurosurgery, to neuroradiology and to its maestro Dr. George Wortzman. This combination, the *specialty* with its precision of technique and almost daily expansion of knowledge and the *specialist* as a role model, served as turning points in a career pathway. Dr. Harwood-Nash very quickly directed his training to the radiological side of neurosciences and, on completion of his formal training program, joined the staff of The Hospital for Sick Children. Here he recognized at once a gap in the spectrum of knowledge of neuroradiology in the field of paediatrics. With characteristic energy he began to cultivate a third-generation tree of knowledge, which—thousands of man-hours and five years later—has blossomed in the form of this monumental work, the world's first complete textbook of paediatric neuroradiology.

The information set forth in this vast display has application well beyond the paediatric field, since, as a result of advances in treatment of patients in their first two decades, the authors and their neuroradiological findings are being encountered increasingly in the adult setting.

It was not until I examined the manuscript of this book that I appreciated the enormous amount of planning, organization, and dedication contributed by Dr. Harwood-Nash and his colleagues, not to mention the self-discipline that is the sine qua non for any such effort.

As one who has watched with great interest the development of Dr. Harwood-Nash's career since his first day as a radiological resident, I am pleased, but not surprised, to see this major accomplishment come into being before its creator has reached the age of forty, at which age, they say, life begins.

R. Brian Holmes, M.D., F.R.C.P.(C)

Professor of Radiology
Dean, Faculty of Medicine
University of Toronto
Toronto, Ontario, Canada

PREFACE

A CHILD IS NOT MERELY A SMALL ADULT. This oft quoted aphorism is eminently appropriate when applied to the practice of paediatric medicine and in particular to the diseases of the central nervous system and its bony coverings in infants and children. Paediatric medicine now parallels adult medicine in scope and complexity, and this is especially true of paediatric neuroradiology.

Neuroradiology has evolved slowly from the pioneer efforts of Dandy with ventriculography and pneumoencephalography and Moniz with cerebral angiography to the inevitable birth and development of paediatric neuroradiology. The basic principles and practice of adult neuroradiology have had to be modified to deal with the peculiarities of childhood diseases. The complexity of developmental neurological diseases, the prevalence of posterior fossa tumors and hydrocephalus, and the physiology of skull sutures are a few of the many instances that make paediatric neuroradiology different.

The present work deals with the radiological diagnosis of abnormalities of the skull, spine, and their contents in infants and children. The methods by which such diagnoses are made constitute the practice of paediatric neuroradiology. The raison d'être of a book dedicated to this topic, distinct from that of books concerned with adult neuroradiology, is threefold: childhood nervous systems, anatomy, and diseases are peculiarly different, and they change with growth. The smaller size of infants and children demands dissimilar or modified neuroradiological techniques. Affections of the skull and spine and central nervous system are common indications for the admission of a child to hospital.

This book is directed toward the adult neuroradiologist with an interest in children, the paediatric radiologist with a minor interest in neuroradiology, the neurosurgeon whether or not he is required to perform and interpret his own neuroradiology in children, the paediatrician and the neurologist who desire an understanding in objective diagnosis by neuroradiology in children, and particularly the physician who is to become a paediatric neuroradiologist.

Paediatric neuroradiology is essentially an objective science tempered by one's own clinical experience, tinged by imagination, blended with a delicate touch because the margin for error is small.

The formidable task of molding an instructive text, an atlas of radiographs, and a bank of references has, we hope, been achieved without detriment to the value of one or another of these facets. The broad philosophy of this book is to present the normal, a logical and methodical description and analysis of the abnormal, and a consideration of the possible pathological entities in the final specific diagnosis. The nature of the disease so diagnosed in neuroradiology is such that a microscopic diagnosis from surgery or autopsy is usually soon forthcoming, providing an excellent radiographic-pathological correlation. We thus hope to furnish the reader with the facts to fulfill the teaching dictum "understand the normal, recognize the abnormal, identify the site, and know the pathological possibilities." The reader will then be able to proceed from the general to the particular in a practical and intellectual fashion.

The contents of this book are arranged to describe initially the details of normal embryology and radiographic anatomy of the central nervous system and its bony coverings. Within each chapter, particular attention is given to succinct prose; we have elected to provide many headings and subheadings as well as lists and step-by-step accounts of procedure protocol or natural history of diseases; and we have included tables showing differential diagnoses, radiographic signs, and the like, with the hope that continuity, interest, and intellectual understanding will be preserved.

The gross *anatomy* of the skull, spine, and central nervous system structures is sufficiently different in infants and children to merit detailed description, in both routine and special neuroradiological procedures. To appreciate changes from the normal, the examiner must pay meticulous attention, first, to the delicate *techniques* of neuroradiology in infants and children, second, to the spectrum of *procedures* and their variations for the adequate demonstration of structures and diseases, and, third, to the awareness of possible *com-*

plications of such techniques in general and of those peculiar to children.

Subsequent chapters follow a pattern parallel with the clinical assessment of the patient and deal with pathological changes that occur in hydrocephalus, head injuries, benign and malignant intracranial neoplasms, and mass lesions of the spinal canal. The book is patient oriented, written by clinical neuroradiologists. Our principles and practice of the art of paediatric neuroradiology are based on a large case experience and have been modified and improved over nine years. These principles continue to undergo change even while the book is being written. Just as a neuroradiological study shows a disease at a point in time, so our book presents our knowledge at the present time. Computed tomography, needless to say, is such an exploding discipline that the text had to be updated day by day. There is a minor but unavoidable duplication of specific entities. The text, however, makes their relative significance quite clear.

With few exceptions, the radiographic illustrations in the book are derived from case records of patients referred to us at The Hospital for Sick Children. Occasionally, on seeing an illustration, the reader will have a feeling of déjà vu. Such repetition allows for a more thorough and thoughtful discussion. The descriptions and illustrations of the neuroradiological diagnostic philosophies and investigative techniques in the book are those in use at The Hospital for Sick Children. We readily acknowledge that they may not correspond in part or in whole with those at other centers; we believe them to be correct, however, due to the large patient volume available to us, and thus they provide the reader at least a comprehensive basis for intellectual dissection.

The Hospital for Sick Children has 760 active care beds. The department of radiology performs over 100,000 examinations a year. The division of neuroradiology performed less than 600 special procedures in 1968, but 1,500 in 1975. A shared computed tomographic unit has given way to our own total body machine. Virtually all the statistics contained in this book are our own; the majority represent the experience of *nine* years of practice, during the period 1968 to 1976 inclusive. These are compared and contrasted with the few relatively important comprehensive reports available. Many disease entities discussed herein have, unfortunately, no such additional data. We hope thus to provoke other writers to augment our data with theirs.

In trying to maintain a proper balance between experienced opinion and objective measurements and statistics, we consider that, in the practice of paediatric neuroradiology at least, the dogmatic adherence to percentages and measurements of radiographic anatomical detail is not always valid. A number of diagnostic conclusions arise from purely subjective assessments of a neuroradiological examination, and these are difficult to detail in objective terms. A great variation exists in the normal skull and its contents between infants and children of different ages and indeed within the same age group. The student of paediatric neuroradiology will often have to rely on this general subjective assessment rather than on the possible deviation from a specific set of figures and measurements.

This hospital is blessed with a pleasant and effective personal liaison between its component medical disciplines, particularly so between ourselves and the staff of the clinical neuroscience services and anesthesiology. The present work therefore reflects the influences of many of these physicians and surgeons— and to them collectively must go our sincere appreciation and respect—in particular, Dr. E. Bruce Hendrick, Dr. Harold Hoffman, and Dr. Robin Humphreys, who supplied the majority of patients illustrated in this book. Dr. Robert Creighton, Anesthesiologist, Dr. David Gilday, Head of Division of Nuclear Medicine, and Dr. Bernard Reilly, Radiologist-in-Chief, have contributed to the manuscript and we give them our sincere thanks. Dean Brian Holmes, who unconsciously provided the stimulus for this book, graciously wrote the Foreword.

Within the Department of Radiology, however, there are three groups of people who are an integral part of this book and to whom we are greatly beholden.

The first is a group made up of the composite of a person. Dr. Bernard Reilly has been many people to us. He is an amalgam of contributor to the book, supporter, politician, protector, critic, teacher, intellect, and friend. With him we have heavily invested in the product of that pure water from Strath Spey, originally so well doctored in the nineteenth century by the Grant brothers of Glenlivet and Glenfiddich. Dr. Reilly's encouragement could well have been

> Wha first shall rise to gang awa
> A cuckolde coward loun is he!
>
> Wha first beside his chair shall fa
> He is the king amang us three.

Robert Burns would have been proud of us.

The second group is a large number of technologists and nurses who cared for and worked on so many ill children. Their products, the radiographs of the head and spine, are what this book is about; and these radiographs are good. Mrs. Chris Montgomery initially and now Miss Ilze Priverts, our supervising technologists, started with us, continue with us, and barring uncontrollable circumstances will still be with us. Editorial secretaries, initially Margaret Rutherford, and especially Lora Klimovitch, correctly deciphered atrocious handwriting and mumbled dictation and worked long and hard. Our own secretary, Gail Lopes, was and is willing to take on any task and made order out of chaos.

The third and overwhelming group is our clinical neuroradiological fellows. In chronological order they are Drs. David Breckbill, Joseph Thompson, Martha Chaplinsky, Donald Hardman, Augustus O'Gorman, Krishna Rao, Paul Berger, John Murray, Donald Kirks, and presently David Boldt and Jonathan Barry. Many of the studies were performed and diagnoses made by them. Their efforts, ideas, and criticisms spawned the statistics, radiographs, references, thoughts, and words that made this book possible. Their irreverent and often iconoclastic arguments made us honest, stimulated us, and kept us desperately trying to stay ahead. They are good people and we are better and thankful for having had them with us. Dr. Boldt and Dr. Barry, willing "galley slaves," will never want to read another textbook.

Mary Casey, medical artist without compare, provided all the line drawings; and Eva Struthers and her staff photographed and often improved upon the many thousands of radiographs we gave them. Their expertise and hard work are evident in virtually every page of this book.

The production of this book would have been impossible without the great generosity of the Physicians and Surgeons Foundation, Incorporated, of Toronto.

The bulk of the manuscript for the book was written during 1975, the centennial year of The Hospital for Sick Children; and we dedicate the book, in part, to this hospital. We also dedicate the book in part to those children who, by their own diseases, gave us experience to better manage present and future children with similar afflictions. Finally, we dedicate the book in part to the acknowledgment and sharing of our families—who truly understand why and how it was written.

We hope that the format and contents of this book will provide a logical, concise, and accurate treatise for the radiological diagnosis of diseases of the central nervous system in infancy and childhood. We also hope that the book will be comprehensive enough to detail and yet fill the entire spectrum of paediatric neuroradiology. It is a large book. It is an indication that paediatric neuroradiology can be a full-time and even a lifetime occupation.

Derek C. Harwood-Nash
Charles R. Fitz

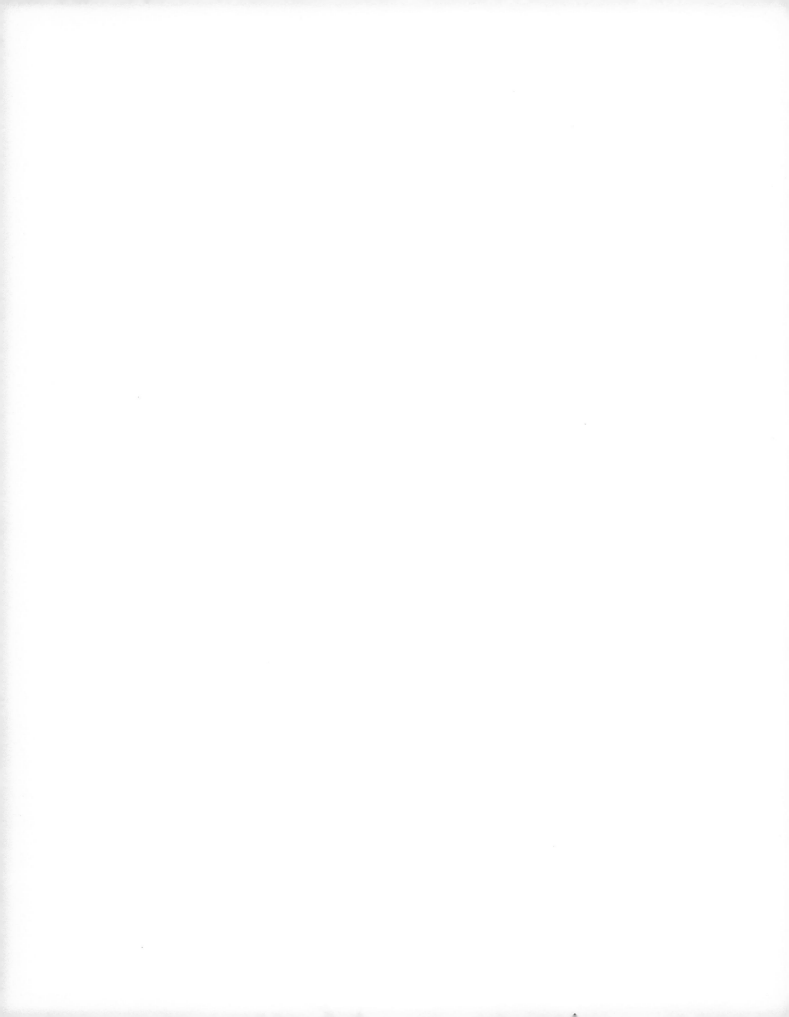

INTRODUCTION

In the Fall of 1967, the opportunity presented itself to design a new in-patient department of radiology at The Hospital for Sick Children. Carte blanche was limited only by the square footage available in the proposed new wing. To be considered were not only the architectural and topographic details related to patient flow and patient load but also the philosophical demands of the development of paediatric radiology in our hospital over the ensuing ten years. The one feature, for weal or woe, unique to this hospital was size. There were 820 active treatment beds filled on a referral basis by children from a watershed area with a population of almost 4 million. Yet largeness creates its own problems. To wallow in volume is easy. The amount of interesting case material and the intellectual stimulation of the hospital as a whole can foster insularity. A life dedicated to patient care, consultation, and education within a monolithic institution such as this might be fulfilling; but there is an obligation to share.

Also, because of patient volume, divisionalization into specialties within paediatric radiology was not only desirable but inevitable. Though the passing of the generalist may be lamentable, the knowledge explosion has made it impossible for one man to be an expert in all facets of paediatric radiology. No matter how much we would like to retain versatility as an ideal in radiology or in the practice of medicine as a whole, specialization means that patients get the best available facilities for diagnosis and treatment. So the omniscient clinician has been replaced by a team of experts all acting in cooperation for the good of the patient.

In deciding which segment of the department would be most productive, not only in patient care and academic excellence but also in the promulgation of new ideas, there were two possible approaches: We could pick the area of interest, invest in the appropriate equipment, and then find the right individual to run that segment of the department. On the other hand, we could find the individual, give him or her the space and equipment required, and then stand by for take-off. We chose the latter and were in the enviable position of not having to look far. Dr.

Harwood-Nash was obviously a man in search of a challenge.

In 1967 paediatric neuroradiology was ripe for development. This is not to say that the other departmental subdivisions were neglected. Far from it. All the subdivisions have been developed in an atmosphere of healthy competition and each radiologist has a major interface with a clinical division or department. It was just that I had the right man in the right place at the right time and he was straining at the bit.

During the almost three years before the new department became a complete reality, Dr. Harwood-Nash and his colleagues made the most of a makeshift special procedures room, working in cramped quarters while the new area was taking shape. Around him grew a team of nurses and technicians with a morale and esprit de corps that carried them through all the frustrations of equipment breakdowns and building delays.

Into a space of 4,000 square feet were planned three large special procedures rooms, one for pneumoencephalography and ventriculography and two for arteriography. Two rooms for skull radiography and one for polytomography were immediately adjacent. Two automatic processors were installed, one at each end of the area; and in the large viewing and consulting section there was an electronic subtraction unit. From the hub of this division, which was the nursing station, we could survey a well-equipped and roomy special procedures area. But we had to be adaptable to new trends and developments. When CT scanning hove onto the horizon, one of the angiography rooms had to be torn apart and redesigned to hold the scanner. CT head scanning is now an integral part of neuroradiology and is, as yet, in its infancy.

A practical problem in performing neuroradiological procedures on a patient population with a span stretching from birth to prematurity to the age of 18 is finding equipment that will fit all sizes. As an example, it was soon evident that there was no marketed pneumoencephalography chair in which an anesthetized infant could be adequately examined and monitored. One had to be created. Consultation with the engineers at Elema Schonander resulted in the production of a prototype of the special infant chair.

The precision and attention to detail that went into the planning and equipping of the Division of Neuro-radiology are typical of Dr. Harwood-Nash's approach to life in general. However, the intellectual stamina and self-discipline required for the long weeks and years that go into the production of a definitive work such as this are not qualities given to too many. They were obvious within the first year. In the tiny office that he shared with two other radiologists, Dr. Har-wood-Nash had a blackboard on which soon appeared a list of ten topics to be presented and published within twelve months. One by one they were methodically ticked off. The archives of the department and the hospital were scoured late into many evenings to find the mother lode of clinical material and radiographs before the latter went to the silver reclaimers. There were radiographs going back almost twenty years, and each one of neuroradiological interest was retrieved and inspected. As the book grew over the succeeding years, so did a large and superbly documented teaching collection for our residents and fellows.

Though other textbooks have emanated from The Hospital for Sick Children, the production of *Neuro-radiology in Infants and Children* is a first in the Department of Radiology, and we are all proud to bask in its reflected glory. So now in 1976 I can only assure my old friend and colleague that the biggest thrill in the life of any teacher is to be totally out-shone by a former pupil.

Bernard J. Reilly

CONTENTS

Intracranial infection

Historical recordings of intracranial infection have been predominantly of dural empyema and brain abscess (Gurdjian, 1969). Lebert (1856) and subsequently Gross (1866, 1873) provided the most detailed case reports of intracranial suppuration during the eighteenth and nineteenth centuries, culminating in a comprehensive treatise of the clinical and surgical approach to cerebral and nervous system suppuration by MacEwen in 1893.

Although reports of these infections in children were few, Wyss in 1871 had seventeen cases, MacEwen in 1893 had fourteen, and Holt in 1898 included his five cases in a review of thirty-two children under the age of 5 collected from the world literature. Holt's report emphasized the otitic origin of childhood intracranial suppurations. Infantile intracranial abscesses, however, were even less commonly reported. Sanford in 1928 reviewed the reports of nineteen infants having cerebral abscesses, seventeen of whom were discovered at autopsy. Hoffman and co-workers in 1970 added six infants, all under the age of 3 months, to reports of seventeen infants from this age group in the literature.

In a paediatric hospital, many infants and children with intracranial inflammatory processes are recognized and diagnosed clinically and are treated medically. The child with focal or progressive neurological signs or both, however, in whom a surgically treatable collection of pus is suspected *must* receive an urgent and complete neuroradiological assessment.

Classification of inflammatory processes

It is practical to subdivide inflammatory processes of the intracranial cavity into either diffuse or focal, involving either the brain tissue or the dural covering (Davis and Taveras, 1966). Due to the frequent combination of meningitis and encephalitis, meningitis is included as an inflammation of the brain tissue.

Inflammatory lesions of the skull and mastoids are discussed in Chapters 2 and 3.

Intracranial infections can be classified as follows:

Diffuse
  Meningoencephalitis
    Encephalitis (acute or chronic)
    Meningitis
  Ventriculitis
  Arachnoiditis
  Vasculitis
    Arteritis
    Mycotic aneurysms
    Cerebral venous and dural sinus thromboses
Focal
  Dural empyema and effusions
  Abscesses
  Parasites
  Granulomas

Neuroradiological diagnostic procedures

In paediatric neuroradiology, intracranial infection and its sequelae can be demonstrated in many forms. Cerebral edema (the brain's acute reaction to infection), focal mass effects (caused by suppurative foci), and late development of hydrocephalus due to CSF pathway obstruction can all result in *split sutures*. The more indolent inflammatory processes, however, whether indolent by nature of the character of the pathogen or by ineffective antibiotic therapy of the inflammation, do not necessarily result in split sutures. Local chronic or cystic inflammatory processes (as with some parasitic infections), or coarctation of the temporal ventricular horns, for example, can lead to *local expansion* of the related bony vault. Granulomatous lesions of the brain per se and inflammatory vasculitis do not usually exhibit radiographic abnormalities of the skull.

It cannot be stressed too strongly that the clinical presentation of the child, the acuteness of the presentation, the CSF abnormalities (if known), and the presence of unilateral seizures or EEG abnormalities or both must all be carefully considered and discussed prior to initiating a neuroradiological sequence of events. If an *acute* abscess or a focal encephalitis is suspected, a full series of radiographs of the skull and as complete a set of cerebral angiograms as are needed should be obtained without delay. The angiograms may demonstrate a mass lesion, arterial abnormalities associated with meningoencephalitis, various venous occlusions, or a combination of these abnormalities.

In the child with an intracranial or a distant inflammatory process and in whom a bleeding mycotic aneurysm is suspected along with a subarachnoid hemorrhage, bilateral carotid and vertebral angiography should be performed. In the child whose clinical presentation is *less acute,* the course of action can be indicated more completely via brain scans—including rapid and delayed imaging—and computed tomography (Chapter 8). Conventional tomograms are necessary for the child whose intracranial infection is suspected to originate in one or the other petrous bone, such as infection due to a fracture, mastoiditis, or an infection occurring in the frontal sinuses.

Depending on the degree of raised intracranial pressure, suspected postinflammatory chronic hydrocephalus in a child necessitates an initial ventriculogram or pneumoencephalogram. If any significantly increased intracranial pressure is present, it is essential to perform ventriculography rather than pneumoencephalography. The child with dilated ventricles, dilated sulci, or both, and without head enlargement or split sutures, could have an underlying abnormality such as mild extraventricular obstructive hydrocephalus (EVOH), superficial or deep cerebral atrophy, or even a combination of these. Cerebral inflammation can create either hydrocephalus or cerebral atrophy in varying degrees of severity. In attempts to differentiate between these two entities, CSF scans are most valuable.

Radionuclide studies and computed tomography also are becoming more valuable in early neuroradiological assessment of the child with a suspect intracranial infection. They help with the decision whether further neuroradiological investigation should be performed and, if so, which study first. As a general rule, surgical treatment of virtually all forms of intracranial pathology ought not to be planned on the basis of radionuclide studies and computed cranial tomography alone.

DIFFUSE BRAIN INFECTIONS
Meningoencephalitis and meningitis

The two inflammatory processes meningoencephalitis and meningitis may coexist. The former displays certain neuroradiological signs of the latter, and vice versa. Either may be bacterial (e.g., caused by *Haemophilus influenzae* or *Diplococcus pneumoniae*) or viral (caused by mumps or herpes simplex).

Encephalitis

Encephalitis in the *acute* stage may be focal rather than diffuse and will commonly produce a focal mass effect. Herpes simplex is most often the cause of focal encephalitis (Radcliffe et al., 1972). Diffuse brain swelling, such as that occurring with *Haemophilus*

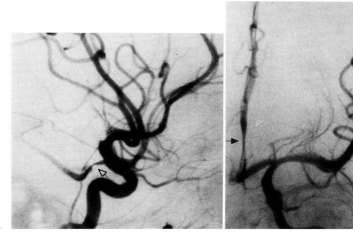

A **B**

Fig. 13-1. **Inflammatory cerebral edema.** Diffuse bilateral frontal encephalitis and edema have produced transtentorial cerebral herniation with depression and partial occlusion of the posterior communicating and posterior cerebral arteries (**A,** arrow) and interhemispheric compression of the anterior cerebral artery (**B,** arrow). It is the depression of the posterior communicating artery, however, rather than of the anterior choroidal artery, that reflects the uncal herniation.

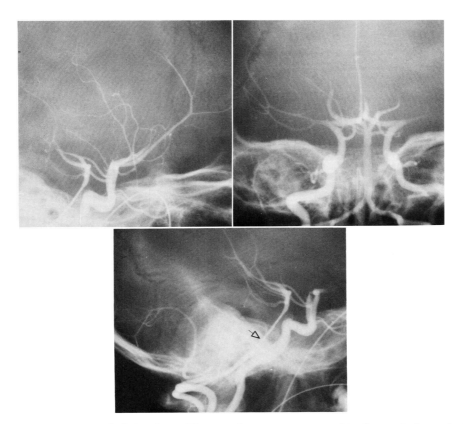

Fig. 13-2. Severe encephalitic edema. This may be so severe as to virtually preclude cerebral flow. Note the small narrowed cerebral vessels and the basilar artery tightly compressed against the clivus (arrow). There is reflux of contrast from the right internal carotid injection across to the other side and down the basilar artery.

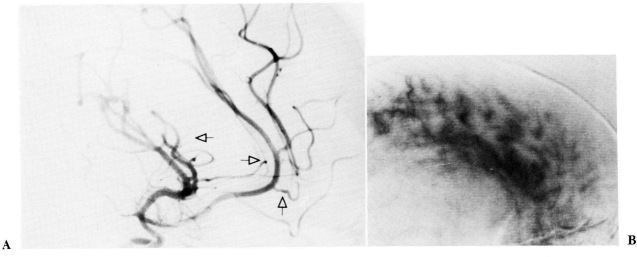

A

B

Fig. 13-3. Temporal lobe encephalitis. A, Displacing the middle cerebral artery anteriorly and superiorly due to herpes simplex. Associated compression irregularities and occlusions of the peripheral cerebral arteries can be seen (arrows). B, Displacing the cerebrogram superiorly and anteriorly due to a similar infection in the temporal lobe of another child.

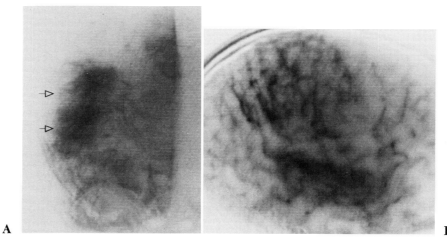

A   B

Fig. 13-4. Cerebrogram and local encephalitis. A, Prolonged (arrows), in a temporal lobe encephalitis. **B,** Similarly prolonged, in a posterior parietal encephalitis. A normal overlap of anterior cerebral and middle cerebral peripheral branches, however, may produce a similar but normal increased cerebrogram that is less well defined.

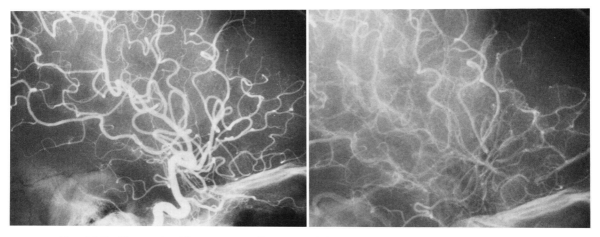

Fig. 13-5. Abnormal pial arteries. Diffuse encephalitis produces dilated small pial arteries, many of which arise directly from the main trunk of a cerebral branch.

influenzae infection, may lead to marked cerebral herniation (Fig. 13-1) or a degree of cerebral edema (Dodge and Swartz, 1965) so severe as to dramatically diminish cerebral blood flow (Fig. 13-2).

The angiographic changes resulting from a focal encephalitis may simulate those resulting from a neoplasm (Margolis et al., 1972):

1. A rapidly developing mass effect frequently situated in the posterior temporoparietal area (Fig. 13-3)
2. A prolonged cerebrogram due to capillary stasis (Fig. 13-4) (we have not observed frank leakage of contrast from capillaries into the sulcal subarachnoid space [Raimondi, 1972])
3. Abnormal dilatation of arteries over the inflamed area, similar to the cerebritis stage of abscesses due to loss of arterial tone

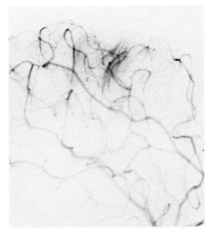

Fig. 13-6. Increased perfusion. An area of focal encephalitis exhibits rapid perfusion of pial vessels in the parietal lobe.

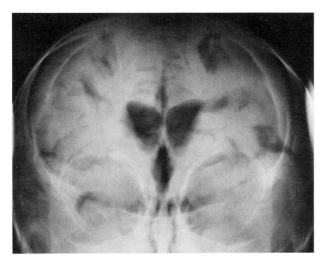

Fig. 13-7. Postinflammatory atrophy. Dilatation of the lateral ventricles and sulci can be seen at pneumoencephalography after diffuse meningoencephalitis.

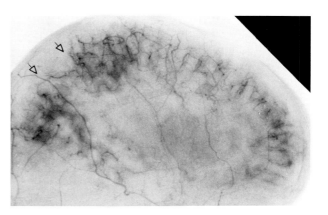

Fig. 13-8. Postencephalitic infarct. An area of absent gyral cerebrogram is due to an occipital cortical infarct (arrows).

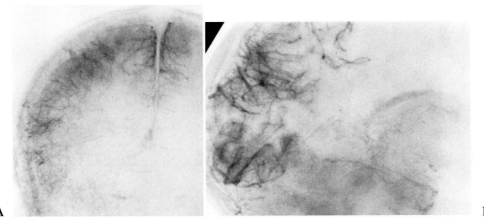

Fig. 13-9. Meningitis. Stasis and dilatation of the pial vessels have created a general cortical cerebrogram (**A**) and a focal occipital gyral cerebrogram (**B**). These changes are similar to the changes seen with encephalitis and probably represent the effects of a combination of the two entities.

4. Small dilated pial vessels arising directly from a large cerebral artery branch (Fig. 13-5) in which the flow is slowed (a similar finding is seen in local areas of contused brain)

5. Increased perfusion (Fig. 13-6) and arteriovenous shunting (Ferris et al., 1968; Radcliffe et al., 1971)

Pneumoencephalography should not be performed on children who have a suspected acute meningoencephalitis, for it may result in tentorial or tonsillar herniation in the face of increased intracranial pressure.

With purulent meningoencephalitis, as with a pneumococcal infection, intra-arachnoid empyema may result. Differentiation between subdural em-pyema and intra-arachnoid empyema by angiography is difficult.

Encephalitis in the *chronic* stage is evidenced at pneumoencephalography by increased size of the ventricles and sulci due to brain atrophy (Fig. 13-7). If the encephalitis is associated with ependymitis, an IVOH may result—particularly if the aqueduct is occluded (Johnson and Johnson, 1968). If the inflammation is severe enough, resultant areas of infarction may lead to development of single or multiple porencephalic cysts. These cysts are seen in infants, particularly after a septicemia and encephalitis with enteric bacilli.

Pneumoencephalography shows just the objective evidence of brain atrophy, not the etiology—whether it be infection, trauma, or cerebral cellular disease.

Angiography may show chronic changes in affected areas of the brain, such as a diminished cerebrogram effect with small irregular pial vessels representing an area of local infarction (Fig. 13-8).

Congenital cytomegalic inclusion disease (Birnbaum et al., 1969), herpes simplex (Schaffer, 1966), and probably rubella (Peters and Davis, 1966; Harwood-Nash et al., 1970; Rowen et al., 1972) are cerebral infections that with toxoplasmosis cause cerebral calcifications in infants. In older children, viral en-

cephalitis may lead to nonspecific calcification (Swischuk, 1973). These effects are demonstrated and discussed in Chapter 2.

Meningitis

Meningitis commonly occurs in the first month of life: two in every 10,000 full-term births, twenty in every 10,000 premature births (Overall, 1970). In the neuroradiology of meningitis, angiographic changes are usually intermingled with the signs of encephalitis (Raimondi, 1972). It is difficult to assess by these changes alone which of the two, meningitis or en-

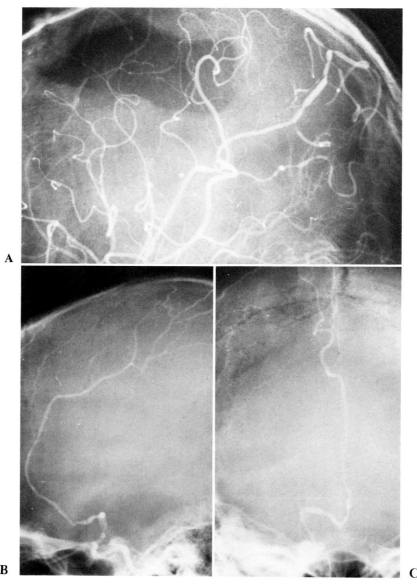

Fig. 13-10. Purulent meningitis. A, Diffuse stenoses and areas of dilatation, particularly in the posterior parietal and angular arteries. **B** and **C,** Occlusion of the middle cerebral artery with stenosis of the supraclinoid internal carotid artery and irregular stenoses and dilatation of the anterior cerebral artery. (**A** courtesy C. Suwanwela, M.D., Bangkok.)

cephalitis, is the dominant condition. Thus the following may present: mass effects, vascular dilatation, subdural effusions or empyema, and hydrocephalus.

Mass effects from focal encephalitis and edema, together with related *large vessel dilatation* (Davis et al., 1970) and an increased gyral cerebrogram (Fig. 13-9), are commonly noted on angiograms of children with meningitis. Vessel narrowing may also be seen, *generally* associated with cerebral edema or *locally* either in concert with the dilatation or alone (Fig. 13-10) (Ferris et al., 1968). These narrowings can develop into occlusions. In a few of our patients with

Haemophilus influenzae or purulent meningitis, we have seen the angiographic changes described by Lyons and Leeds (1967) of vasospasm, stenosis, and occlusion (Fig. 13-11), cerebral infarcts, slow arteriovenous circulation time, and collateral cerebral and meningeal blood supply. Tuberculous meningitis will often lead to a basal arachnoiditis with adhesions and stenosis of the intracranial portion of the internal carotid artery and its proximal branches. Dilatation or, rarely, irregular stenoses of anterior meningeal or posterior meningeal arteries in the subacute or chronic stages of meningitis occur (Fig. 13-12). Similar

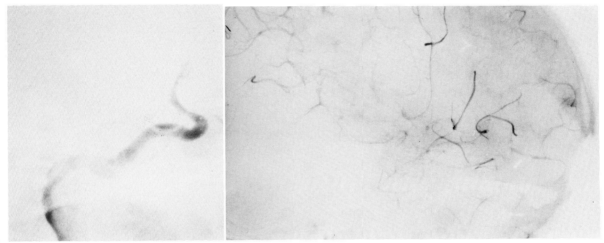

A   B

Fig. 13-11. Meningitis and arterial occlusions. A, Stenosis and occlusion of the supraclinoid internal carotid with *Haemophilus influenzae* meningitis as seen on a lateral carotid angiogram. **B,** Peripheral middle cerebral occlusions with a purulent meningitis.

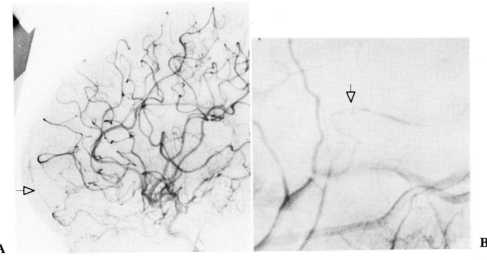

A   B

Fig. 13-12. Meningitis and meningeal arteries. A, Hypertrophy of the anterior meningeal (arrow). Note the diffuse dilatation of the pial vessels. **B,** Irregularity of the anterior branch of the middle meningeal (arrow).

changes can occur in the presence of subdural empyema or effusion.

Postmeningitic *subdural effusions* or *subdural empyema* (Goodman and Mealey, 1969) may occur, developing more commonly in infants than in older children. Effusions occur in 50% of infants with meningitis (Benson et al., 1960). Subdural taps will usually identify such effusional collections but may be negative when the collections are posteriorly placed. Angiography or ventriculography will demonstrate the location of an effusion or empyema. Often no history of infection is found, even in the presence of huge subdural effusions. Intrauterine infections may give rise to subdural effusions, for we have detected these at angiography within a few days of birth.

The development of *hydrocephalus,* particularly in children who have received inadequate antibiotic treatment, is relatively common with meningitis and occurs in 30% of infants surviving neonatal meningitis (Lorber and Pickering, 1966). If an associated ventriculitis exists, an IVOH may develop, particularly at the foramen of Monro or in the aqueduct; EVOH with arachnoiditis in the basal cisterns or around the cerebellum at the tentorium may also result (Chapter 10).

Ventriculitis

Ventriculitis was found in 92% of neonates who died of meningitis (Berman and Banker, 1966). Hydrocephalus, either intraventricular or extraventricular, is a common sequela. Ependymal inflammation is often associated with meningoencephalitis.

This ependymitis may produce a delicate hypervascularity on angiography as well as a positive brain scan, both creating a shadow of the large ventricle. Ventricular bands (Fig. 13-13, *A* and *B*), ventricular wall irregularities, formation of multiple encysted cavities within the ventricular system due to these bands (Fig. 13-13, *C*), or occlusions of the foramen of Monro, aqueduct, or foramen of Magendie may occur (Schultz and Leeds, 1973). Occlusions of the foramen of Magendie may also result from basal arachnoiditis or fourth ventricular ependymitis, causing an IVOH, usually seen in infants and associated with dramatic fourth ventricular dilatation (Chapters 6 and 10). A similar finding may occur when birth trauma or head injuries result in subarachnoid hemorrhage with occlusion of the foramen of Magendie by posttraumatic basal adhesions.

Ventriculography is the method of choice for investigating the sequelae of ventriculitis. The findings may be so bizarre that only in the event of an autopsy can the true geography of the cysts and bands become apparent.

Arachnoiditis

Arachnoiditis is difficult to diagnose neuroradiologically. Nonfilling with air of the cisterns or subarachnoid space over the cortex during pneumoencephalography does not necessarily indicate a pathological obstruction to CSF flow. Air may not pass where CSF will. For example, *only when* a normally filling cistern has been previously identified by pneumoencephalography can the presence of arach-

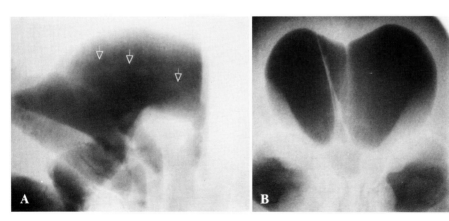
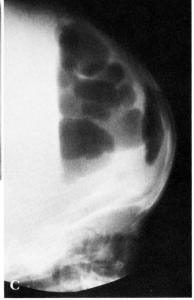

Fig. 13-13. **Ventriculitis. A,** Multiple slender intraventricular adhesions (arrows) within the body and posterior aspect of the lateral ventricles. **B,** Localized thick ventricular band in one frontal horn. **C,** Multiple ventricular bands forming loculations within dilated hydrocephalic ventricles.

noiditis around the optic nerves be inferred from non-filling of the chiasmatic cistern. Postmeningitic basal arachnoiditis with a vasculitis may lead to stenosis or occlusion of the arteries at the base of the brain.

We believe that an arachnoiditis leads to sequestration of various parts of the subarachnoid space, especially in the basal cisterns, creating a state of affairs as a result of which an ingress of CSF is permitted but no egress—ergo, an *arachnoid cyst* (Chapter 15). These cysts are frequently associated with hydrocephalus per se and may indeed be big enough to cause IVOH.

The main effect of arachnoiditis is obstruction of CSF flow somewhere along the extraventricular CSF pathway sufficient to produce an EVOH.

Inflammation of the cerebral vessels
Arteritis

Ferris and Levine (1973) have provided an excellent classification of cerebral arteritis occurring in all age groups*:

Bacterial arteritis
  Meningitis
  Cavernous sinus thrombophlebitis
  Osteomyelitis
  Abscess
  Embolism
Tuberculous arteritis
  Meningitis
  Tuberculoma
Mycotic (fungal and yeast) arteritis
  Tuberculous type
  Hyphal type
Syphilitic arteritis
  Meningovascular syphilis
  Gummatous meningitis
Necrotizing angiitis
  Periarteritis nodosa
  Hypersensitivity angiitis
  Rheumatic arteritis
  Temporal arteritis
  Allergenic granulomatous angiitis
  Wegener's granulomatosis
Carotid arteritis
Collagen disease arteritis
  Lupus erythematosus type
    Lupus erythematosus
    Scleroderma
    Dermatomyositis
    Rheumatoid arthritis
  Thrombotic thrombocytopenic purpura
Miscellaneous
  Rickettsial arteritis
  Viral arteritis
  Cysticercosis
  Radiation arteritis
  Chemical arteritis
  Acute hemorrhagic leukoencephalitis
  Sarcoidosis

*Modified from Ferris, E. J., and Levine, H. L.: Cerebral arteritis: classification, Radiology 109:327, 1973.

The many forms of angiitis that can occur in the brain are rare. They are not usually examined neuroradiologically in children; rather the diagnosis is made clinically or at postmortem examination. Granulomatous angiitis of the central nervous system (Peison and Padleckas, 1964), giant cell arteritis (Wagenvoort et al., 1963; Andrews, 1966), and rheumatoid vasculitis (Sievers et al., 1968) are common varieties. We have performed cerebral angiography on children with clinical diagnoses of temporal arteritis and also migraine; but, as yet, we have not identified any intracranial arterial abnormality associated with these latter two conditions.

The carotid arteritides (the largest group), about which we have very little information, are infections in children presenting with stroke (Shillito, 1964; Harwood-Nash et al., 1971; Hilal et al., 1971; Isler, 1971). These children have occlusions and/or irregularities of the cerebral arterial lumina in the absence of any predisposing clinical abnormality.

Bickerstaff (1964) theorized a relationship between arteritis and a past history of severe upper respiratory tract infections in some patients who developed an inflammatory response in the supraclinoid internal carotid arteries and branches. We support this contention (Harwood-Nash et al., 1971). Objective evidence of cervical internal carotid narrowing and intracranial arteritis has been present in our series. Shillito (1964) operated upon two such children and found nonspecific inflammatory changes in the vessels. These entities are discussed more fully in Chapter 14.

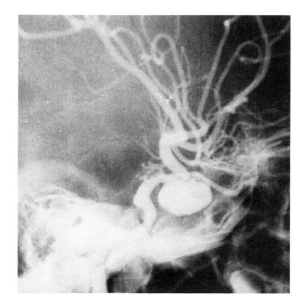

Fig. 13-14. Intracavernous carotid aneurysm. This was located proximal to the origin of the ophthalmic artery subsequent to a carotid sinus thrombosis. (Courtesy C. Suwanwela, M.D., Bangkok.)

Inflammatory vasculitis associated with meningitis and encephalitis has been discussed in the preceding pages of this chapter and will not be repeated. The arterial abnormalities seen at angiography are due to inflammatory exudate, granulation tissue, arterial wall edema, and adventitial fibrosis, or to a mixture of these factors.

Mycotic aneurysms

In the preantibiotic era, a third of intracranial aneurysms in children were mycotic (McDonald and Korb, 1939); however, more recent series (Matson, 1965) and our own (Thompson et al., 1973) indicate an incidence of 10%, though admittedly all three series are small.

The routes of infection into the vessel wall are an infective microembolus to the vasa vasorum (probable), an infective embolus in the lumen with thrombosis (unlikely), or a paravascular infection (possible) (Hannesson and Sachs, 1971). The inflammatory process initially involves the artery by endothelial swelling and proliferation, fibrinoid necrosis of all or part of the wall, intimal cellular swelling and hyperplasia, and infiltration of adventitia with chronically inflammatory cells. The necrosis leads to weakening and even rupture of the arterial wall.

These aneurysms, more correctly called septic rather than mycotic, may thus arise from infected cerebral vascular emboli (usually originating from subacute bacterial endocarditis) or be associated with purulent

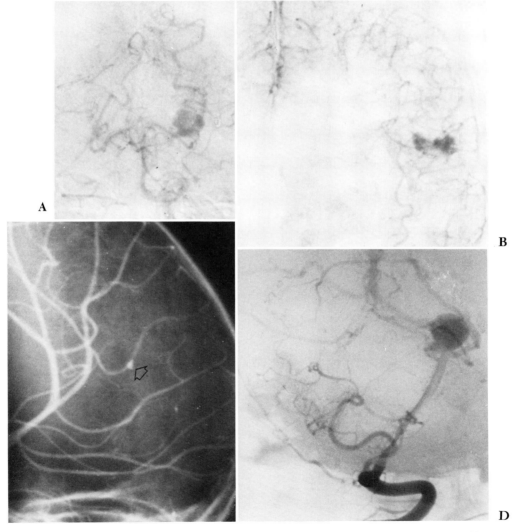

Fig. 13-15. Septic cerebral aneurysms. A, On the left posterior cerebral. **B,** On the left middle cerebral. **C,** On a branch of the anterior cerebral (arrow) in a patient with subacute bacterial endocarditis. This aneurysm subsequently bled. **D,** On the basilar tip. (**A** and **B** courtesy B. Annis, M.D., La Crosse, Wis.; **C** and **D** from Thompson, J. R., et al.: Am. J. Roentgenol. Radium Ther. Nucl. Med. **118:**163, 1973.)

meningitis (Ojemann et al., 1966; Hannesson and Sachs, 1971; Thompson et al., 1973); or they may occur concomitantly with other adjacent areas of infection as occur in cavernous sinus thrombosis (Fig. 13-14), osteomyelitis of the skull (Suwanwela et al., 1972), and mycotic infection (Morriss and Spock, 1970). It is interesting to note that, in our experience, abscesses have tended to occur with congenital heart disease whereas aneurysms have occurred with subacute bacterial endocarditis.

In the supratentorial arteries these aneurysms may be multiple (Fig. 13-15, A and B) (Bigelow, 1955; Thompson et al., 1973) and peripheral (Fig. 13-15, C); however, they may also be found at the basilar tip, as occurred in a 2-year-old boy with documented *Diplococcus pneumoniae* meningitis followed by bacterial endocarditis (Fig. 13-15, D). Which infection caused the intracranial aneurysm in this boy is a moot point.

Mycotic aneurysms may change in size and shape between successive angiograms (Roach and Drake, 1965; Cantu et al., 1966). As with the investigation of any aneurysm therefore, all vessels must be studied by angiography—including both vertebral arteries, if no retrograde filling is seen from the first vertebral injection. Both PICAs also must be visualized.

We have not seen an abscess and a septic aneurysm in concert. One aneurysm bled massively into the frontal lobe.

Although we have had no experience with this type, fusiform aneurysms can occur in syphilis (Blackwood et al., 1966).

Most cerebral aneurysms occurring in children tend to be large (Fig. 13-16) (Thompson et al., 1973) and have an irregular lumen (Fig. 13-15). It is difficult therefore to relate with any accuracy the criteria applied to differential diagnosis between septic and berry aneurysms in adults and children. Suffice it that peripheral aneurysms in children are probably septic. Furthermore, could it be that most aneurysms in children are indeed septic and that very few are truly "congenital"?

Venous thromboses

Cerebral venous and dural sinus thromboses may be associated with local septic conditions or with generalized infections, trauma, or intracranial neoplasms; or they may be primary and aseptic. A thrombosis of a cortical vein, dural sinus, or both may occur. Clinical signs and symptoms in children are often quite difficult to evaluate. The clinical presentation depends on the location and the degree of involvement, on the general clinical state of the patient, and on the underlying cause (if it can be determined). In many children the thrombosis may be subclinical.

Morgagni in 1761 was probably the first medical writer in history to refer to sinus thrombosis as an entity. Byers and Hass (1933) presented their experience with fifty infants and children who had had dural venous sinus thromboses before the era of antibiotic treatments. Their clinical description is remarkably concise. Over half their cases were ascribed to concurrent infections; the other half were associated mainly with severe dehydrating and debilitating conditions. Kalbag and Woolf (1967) in their monograph on intracranial venous thromboses reported thirty cases of all ages from a clinical, pathological, and radiological viewpoint. Greitz and Link (1966) considered aseptic thromboses of intracranial sinuses in all age groups. Vines and Davis (1971) discussed in detail the clinical and radiological correlation in such thromboses (Yaşargil and Damur, 1974).

In brief, the entities that may be associated with intracranial venous thromboses in children are as follows:

Inflammatory
  Meningitis
  Encephalitis
  Brain abscess
  Subdural empyema
  Mastoiditis
  Face and scalp cellulitis
  Septicemia
  Tolosa-Hunt syndrome (Tolosa, 1954)
Aseptic
  Primary idiopathic
  Severe dehydration in infants
  Trauma (by direct injury, associated with subdural
    hematoma, or after craniectomy)
  Neoplasms (of brain or meningeal deposits)
  Hematological disorders (polycythemia, those
    occurring after cardiac bypass procedures, platelet
    abnormalities)

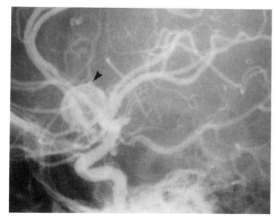

Fig. 13-16. Septic aneurysm. This occurred on the middle cerebral artery (arrow). (From Thompson, J. R., et al.: Am. J. Roentgenol. Radium Ther. Nucl. Med. **118:**163, 1973.)

Inflammatory thrombosis is associated with an inflammation of the endothelial lining of the sinus; whereas aseptic thrombosis is not (Byers and Hass, 1933; Krayenbühl, 1966b).

The sequelae of such thromboses may range from minor changes (e.g., unconsciousness), through hemi-paresis, subarachnoid hemorrhage, and seizures, to severe coma with cerebral edema and death (Byers and Hass, 1933; Krayenbühl, 1966b; Gabrielsen and Heinz, 1969).

NEURORADIOLOGY OF VENOUS THROMBOSES. It is unusual for infants and children to be neuroradiological-

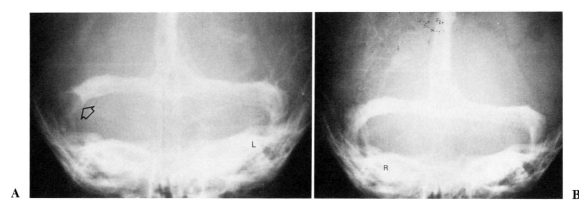

Fig. 13-17. Right transverse sinus pseudothrombosis. A, A left carotid injection fills the right transverse sinus, which has a pseudo-occlusion (arrow) in it due to dilution by the vein of Labbé. B, A right carotid injection fills the normal sinus completely.

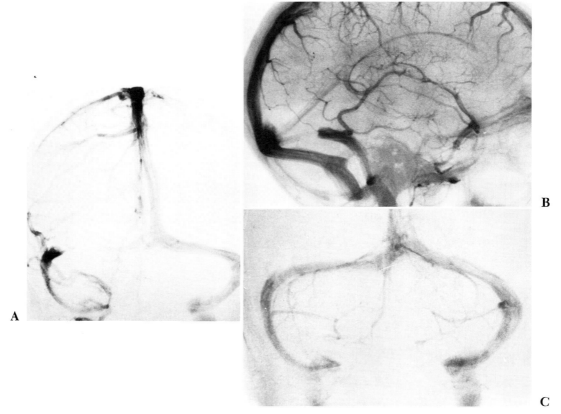

Fig. 13-18. Right transverse sinus pseudothrombosis. A and B, A right carotid arteriogram depicts a thrombosed sinus. C, A vertebral arteriogram demonstrates venous drainage into this apparently occluded sinus.

ly investigated for cerebral sinus thromboses per se. Such thromboses are generally identified during investigation for associated abnormalities as just detailed. In some children, cerebral venous thromboses may cause sudden hemiplegia as a complication of one of these underlying conditions.

GENERAL. The sagittal sinus in infants is often not a fully formed single venous channel but may be composed of interlocking veins close to the midline. The anterior portion may be absent or may drain anteriorly. In most children the sinus is fully formed only after 9 to 12 months of age, when the portion between the fontanelles becomes a single well-formed

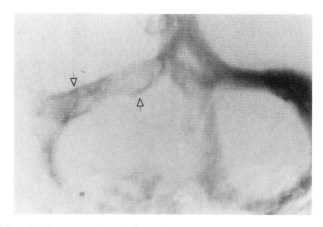

Fig. 13-19. Recanalized thrombosis. A right transverse sinus thrombosis has recanalized by intradural collateral channels (arrows) around the thrombus. Note the vertical central persistent occipital sinus.

channel. Similarly, the mobile lambdoid suture may be compressed inward and impinge on the sinus itself (Chapter 2). Though this compression of the suture occurs quite normally, in some children the sinus may be partially obstructed and the obstruction may presumably go on to produce in concert with infection a thrombosis. Such compression is commonly seen in children under the age of 2 months.

We have found a large left transverse sinus involved in at least 75% of children having thromboses, the left being normally larger than the right in at least 50%. The vein of Labbé may normally be quite large in infants. If contrast fills the transverse sinus on the side opposite the injection during carotid angiography, dilution of the contrast with unopacified blood from the vein of Labbé (Fig. 13-17) or the cerebellar veins (Fig. 13-18) into this sinus will produce a spurious occlusion.

Bilateral carotid and vertebral angiography is therefore essential in assessing sinus patency. As a rule, vertebral angiography alone gives poor filling of the transverse sinuses. On carotid angiography a poorly visualized inferior sagittal sinus is a normal phenomenon.

Differentiating a thin but normal transverse sinus from a recanalized previously thrombosed sinus is often difficult. Thin intradural falcine collateral venous channels or recanalized pathways may be visualized around a dural thrombosis (Fig. 13-19). Because the underlying thrombotic process may be seriously aggravated, however, direct sinus venography should not be performed in children. Neither do we advocate retrograde venography, for it lacks diag-

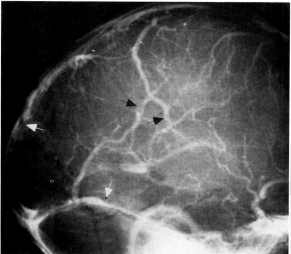

A

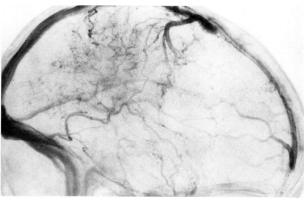

B

Fig. 13-20. Cortical venous thrombosis. A, Focal filling defects due to thrombosis (black arrows) are associated with partial transverse and sagittal sinus thromboses (white arrows). B, Tortuous collaterals. A diffuse cerebral blush in the parietal lobe is probably due to dilated tiny pial veins.

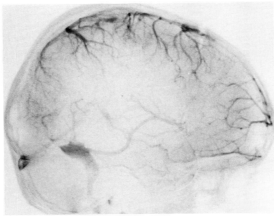

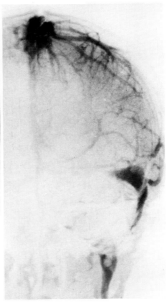

Fig. 13-21. Transverse sinus thrombosis. Occlusion of the medial half of the left sinus was subsequent to a meningitis.

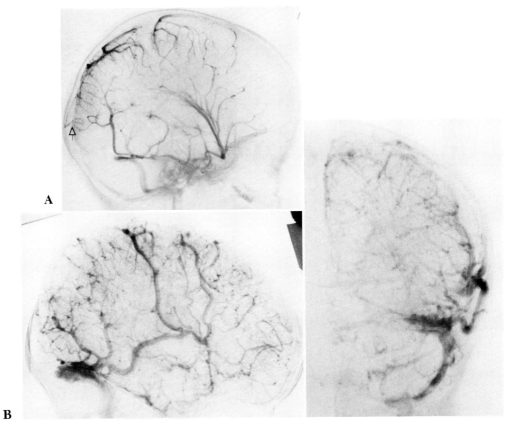

A

B

C

Fig. 13-22. Sagittal sinus thrombosis. A, Patchy, in an infant. Note the connection between a cortical vein and an extracerebral cranial or scalp vein (arrow). B and C, With transverse sinus and cortical venous thromboses and reversal of flow inferiorly via the vein of Labbé.

nostic accuracy in children due to both inadequate filling of the sinuses and the many anatomical variations. Furthermore, a false-positive result in venography is common.

An adequate volume of contrast in catheter arteriography, along with a sufficiently prolonged radiograph timing well past the normal venous filling phase is as essential as the procurement of good subtraction films. In our experience, these measures will ensure optimal angiograms in cases of suspected sinus thrombosis.

Focal filling defects with partial occlusions are not seen so commonly in the sinuses as in the cortical veins (Fig. 13-20, A). Tortuous collateral veins around sites of cortical vein thrombosis are frequently present (Fig. 13-20, B). Venous occlusive phenomena may be associated with regional infarcts and localized arteriovenous shunting as well (Greitz and Link, 1966; Gabrielsen and Heinz, 1969).

Neuroradiological detection of sinus thrombosis in children occurs more often in the transverse sinus (Fig. 13-21) than in the sagittal sinus (Fig. 13-22). A generalized arteriovenous circulatory delay sometimes develops; reversal of contrast flow in larger patent cortical veins away from the thrombosed sagittal sinus may also be observed (Fig. 13-22, B and C) (Vines and Davis, 1971). We have not seen thromboses of the vein of Galen or of the internal cerebral veins, conditions said to be fatal.

The term "otitic hydrocephalus" is a misnomer. The entity originates in a child as otitis media. A subsequent thrombosis of a dominant transverse sinus, together with cortical venous thromboses, leads to severe intracerebral edema and diffuse cerebral ischemia. If death does not supervene, residual cerebral atrophy results from this ischemia. Thus ventricular enlargement in such cases is due to atrophy, not to hydrocephalus per se. A concomitant hydrocephalus caused by subsequent postinflammatory arachnoiditis obstructing the CSF pathways or obliterating the arachnoid villi may be present but is certainly not due to chronic venous obstruction.

TRAUMA. *Acute* thromboses may result from occlusion of the sinus by a fracture, depressed or otherwise; by association with an area of cerebral contusion or laceration; or by the presence of an extradural hematoma (Chapter 12).

Chronic thromboses may result from compression and occlusion of cortical veins or sinuses contiguous with a chronic subdural hematoma and may occur along with the development of irregular tortuous abnormal veins that either were previously normal but have altered or are collateral pathways for blood flow.

INFECTION. Meningoencephalitis (Fig. 13-20, B), brain abscesses, or dural empyema may be an associated factor in venous and sinus thromboses (Fig. 13-23). Poor filling of the veins, the sinus, or both may ensue from a generalized or localized mass effect. The examiner should rely more on focal venous irregularities or sudden occlusion of the veins or sinuses than on the generalized nonfilling of a particular vessel.

When investigating a possible *cavernous sinus thrombosis*, the examiner may find the intracavernous portion of the internal carotid artery to be narrowed on an angiogram along with nonfilling of the cavernous sinus in the venous phase (Fig. 13-24). For the latter to be seen, meticulous subtraction or orbital venography is necessary.

The venous abnormalities associated with a subdural empyema, particularly those at its edges, are similar to the angiographic findings in a subdural hematoma (Chapter 12).

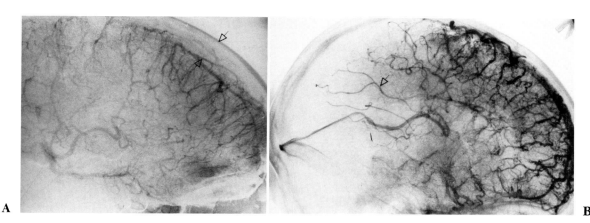

Fig. 13-23. Sagittal sinus thrombosis. A, Associated with a subdural empyema in the frontal region (arrows). **B,** Posterior, associated with cortical venous thrombosis and a parieto-occipital abscess over which there is delayed filling of the posterior middle cerebral artery branches (arrow).

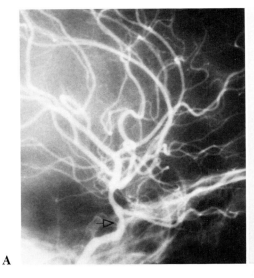

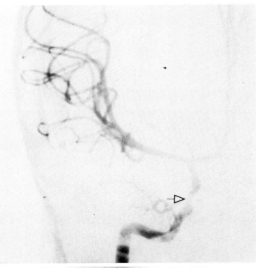

Fig. 13-24. Cavernous sinus thrombosis. Marked stenosis of the intracavernous portion of the internal carotid artery (arrows) (**A** and **B**) caused nonfilling of the sinus (**C**) in a patient with classical signs and symptoms.

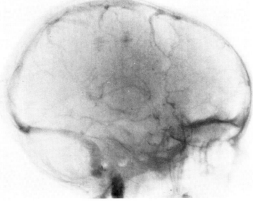

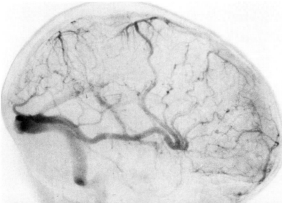

Fig. 13-25. Polycythemia and venous occlusion. A, Sagittal sinus thrombosis in a child with polycythemia due to a transposition of the great vessels. **B** and **C,** Marked cortical venous sludging in another patient with a similar condition and gross polycythemia. A large frontal abscess subsequently developed in this patient.

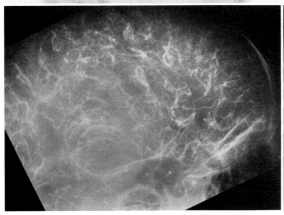

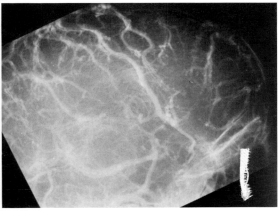

In *mastoiditis* (Macpherson and Dunbar, 1965) the venous occlusion occurs at the sigmoid sinus first and then extends back in a retrograde fashion along the sinus to the junction of the sinus and the vein of Labbé (if this vein is present). If the vein of Labbé is absent or small, the thrombosis may extend back to the torcular. Occlusion of the transverse sinus in mastoiditis may be relatively abrupt or greatly attenuated due to partial obstruction of the lumen or some recanalization. Collateral circulation through the occipital and basal veins is customarily seen. Since diagnosis of a thrombosis is valid only in a dominant sinus, identification of the other transverse sinus by i`,silateral carotid angiography is important. Anatomical variations, as mentioned, may mimic thromboses in a nondominant sinus.

NEOPLASMS. Tumors of the cranial vault (e.g., teratoma) and of the petrous bone (rhabdomyosarcoma, lymphoblastoma) may directly occlude a sinus. Histiocytosis, not really a neoplastic process, can mimic this type of sinus occlusion. A secondary subarachnoidal seeding of cerebral neoplasms (e.g., medulloblastoma, ependymoma) may lead to local cortical venous thrombosis.

HEMATOLOGICAL CONDITIONS. If severe and prolonged as in congenital heart disease, polycythemia can be associated with a remarkable profusion of dilated cortical veins through which blood flows quite slowly (Fig. 13-25). Sludging and thrombosis occur, leading to infarcts that may become secondarily infected and thus create a possible abscess.

Severe dehydration in infants leads to a state of hypercoagulation and relative polycythemia and may result in cortical venous thrombosis, sinus thrombosis, or both.

Even in the present-day era, we have not seen a child with an identified relationship between the taking of contraceptive pills and venous occlusive disease (Doll and Vessey, 1968); neither have we as yet seen cortical venous abnormalities in any drug-addicted child.

PRIMARY ASEPTIC THROMBOSIS. The many conditions in adults that lead to primary aseptic thrombosis (Greitz and Link, 1966; Gabrielsen and Heinz, 1969; Heinz et al., 1972) do not happen in children. Cortical venous thromboses have been detected during investigation of some children with seizures or sudden strokes. These thromboses may be involved with a cerebral arterial disease of unknown origin (Taveras, 1969; Harwood-Nash et al., 1971; Hilal et al., 1971). There may be some relationship to a previous generalized inflammatory disease in these cases, or to a local and severe upper respiratory tract infection (Bickerstaff, 1964; Shillito, 1964; Harwood-Nash et al., 1971). In many cases the diagnosis of primary aseptic cortical vein or dural sinus thrombosis is made by exclusion of other possible causes.

FOCAL INFECTIONS
Dural empyema and effusions

Extradural empyema. Extradural empyema is uncommon but may occur after craniotomy as a postoperative complication or after severe cranial fractures. This infection is usually recognized clinically and rarely requires a neuroradiological investigation. A chronic form, due to either a craniotomy or a posttraumatic event associated with a frontal sinus infection (Fig. 13-26), may occur in association with osteomyelitis of the skull. The latter association is a more frequent cause. The chronic extradural empyema barely qualifies for the name empyema: since its suppurative element is the minor portion of the lesion, it is more a low-grade granulomatous condition in the extradural space than a collection of pus.

Subdural empyema and effusions. Subdural empyema is a purulent bacterial infection situated between the dura and the pia. It is commonly associated with meningitis, otitis media, or frontal sinusitis in older children or with an underlying brain inflammation like an abscess.

In The Hospital for Sick Children (HSC) series, twelve (9%) of the 135 children with a brain abscess had an associated overlying subdural empyema. In addition, we had another ten children not included in the series with a subdural empyema only.

Subdural effusions as a sequela of meningitis are usually diagnosed and treated by subdural taps; they rarely require neuroradiological investigation (Goodman and Mealey, 1969). They are commonly asso-

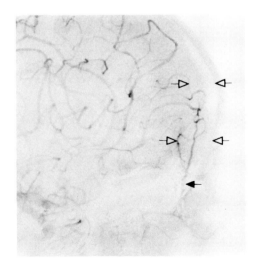

Fig. 13-26. Extradural empyema. Chronic frontal sinusitis with a pancake extradural empyema (open arrows) is fed by a hypertrophied anterior meningeal artery (solid arrow).

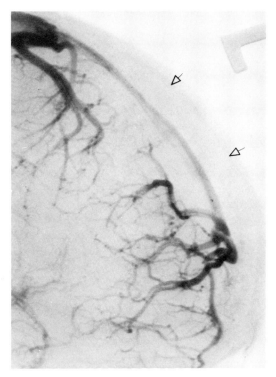

Fig. 13-27. Extradural empyema. In the frontal region there is displacement of the anterior sagittal sinus away from the inner table (arrows).

ciated with inadequately treated *Haemophilus influenzae* meningitis; they contain proteinaceous yellow fluid and may develop membranes. No hemosiderin is found in either the membranes or the fluid, which factor differentiates a subdural effusion from a subdural hygroma resulting from a posttraumatic event.

A subdural empyema usually occurs in children who have pneumococcal meningitis (Farmer and Wise, 1973) or otitis media; in adults, 80% of subdural empyemas arise from a frontal sinus infection (Woodhall, 1966).

The commonest site of subdural effusions is over the parietal convexity. Subdural effusions are more often bilateral, whereas subdural empyemas tend to occur unilaterally in the middle fossa and low convexity or in the posterior fossa, either laterally or beneath the tentorium. Interhemispheric collections of pus may also occur in children (Wilkins and Goree, 1970).

NEURORADIOLOGY OF DURAL EMPYEMA AND EFFUSIONS. During neuroradiological investigation of a child for suspected brain abscess, a significant collection of subdural fluid may be found. The initial clinical diagnosis is usually of the underlying cerebral infection, not of the subdural collection.

An extradural empyema has a similar appearance to its subdural cousins; only when a sinus is displaced from the inner table is differentiation possible (Fig. 13-27). An overlying osteomyelitis, frontal sinusitis, or surgical defect is usually present.

An infant in either the acute or the recovery stage of meningitis, particularly an infant with a fluctuating temperature who has an enlarging head, may also have a subdural effusion or empyema. These infections may be encountered during the subdural tap prior to ventriculography or at angiography when a single or bilateral subdural collection is discovered.

Pneumoencephalography, performed in the absence of raised intracranial pressure to evaluate mild head enlargement or investigate postmeningitic seizures, may reveal a subdural effusion that commonly depresses the upper angle of the ventricles and flattens the medial border—as occurs in a subdural hematoma. Similar findings are seen during ventriculography in infants for investigation of marked chronic enlargement of the head. Concomitant hydrocephalus may be present, but the head enlargement may be due solely to the effusions. If the effusions are tapped, instilled air will demonstrate their size and extent (which at times may be considerable) (Fig. 13-28).

As it is in the investigation of *all* suspect intracranial inflammations, cerebral angiography is the procedure of choice for identifying a suspect subdural fluid collection. Angiographic findings associated with effusions and empyema are similar to those associated with a subdural hematoma. Hypertrophy of the falcine branch of the anterior meningeal artery (Figs. 13-12, A, and 13-26) (similar to that occurring in meningitis and chronic subdural hematoma and extradural hematoma) may also be present in subdural empyema or effusions, together with similar hypertrophy of the tentorial artery in tentorial or interhemispheric subdural empyema (Fig. 13-29).

Effusions, usually in the parietal region, are commonly large and biconvex if chronic (Fig. 13-30, A) but may be concave and thin in both acute and chronic collections (Fig. 13-30, B). A well-defined area of contrast medium persistence may be seen circumscribing the mass; it represents the rim or capsule of the collection at the junction of the capsule with normal brain tissue (Fig. 13-30, C). This visible junction is the hypervascular portion of the capsule, similar in part to that seen in a chronic subdural hematoma. In effusions and empyema, however, the rim is often more irregular than the rim of a subdural hematoma (Ferris and Ciembroniewicz, 1964) —being more pronounced in empyema than in effusions.

As in the investigation of a subdural hematoma, to identify the presence and extent of the subdural fluid collection, oblique angiographic projections may

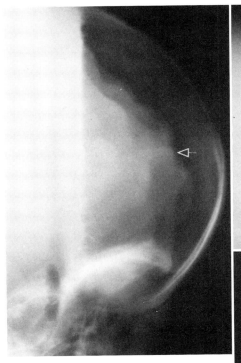

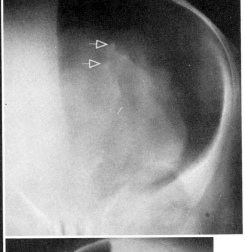

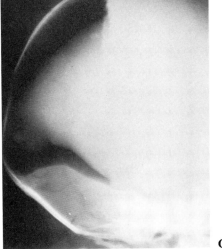

Fig. 13-28. Subdural effusion. Air has been inserted into a panhemispheric effusion and is visualized in the brow-up (A and B) and brow-down (C) positions. Note the nipplelike peaks on the inner surface caused by bridging veins (arrows).

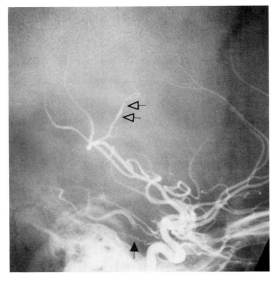

Fig. 13-29. Hypertrophied tentorial artery. A huge fronto-parietal abscess caused depression and stenoses of the middle cerebral vessels, stenoses and dilatation of the distal branches (open arrows), and a hypertrophied tentorial artery (solid arrow) which fed an associated extensive interhemispheric and supratentorial subdural empyema.

be necessary. The empyema or effusion may also be loculated (Fig. 13-30, C), a finding not so common in subdural hematomas.

Associated dilatation and narrowing of the cerebral arteries near the subdural abscess may take place (Fig. 13-29), probably due to spasm. There may be local irregular arterial or pial capillary dilatation similar to that in cerebritis (Fig. 13-30, B) or cerebral trauma, probably due to local loss of arterial tone. Though uncommon, associated arterial occlusions and arteriovenous shunting also may occur (Ferris et al., 1968).

The subdural mass effect, together with the commonly associated underlying cerebral edema or even abscess, may often pose a diagnostic problem since the vascular displacement and abnormalities may be quite bizarre. Suffice it that the examiner should bear in mind the mass effect of all three conditions (empyema or effusions, edema, and abscess) in

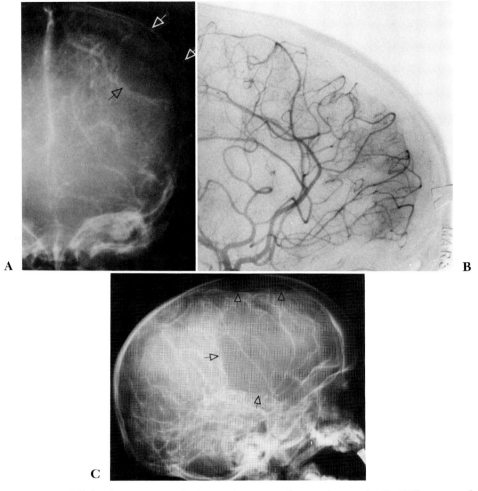

Fig. 13-30. Subdural empyema. A, Large biconvex chronic (arrows). **B,** Diffuse pancake frontal, with dilatation and stasis of the underlying pial vessels indicating an associated cerebritis. **C,** Large loculated frontoparietal, with a sharp but irregular border (arrows).

making an assessment. Similarly, the examiner should not lose sight of the fact that on the angiogram a concomitant hydrocephalus may cloud the local mass effect of the empyema by the general mass effect of the large ventricles.

The cause of some large infantile subdural fluid collections (Fig. 13-31, *A*) is unclear. Examination of the fluid may not decisively reveal whether the collection is postmeningitic or posttraumatic. We have found in the subdural fluid collection of some infants a substance similar to CSF. In these children we can only surmise that there has been a tear in the arachnoid, with a resultant CSF collection between the dura and the arachnoid. These are not arachnoid cysts. Subdural effusions in neonates, possibly being present in utero, may be so huge as to simulate *hydranencephaly*—except that in effusions the cortical vessels are intact, albeit compressed inwardly and

inferiorly toward the base of the skull (Fig. 13-31, *B* to *D*).

Brain abscesses

The spectrum, occurrence, and treatment of intracranial abscesses have evolved over the last century. Gurdjian (1969) termed the first phase during this period the "otologic era" of intracranial suppuration, when uncontrolled infections of the otitic and paranasal sinuses were assumed to be the only routes of intracranial infection. Then came the "neurosurgical era," spanning the World Wars, when the techniques of surgical localization, isolation of the suppuration, and even excision of the abscess were being developed. Finally, the advent of the present "antibiotic and antibacterial era," in conjunction with refinements of neurosurgical techniques, has led to better treatment as well as changes in the clinical presentation

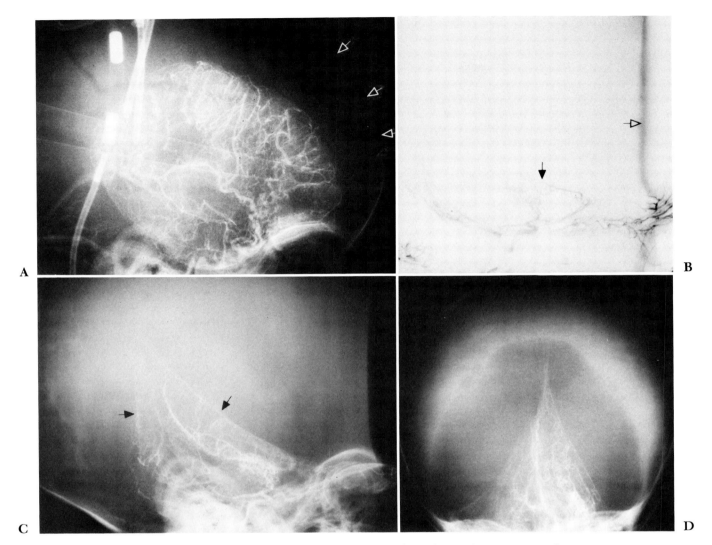

Fig. 13-31. Massive subdural hygromas. A, Panhemispheric (arrows), compressing the cerebrum. **B** and **C,** Enormous infantile bilateral in another infant. A previous attempted ventriculogram shows the air-fluid level in the hygroma (**B,** open arrow). A lateral carotid angiogram reveals the middle cerebral artery, posterior cerebral artery, and entire cerebrum compressed into a triangular shape (solid arrows). **D,** Bilateral, compressing the brain tissue. The AP projection demonstrates the full complement of cerebral arteries in the same patient as in **B** and **C,** which differentiates this hygroma from hydranencephaly. (**A** courtesy D. Hardman, M.D., New Haven, Conn.)

of some abscesses. Drug-resistant organisms are mainly responsible for these changes, but inadequate antibiotic therapy can also cause some abscesses to present chronically.

The three eras of evolution, however, relate to surgical management; there has been little comparative change over the last twenty years in the sites of the initial infections or in the sites of the resultant intracranial abscesses (Garfield, 1969).

Although intracranial suppuration in adults has received much attention over the years, relatively little has been paid this condition in infants and children. It is valid to compare and contrast the spectrum of the disease between adults and children. Predominantly adult cases are reported by Krayenbühl (1966a), Garfield (1969), Gurdjian (1969), and Morgan and co-workers (1973). The perspective of the paediatric age group is provided by the combined experiences of Nestadt and co-workers (1960), Arseni and co-workers (1966), Wright and Ballantine (1967), and Eberhard (1969) as well as by our own experience with 135 cases occurring in the last eighteen years (which we now report here). A group of thirty children previously published by McGreal in

Table 13-1. Intracranial infection: summary of selected cases from the literature

	Nestadt et al. (a)	Arseni et al. (b)	Wright and Ballantine (c)	Eberhard (d)	Combined (a, b, c, d)	HSC series (e)	Total (a, b, c, d, e)
Cases	35	81	30	26	172	135	307
Sex	—	M > F	M > F	M = F	—	M > F	M > F
Under 1 year of age	5	3	2	1	11 (6%)	31 (23%)	42 (14%)
Peak ages	—	10-15	15-17	11-15	13	0-1	—
Source							
Otitis	18	37	11	4	70 (41%)	36 (27%)	106 (35%)
Congenital heart disease	4	5	4	7	20 (12%)	19 (14%)	39 (13%)
Sinus	3	5	3	3	14 (8%)	4 (3%)	18 (6%)
Chest	0	3	2	0	5 (3%)	4 (3%)	9 (3%)
Skull fracture	0	12	0	3	15 (9%)	12 (9%)	27 (9%)
Miscellaneous	5	9	5	0	19 (11%)	24 (18%)	43 (14%)
Unknown	0	10	5	9	24 (14%)	26 (19%)	50 (16%)
Meningitis	—	—	—	—	—	13 (10%)	13 (4%)
Site							
Multiple	1	7	1	8	17	7	24
Frontal	9	17	9	13	48 (28%)	45 (33%)	93 (30%)
Temporal	10	27	7	9	53 (30%)	38 (28%)	91 (30%)
Parietal	10	4	4	11	29 (17%)	31 (23%)	60 (20%)
Occipital	0	2	1	2	5 (3%)	17 (13%)	22 (7%)
Posterior fossa	10	23	8	1	42 (24%)	19 (14%)	61 (20%)

1962 is included as part of our 135 children from the HSC series.

Statistics of brain abscesses

To provide an accurate statistical perspective of most facets of intracranial abscesses in infants and children, results of the reports by Nestadt and co-workers (1960), Arseni and co-workers (1966), Wright and Ballantine (1967), and Eberhard (1969) are listed in Table 13-1 first separately and then combined, for comparison with our HSC series of 135 children. Finally, a tabulation of data on the 307 infants and children from all the series is given.

Age. A majority of our 135 infants and children were boys (ninety-one or 67%), a factor in nearly every series.

Of all the series, ours noted a surprising preponderance of abscesses under the age of 1 year (Fig. 13-32). Most were in boys. This discrepancy may be due to the presence of a large and active neonatal unit at our hospital.

A slight increase of brain abscess incidence occurred in the early teen-age period (ages 11 to 13) of other series. This was not so in our series, the incidence remaining fairly constant throughout childhood (Fig. 13-32).

Site. Single abscesses were found in 128, and multiple abscesses in seven, children. Frontal lobe involvement was the most common (33%). The temporal and parietal lobes (28% and 23% respectively) were sites for infection more often than the

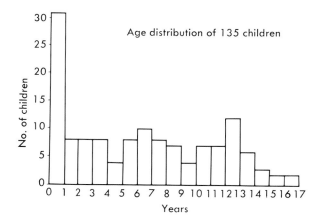

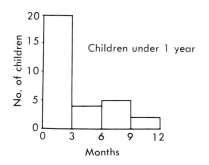

Fig. 13-32. Age and brain abscesses.

posterior fossa and the occipital lobe (14% and 13% respectively). Most posterior fossa abscesses were discovered at autopsy and occurred in younger age groups and in children with multiple abscesses. These figures are in general agreement with figures of the combined series (Table 13-1).

An associated subdural space empyema of significant volume was found in twelve (9%) of the 135 children. In addition to these 135 children having abscesses, an additional ten had a subdural empyema only.

Microorganism. The type of infecting microorganism varied, but certain organisms were found more frequently than others (Fig. 13-33). Hemolytic *Streptococcus* and pyogenic *Staphylococcus* were by far the most common, followed by *Streptococcus viridans* and *Escherichia coli.* Gram-negative enteric organisms were commonly involved in infants. Whereas multiple organisms were present in many abscesses, in ten children (7%) no organisms at all were found. Most of these latter children had been given antibiotics elsewhere before admission to our hospital.

Rare organisms that did occur in our series were *Aspergillus fumigatus* in one child (Conen et al., 1962), *Nocardia asteroides* in another (Turner and Whitby, 1969), and *Clostridium perfringens* in a third. This last child first presented radiographically with air in the subdural space (Norrell and Howieson, 1970). *Pseudomonas aeruginosa* was found in an abscess in another of our infants (Wise et al., 1969). Actinomycosis of the brain has been described in no fewer than seventeen cases (Bolton and Ashenhurst, 1964), of whom three were children. No actinomycotic infections occurred in our series.

In children with an inherently or iatrogenically impaired immunological response, a wide variety of yeasts, fungi, protozoans, and viruses as part of a generalized infection, may involve the brain (e.g., *Cryptococcus neoformans* meningitis) (Lehrer et al., 1967).

Development. The pathological process by which an abscess may form begins with inflammation, is associated with leukocytic infiltration, edema, and necrosis of brain tissue, and results in a central collection of pus. If the process is *acute,* the encephalitis and edema together with isolated foci of suppuration can create a poorly localized area of swelling. If the process is *chronic,* the abscess will have a granulomatous capsule surrounding the pus with compressed edematous brain tissue adjacent to that. The layers of a chronic abscess may be arbitrarily divided into a central locus of pus, a granulomatous layer, a region of hyperemia and fibrosis, and finally an external layer of gliosis (Gurdjian, 1969). The involvement is usually quite extensive in children, and satellite areas of inflammation and suppuration may be present. The pus may rupture into the subdural space or into the ventricular system.

Infantile abscesses

Incidence. In our series, 23% (thirty-one) were infants under the age of 1 year (Fig. 13-32). This differs markedly from the 6% total of other reports given in Table 13-1 and alters the total series incidence to 14%. Of these thirty-one children, twenty were under the age of 3 months. The youngest, a premature infant, died at 4 days of age. The cerebral abscess was found at autopsy. In only sixteen of these thirty-one infants (nine being less than 3 months old) was the abscess identified before death. Six of the nine infants under the age of 3 months

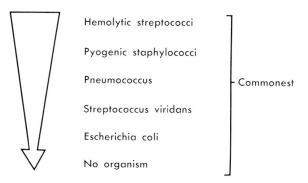

Fig. 13-33. Infecting organism and brain abscesses.

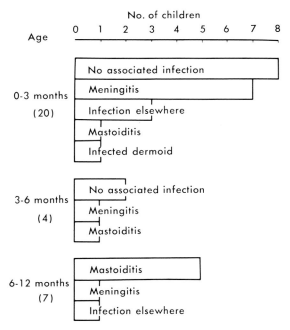

Fig. 13-34. Origin of infection in thirty-one children under 1 year of age.

who were diagnosed clinically have been reported by Hoffman and co-workers (1970). Eberhard (1969) reviewed the literature and reported seventeen infants under the age of 3 months with abscesses; these, combined with Hoffman and co-workers' six and our newly reported fourteen, give thirty-seven such infants under 3 months overall.

Origin of infection. In our infants under 3 months of age, the origin of infection was usually meningitis or was unknown (Fig. 13-34). Mastoiditis was a more common source in infants between the ages of 3 months and 1 year. In no infant was a cerebral abscess associated with congenital heart disease.

Presenting signs. In our experience, infants under 1 year of age having abscesses presented with large heads. The abscess was often entered during attempted needling of the ventricles as part of the ventriculography procedure to assess possible hydrocephalus. Such infants had relatively few local clinical signs besides a raised leukocyte count, usually with no raised temperature. The wide fontanelles and open sutures allowed the heads to enlarge from the mass effect of the abscess.

The poor reaction by infants to this type of infection was explained by Hoffman and co-workers (1970), who stated that the M fraction of the immunoglobulins does not cross the placenta barrier and that M fraction production in infants reaches normal levels only after several months. Therefore the somatic antigen and the gram-negative bacillus do not encounter the specific bactericidal action of the M fraction at this early age, accounting for the high incidence of intracranial infection in infants under 3 months of age.

Sources of infection

Most previous reports considered patients of all ages. Evans (1931) found otitis media to be a source of intracranial suppurations in 83.5% and the paranasal sinuses a source in 9.1%. Courville (1944), however, implicated otitis media in only 46%. In 1936, Charrier and Ferradou reported that 56% of 260 patients of all ages had metastatic lesions from extracranial sources. In more recent years, Krayenbühl (1966b) stated that in 130 cases of abscess, 38% were due to a distant source (half of these originating from within the thorax) and 28% were due to ear, nose, and throat sources (12% being from the mastoidal region). Garfield (1969), on the other hand, stated that only 22% of his series had infections arising from thoracic or other distant sites whereas 57% had infections from ENT sources. Gurdjian (1969) and Morgan and co-workers (1973) both reported a lesser proportion of thoracic than ENT sources.

Congenital heart disease as a distant source of

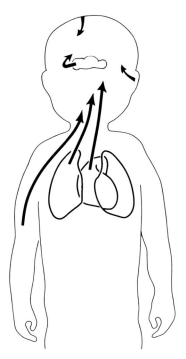

Fig. 13-35. Various extracranial sources of infection in brain abscesses.

intracranial infection is uncommon at all ages. In 1952, Clark and Clarke reported a total of ninety-five collected and personal cases having congenital heart disease as a source of infection; Newton in 1956 included seventy-two recorded and seven personal cases of abscess associated with congenital heart disease. Neither series was confined to the paediatric age group.

Among children, we have found in The Hospital for Sick Children series the following sources of infection (Fig. 13-35) leading to intracranial abscesses*:

> *Cranial sources*
>   Otitis
>   Facial sinuses
>   Fractures
>   Thrombophlebitis
>   Miscellaneous (postsurgical, osteomyelitis of the skull, etc.)
> *Intracranial sources*
>   Meningitis
>   Infected dermoid
> *Blood-borne metastatic infections*
>   Congenital heart disease
>   Pulmonary infections
>   Miscellaneous
> *Unknown sources*

*The statistical material given in the ensuing discussion is based largely on our own study of 135 children having brain abscesses seen over the last eighteen years at The Hospital for Sick Children, Toronto (Table 13-1).

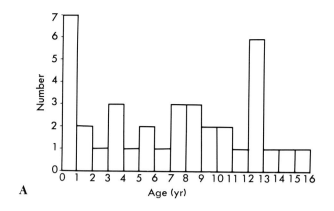

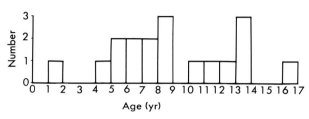

Fig. 13-36. Brain abscesses due to mastoiditis (A) and congenital heart disease (B) at varying ages. (These statistics are drawn from the HSC series.)

Cranial infections

Otitis. Acute and chronic inflammations of the mastoid and middle ear complex occur frequently in children. Rarely in the present day and age does the inflammation extend into or through the dural coverings, but this route is still common in children whose brain abscess is in the temporal lobe. Abscesses having an otitic origin accounted for 27% of the HSC, 41% of the combined, and 35% of the total series (Table 13-1).

No specific age group had a preponderance of abscesses due to mastoiditis, but infants under 1 year of age and children from 7 to 12 years showed a slightly increased incidence (Fig. 13-36). The relatively poorer resistance to infection in the infant age group may outweigh the less well-developed mastoidal air cell complex, which in the older child allows a more extensive spread of the inflammatory process.

Inflammatory otogenic complications are meningitis, venous sinus thrombophlebitis, and abscesses of the brain or dural spaces. One or more of these can occur in children. The nature of such complications is determined by the inflammation's character and pathway of extension.

Inflammation of the petrous bone commonly begins

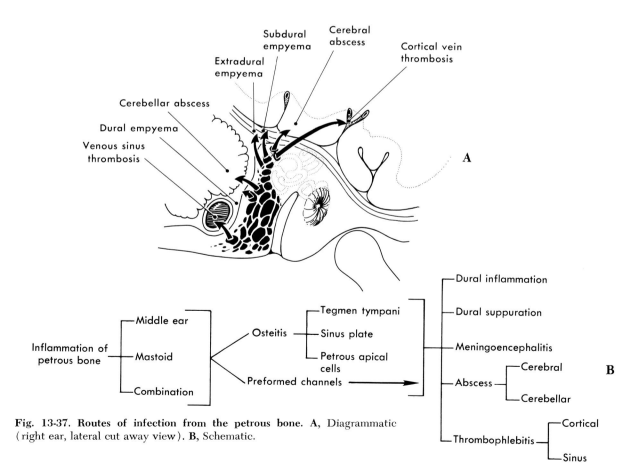

Fig. 13-37. Routes of infection from the petrous bone. A, Diagrammatic (right ear, lateral cut away view). B, Schematic.

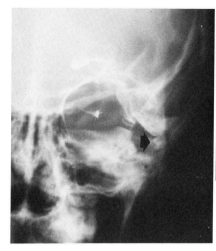
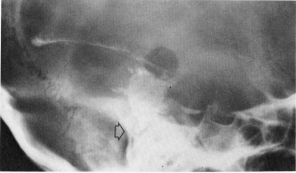

Fig. 13-38. **Brain abscess and mastoiditis.** Sterile barium placed in a temporal lobe abscess depicts the extension of the abscess from the middle ear through the posterior tegmen (arrows).

in the tympanic and mastoid cavity (Fig. 13-37). If infection occurs, its clinical course of spread depends on many factors—chief among which are inadequate treatment, presence of previous ear infections, degree of pneumatization of the mastoid, and virulence of the organism.

In acute suppurative otitis media (commonly associated with acute rhinitis and pharyngitis, childhood infectious diseases, and rupture of the tympanic membrane), a serous and then a purulent exudation arises, together with an edematous mucosal obstruction of the eustachian tube. If the infection continues, necrosis of the mastoid cellular septa, coalescence of the cells, and osteitis of the mastoid cortex itself result. The inflammatory process may spread beyond the confines of the mastoid and into the intracranial cavity. Otitis media in the early acute stage is seldom, if ever, associated with a brain abscess.

Chronic suppurative otitis media may be merely a continuation of an acute suppurative infectious process, especially in infants and children, due possibly to reinfection or to poor treatment or perhaps associated with a cholesteatoma (Chapter 3). A cholesteatoma is a collection of hyperplastic desquamated epithelium in laminae that are permeated with cholesterol crystals; it is a reaction to a chronic middle ear infection.

In infants and young children with acute suppurative otitis media, serious intracranial sequelae may result; but in older children these sequelae often occur with acute exacerbations of chronic otitis media. In older children, complicating osteitis may be associated with a direct bony erosion due to the mass of the cholesteatoma itself.

Common infecting organisms in otitis media are hemolytic *Streptococcus, Pneumococcus, Staphylococcus albus* and *S. aureus, Haemophilus influenzae,* and *Escherichia coli.*

The classical route of direct contiguous spread through the mastoidal complex is especially via the tegmen tympani into the middle cranial fossa (Fig. 13-38) or via the sinus plate into the posterior fossa. The inflammation does not often involve the petrous apex unless the apex is well pneumatized (rare in young children). Osteitis of this region may give rise to localized suppuration or lead to a vasculitis of the neighboring brain stem, thus resulting in Gradenigo's syndrome (Wintrobe et al., 1970).

Preformed anatomical pathways not uncommonly assist in the spread of infection from within the mastoidal air cells into the intracranial cavity. These pathways are the perineural spaces, the internal auditory canal, the perilymphatic and endolymphatic ducts, the tympanic suture lines, and skull fractures.

Extension of the inflammation (which arises within the mastoidal complex) along the venous channels and into the dural sinuses leads to a sequence of events in younger children who have intracranial complications due to otitis media. Venous thrombosis of the dural veins and sinuses and of the cortical veins, as well as meningitis and ultimately a brain abscess, can result if the infection is allowed to continue. Most of the children, however, present with meningitis prior to the brain abscess stage; but in very young children the clinical signs of brain abscesses may be minimal.

It therefore behooves the neuroradiologist to recognize, if possible, the otological component of the infection (Chapter 3) and the potential intracranial sequelae. These sequelae can occur singly or in combination and may present as chronic localized dural collections of pus or as acute localized (Fig. 13-38) or diffuse areas of cerebral inflammation.

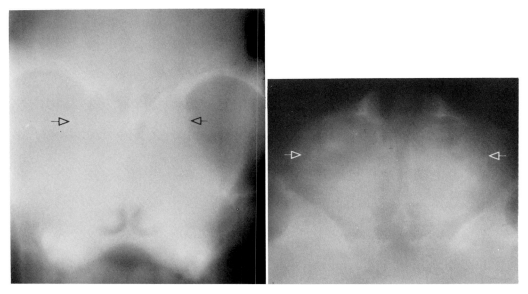

Fig. 13-39. Ethmoidal sinusitis. Huge ethmoidal mucoceles (arrows) seen on coronal and axial tomograms in an infant bulge with the orbits and may erode through the floor of the anterior fossa, producing inflammatory intracranial sequelae.

Facial sinuses. Brain abscesses due directly to infection spread from facial sinuses occurred in nineteen children (14%). This incidence closely agrees with that of the combined series (Table 13-1). Most children with such abscesses were over 8 years old, an age when the facial sinuses are better developed than in younger children.

According to Nager (1966), intracranial complications occur more commonly from exacerbation of a chronic than of an acute sinusitis. The frontal sinus is by far the most commonly implicated (Fig. 13-26); rarely are the ethmoidal (Fig. 13-39) and sphenoidal sinuses involved (Nelson et al., 1967).

Various routes by which a brain abscess can occur are (1) an osteitis or osteomyelitis of the inner table of the skull, progressing to a leptomeningitis, then to an abscess via perivascular channels or (2) a retrograde thrombophlebitis, thromboarteritis, or cortical vein thrombosis.

Although most sinugenic abscesses are in the frontal lobe, distant brain abscesses may develop from venous thrombotic spread. Such thromboses are more often associated with meningitis or abscesses than with facial sinusitis.

Fractures. Even if depressed or involving a facial sinus, fractures of the cranial vault rarely cause cranial abscesses. Those involving the petrous bone are more likely to do so. In the twelve children (9%) who had a fracture and a brain abscess, the majority of fractures were of the petrous bone (Fig. 13-40, A and B). In all fractures the tegmen tympani was involved.

By its contiguity, the temporal lobe is involved in many inflammatory processes via the fracture defect. Recurrent, especially pneumococcal, meningitis more commonly results from infected petrous fractures than do abscesses; however, meningitis usually precedes abscess formation. Whether all petrous fractures should be treated prophylactically with antibiotics therefore is a moot point. Penetrating wounds, spikes, bullets, etc. with a concomitant fracture may also lead to an abscess.

Thrombophlebitis. Facial thrombophlebitis associated with inflamed facial soft tissue, frontal or ethmoidal sinusitis, or orbital cellulitis may extend into the cavernous sinus. This extension rarely occurs in children; even rarer is association of a facial thrombophlebitis with a brain abscess.

Miscellaneous. Postcraniotomy or postcraniectomy complications rarely include intracerebral inflammation or brain abscesses in the present day and age of surgical sterility and antibiotic umbrellas (Gurdjian, 1969). If these complications do occur, it is in those children with severe traumatic morcellation of the skull in whom emergency surgery is performed under less than ideal circumstances.

Osteomyelitis of the cranial vault (other than of the sinuses) (Fig. 13-40, C and D) usually gives rise to extradural inflammatory granulomatous tissue or small extradural abscesses rather than to brain abscesses.

Intracranial infections

Meningitis. It is obviously quite difficult to decide in some children which comes first, the meningitis

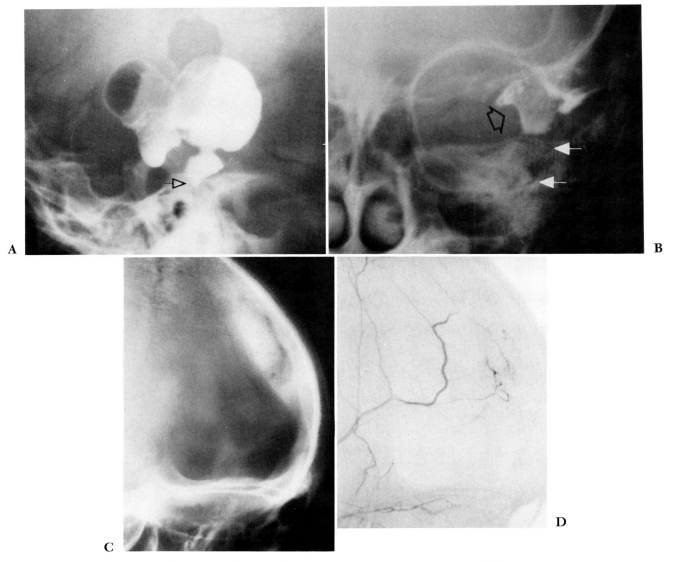

Fig. 13-40. Abscesses and petrous bone fractures. A, An acute temporal lobe abscess surgically tapped and containing barium connects through a fracture in the tegmen (arrow) with the petrous bone. **B,** Shrinkage of the abscess a year later (open arrow). The fracture of the petrous bone is faintly visible (solid arrows). **Osteomyelitis. C,** Chronic, with dense sclerosis of the frontal bone. **D,** On a selective external carotid angiogram a diffuse area of vascularity within the inflammatory tissue can be seen.

or the abscess. In our judgment, meningitis antedated the development of the abscess in thirteen infants and children (10%)—most of whom were under the age of 3 months. The organisms isolated in these cases were quite varied, ranging from *Pneumococcus* and a gram-negative enteric bacillus (which was the commonest) to *Staphylococcus.*

In neonates, meningitis due to gram-negative enteric bacteria will often cause severe hemorrhagic cerebral necrosis rather than abscesses (Cussen and Ryan, 1967).

Even though a few children with temporal lobe abscesses and petrous bone disease did have some local meningitis, the abscess was the dominant clinical presentation.

Abscesses tend to rupture into ventricles more often than into the subarachnoid space. This is graphically shown by barium instillation into an abscess cavity with subsequent intraventricular rupture and ependymal capture of the micropaque particles (Fig. 13-41). An intraventricular loculation of pus, ventriculitis, and meningitis usually all result. Furthermore, the general effect of a purulent meningitis (i.e., cerebral edema, ventriculitis, arachnoiditis with ob-

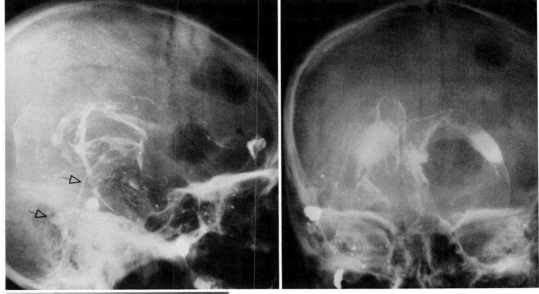

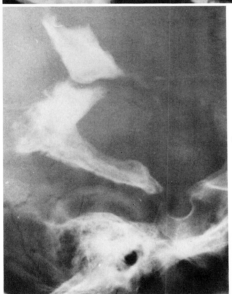

Fig. 13-41. Intraventricular rupture of abscesses. A and **B,** Rupture of a left frontal lobe abscess (solid arrow) into the ventricular system and down into the cervical subarachnoid space. The aqueduct and fourth ventricle (open arrows) are clearly evident. There is still a considerable shift of the ventricular system to the right as seen on an AP projection (**B**). The ependyma of the ventricles has taken up the barium. **C,** A parietal abscess in another child has ruptured into the occipital and temporal horns.

struction of the cerebrospinal fluid pathways resulting in hydrocephalus) may, together with a brain abscess, create severe and dramatic effects on the clinical status of the patient. In addition to these general effects, the inflammatory process due to meningitis causes local effects on cerebral vessels themselves, varying from focal constriction to regional dilatation and occlusion.

Infected dermoid. This is a rare but dramatic combination of an intracranial dermoid with a cutaneous stalk connection which becomes infected (Fig. 13-42).

Blood-borne metastatic infections
Congenital heart disease

INCIDENCE. Although it is difficult to assess, Clark (1966) estimates that brain abscesses occur in 3% to 4% of all children having congenital heart disease (CHD). Our own approximate figure is 2%. For the last five years, however, we have thought the incidence was even lower, due probably to earlier and more successful treatment of cyanotic CHD in infants and children.

Conversely, in children having brain abscesses the incidence of associated cyanotic CHD is 14% (nine-

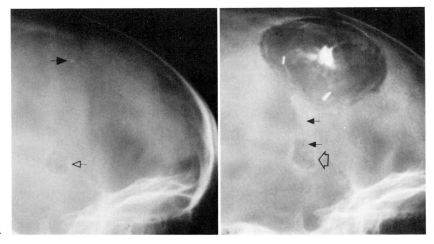

Fig. 13-42. Infected dermoid. A, An intradiploic dermoid (open arrow) with an intracranial component containing a distant calcification (solid arrow). B, Evacuation of the intracerebral abscess and instillation of barium in the upper frontoparietal region at the site of the calcification. A faint dermoid track can be seen (solid arrows) extending to the vault defect (open arrow).

teen of 135) in the HSC series, and 12% of the combined series (Table 13-1). The age at which these abscesses occur indicates both that they are very rare under the age of 2 (Raimondi et al., 1965; Clark, 1966) and that a peak incidence occurs between 5 and 9 years of age (Fig. 13-36).

MECHANISM. The mechanism by which the abscess arises in the brain depends on the presence of many of the following features:

1. Cyanotic CHD (abscess rarely occurs with a cyanotic septal defect)
2. Polycythemia
3. Small cerebral vessel thrombosis
4. Scattered small areas of cerebral infarction or softening
5. Some degree of chronic hypoxia of the brain
6. Septic emboli to the brain

These septic emboli bypass the lung from such inflammatory foci as respiratory tract infections, suppurative abscesses of the skin, teeth, tonsils, abdomen, etc., or more commonly unknown sites. In this last group, organisms normally found in the respiratory and gastrointestinal tracts may enter the systemic vascular system and cause transitory bacteremia—thus infecting the compromised cerebral tissue.

Subacute bacterial endocarditis in CHD is not a significant causative factor of abscess (Clark, 1966). Only one of our 135 children with brain abscess had subacute bacterial endocarditis, and this was due to rheumatic heart disease.

SITE. Abscesses develop predominantly in the middle cerebral artery area (Fig. 13-43), particularly in the middle and anterior portions of its peripheral branches. One child developed an abscess within the pituitary fossa.

TYPES. In our series, brain abscesses due to CHD were associated with tetralogy of Fallot in 50% and transposition of the great vessels in 20%. Less common anomalies were atrioventricularis communis, truncus arteriosus, and tricuspid atresia with pulmonary stenosis.

This distribution of types of CHD in our series agrees with that in the large series by Raimondi and co-workers (1965) and Clarke (1966). The high incidence of tetralogy of Fallot is probably due to the combination of a child's longer survival and the presence of polycythemia and arterial desaturation. In the 5-to-9-year age group with an abscess, the majority of patients had tetralogy of Fallot.

CLINICAL FEATURES. An abscess associated with CHD may not present clear clinical features. Askenasy and Kosary (1960), Raimondi and co-workers (1965), and Clark (1966) all clearly discussed the difficult clinical assessment and diagnosis of an abscess developing in a child with CHD. The importance of immediate investigative computed tomography and angiography should be strongly impressed on the clinician. Even in the presence of only vague signs and symptoms, angiography is the definitive diagnostic procedure for brain abscess. Prominent angiographic findings in children with CHD and a deteriorating noncardiac clinical state that may be related to the brain are mass lesions such as abscess, extradural hematoma, cerebral infarct, intracranial hemorrhage, a bleeding vascular malformation, or a specific arterial

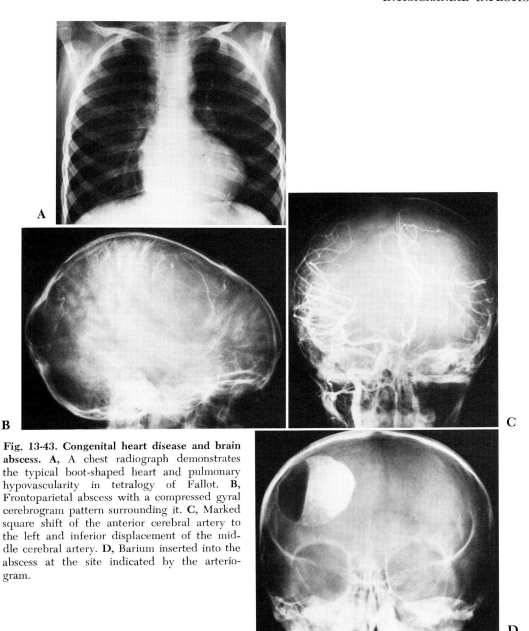

Fig. 13-43. Congenital heart disease and brain abscess. A, A chest radiograph demonstrates the typical boot-shaped heart and pulmonary hypovascularity in tetralogy of Fallot. B, Frontoparietal abscess with a compressed gyral cerebrogram pattern surrounding it. C, Marked square shift of the anterior cerebral artery to the left and inferior displacement of the middle cerebral artery. D, Barium inserted into the abscess at the site indicated by the arteriogram.

or venous thrombosis. In a child under the age of 2 with CHD, intracranial arterial thrombosis causes a neurological abnormality more often than does an abscess.

Pulmonary infections. In only four children (3%) was a chest infection directly related to a brain abscess in the absence of CHD. Two of these children had rare chest infections, one *Nocardia asteroides* and the other *Aspergillus fumigatus.* We had no case of a tuberculoma of the brain.

Miscellaneous infections. In twenty-four children (18%) some form of suppurative inflammation existed elsewhere in the body—ranging from carbuncles,

osteomyelitis, suppurative peritonitis, and infected bones to tonsillitis and caries.

Unknown sources. No detectable source of infection could be found in twenty-six children (19%). Some of their histories mentioned sore throats, inflamed ears, and upper respiratory tract infections; but these common childhood afflictions could not be definitely implicated as causes of intracranial abscess.

Neuroradiology of brain abscesses

During the past seven years the presentation of a child with a brain abscess requiring neuroradiological investigation has changed in emphasis. Previously, ill-defined neurological symptoms, possible presence of papilledema, equivocal suture splitting, and mild or no fever were the order. Now, quicker referral to our hospital, less likelihood of unsatisfactory antibiotic therapy, and availability of more sophisticated neuroradiology and angiography have led to earlier diagnoses of the disease.

Investigation of a suspect local inflammatory process of the brain necessitates urgent neuroradiological attention. In the overall radiological approach to inflammations of the brain (Davis and Taveras, 1966), there is a certain logical sequence of radiography to be followed.

Preliminary radiology. Certain radiographs should always be obtained prior to cerebral angiography.

Chest radiographs. These may reveal pulmonary infections or cardiac abnormalities. The disparity between clinical examinations and radiological examinations, and vice versa, has provided many a peaceful professional entente!

Pneumonia (with or without a pleural effusion), cardiac configuration abnormalities, and pulmonary plethora may all provide evidence of the source infection in a suspect brain abscess.

Skull radiographs. As we have stressed repeatedly, no neuroradiological special procedure or brain scan should be performed without the acquisition first of a recent set of skull radiographs. A full series of posteroanterior, lateral, half-axial and basal views should be obtained.

Among the 135 children in the HSC series, no abnormality was found in forty-five. Among the remainder, however, the following abnormalities were seen—either alone or in concert:

Split sutures	59%
Mastoid disease	33%
Skull vault fractures	6%
Dermoid defect	5%
Frontoethmoidal sinusitis	4%

Split sutures were invariably of the acute configuration. Most changes in the petrous bone suggested chronic mastoid disease.

Intracranial air was seen only once, in the previously mentioned child with an abscess due to *Clostridium perfringens* (Fig. 13-44). Chronic abscesses will rarely produce local thinning of bone (Ferris et al., 1968); but in infants having large abscesses, a considerable part of the hemicranium may bulge outward (Fig. 13-45).

Tomograms. Children who have a suspected or identified temporal lobe abscess and, in addition, a chronic otitis media, previous head injury and suspected skull fracture, or recurrent meningitis should all be subjected to anteroposterior and lateral poly-

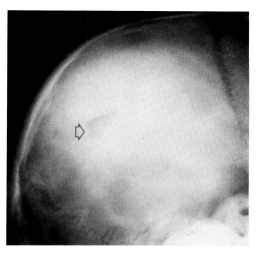

Fig. 13-44. Air in a brain abscess. A posterior parietal abscess (arrow) due to *Clostridium perfringens* contains air.

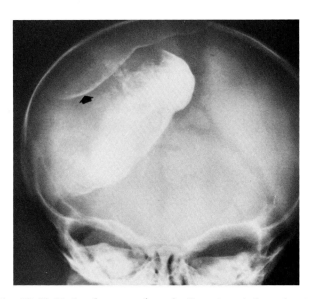

Fig. 13-45. Brain abscess and vault distortion. A huge hemispheric abscess in an infant has been tapped and barium replaced. It is causing markedly split sutures together with a subdural empyema (arrow) and bulging and thinning of the right hemicranial vault.

tomography of one or both petrous bones. The lateral petrous tomograms are most useful for identifying defects of the tegman tympani, which is the commonest site of bony destruction that leads to intracranial infection (Fig. 13-46).

Similarly, for children who have a frontal lobe abscess and either a frontal sinusitis or a frontal fracture, anteroposterior and lateral polytomograms of the frontoethmoidal sinuses should be obtained. In older children a sphenoidal sinus defect may be present in basal fractures and may extend laterally into the sphenoid wings.

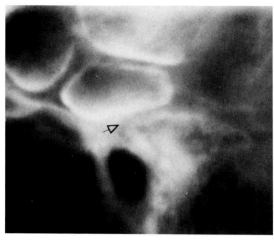

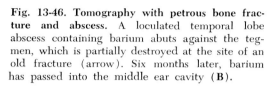

A

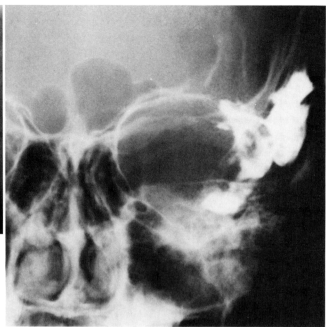

B

Fig. 13-46. Tomography with petrous bone fracture and abscess. A loculated temporal lobe abscess containing barium abuts against the tegmen, which is partially destroyed at the site of an old fracture (arrow). Six months later, barium has passed into the middle ear cavity (B).

Penetrating wounds of the skull may also need tomography to identify the bony breach. Precise delineation of the defects just detailed will allow the neurosurgeon to both treat the abscess and repair the channel of infection satisfactorily.

Isotope studies. After these preliminary radiographs are completed, a brain scan is a most useful diagnostic aid for the clinician (Chapter 9). It localizes the suspect inflammatory focus for the neuroradiologist and enables him to choose on which side to take the initial angiogram. False-negative isotope examinations are rare. Scanning is a sensitive tool in the detection of intracranial inflammatory processes; a positive image can occur before neuroradiological procedures are able to reveal a mass effect (Jordan et al., 1972).

The size, configuration, and character of an abnormal brain scan in the child with an intracranial infection are discussed in Chapter 9. The abnormalities seen on these scans are due to a combination of cerebritis (either perifocal or preabscess), the abscess wall itself, and surrounding cerebral edema. Until a local or general intracranial mass has been ruled out by the clinician and the neuroradiologist, under no circumstances should a cerebrospinal fluid scan be performed. In the presence of a mass effect from any form of intracranial inflammation, the catastrophic sequelae of coning after a lumbar puncture are very real.

Computed tomograms. If available, cranial CT (Chapter 8) is now the screening procedure of choice.

It will demonstrate the area of edema, the shift of ventricular structures, and in chronic abscesses a capsule with a necrotic center. The inflammatory process may be enhanced by injection of contrast medium. The precise diagnosis of a cerebral inflammatory process, however, cannot be made from the computed tomogram alone but must be related to the clinical history and signs. To define precisely the true nature of the lesion and possible vascular sequelae, we follow the computed tomogram with angiography.

Chronic brain abscesses seldom calcify (Fig. 13-47); but if they do, it is usually in a popcornlike fashion and CT can aid in the initial identification of the deposits.

Cerebral angiography. The prime diagnostic technique for identifying the character and precise location of the mass effect and associated vascular changes is cerebral angiography. It is essential for detecting the following intracranial abnormalities:

General
    Ventricular size
    Diffuse cerebral edema
    Regional mass effect, single or multiple
    Gyral swelling and displacement (onion-ring effect)
    Dural mass collections
Focal
    Focal mass effect
    Focal hypervascularity
    Arterial abnormalities
        Major (thrombosis, spasm, dilatation)
        Minor small (dilatation, stasis, thrombosis)
    Cortical venous abnormalities

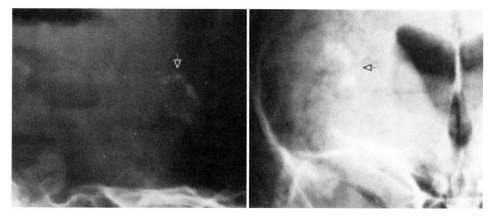

Fig. 13-47. Calcified chronic abscess. Ringlike dense calcifications surround a chronic right frontal abscess (arrows). Such calcifications are rare.

As has been stressed previously—when an abscess is suspected, once the preliminary head and chest radiographs, the CT, and the brain scan have been completed, angiography should be performed immediately. Our practice is to use hyperventilation and magnification techniques during angiography since both are indispensable to the visualization of possible alterations in small cerebral vessels.

Once a brain abscess is suspected clinically, cerebral angiography is the definitive diagnostic procedure. The clinical signs may be vague. A child could present with a few or many of the following symptoms: an infected ear, congenital heart disease, fever, irritability, an alteration in the level of consciousness, focal neurological abnormalities, focal EEG abnormalities (present in at least 95% of abscesses), or a localized abnormality revealed by brain scan. Such a child should be given an immediate angiogram. At this stage the infection may vary from a localized acute suppurative encephalitis to a chronic well-encapsulated abscess. Multiple abscesses, often bilateral, may also occur.

Angiographic abnormalities from a brain abscess itself may be classified thus:

Mass effects
    General edema
    Local vessel displacement
    Perifocal edema
Vascular abnormalities
    Alteration in vessel caliber (dilatation, narrowing)
    Local vascular stasis
    Capsule vascularity
    Arterial occlusions
    Early-filling veins
    Venous or sinus thrombosis or both

To generalize, we may state that abscesses due to otitis media involve the posterior temporal lobe and less commonly the cerebellum and may be associated with subdural empyema or metastatic abscesses of

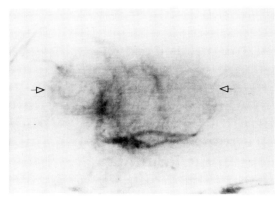

Fig. 13-48. Cerebritis cerebrogram. On a lateral carotid angiogram a large frontoparietal area of cerebritis can be seen with a dense cerebrogram (arrows). This subsequently formed a suppurative abscess.

the parietal lobe. Abscesses due to extracranial metastatic spread occur mainly in the parietal lobe. Brain abscesses are usually found in the white matter adjacent to the gray-matter–white-matter junction (Blackwood et al., 1966)—the area between arteries entering the peripheral gray matter and deep perforating arteries of the white matter being an area of relatively poor vascular supply.

Mass effects. It is difficult to determine whether the mass effect seen by angiography is due to an acute inflammation without a formed suppurative center or to a fully developed abscess. Certain features in the local vessels may indicate a capsule with a central avascular area of suppuration. When hyperventilation and magnification are used during angiography in children, however, an intermediate solid dense and relatively homogeneous blush may be seen in the capillary phase of the lateral view (Fig. 13-48). Such a capillary blush indicates the likelihood of cerebritis rather than a well-

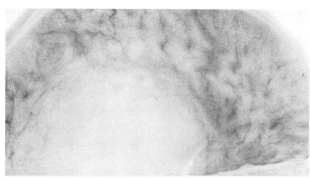

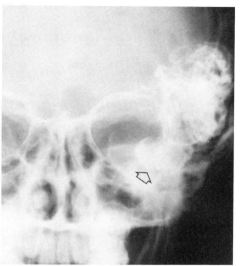

Fig. 13-49. Abscess cerebrogram. Note the large avascular temporal and inferior parietal region with displacement of the normal cerebrogram. A well-formed temporal lobe abscess (arrow) filled with barium now arises from a suppurative ear infection.

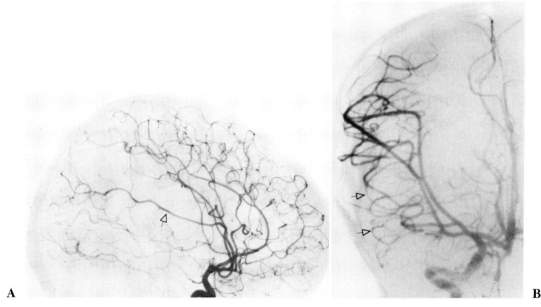

A   **B**

Fig. 13-50. Temporal lobe abscess. A, Marked displacement of the entire middle cerebral—except for the angular branch, which is inapproproately dilated due to loss of autoregulation (arrow). B, This phenomenon is better seen in the AP view, showing the middle cerebral artery displaced medially and superiorly in its proximal portion. Inferiorly, due to a concomitant subdural empyema (arrows), the distal branches are displaced inwardly.

formed abscess with a central necrotic focus; contrariwise, a relatively avascular mass along with clinical indications of infection suggests a better-formed necrotic center than in cerebritis (Fig. 13-49). These two observations are by no means exclusive and may merge one with the other.

GENERAL EDEMA. A contiguous cerebral edema is commonly present in both the acute stage and the chronic stage of an abscess but is more prominent in the acute stage. Thus the mass effect may be far larger than the actual suppurative cavity. Furthermore, with the extensive inflammatory changes that occur, particularly in infants, a concomitant ventriculitis may result in *hydrocephalus* (either IVOH or EVOH)—which may also alter the mass effect of the abscess on an angiogram.

LOCAL VESSEL DISPLACEMENT. Whatever the stage of maturation of the infection, local vessel displacement tends to be considerable (Fig. 13-50). In the lateral view, arteries may be displaced around the

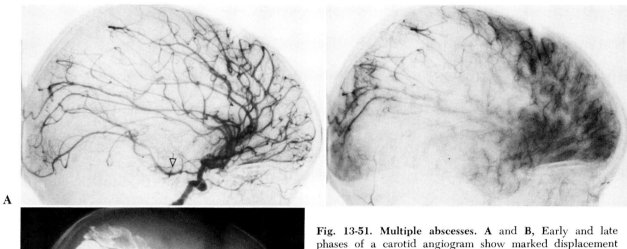

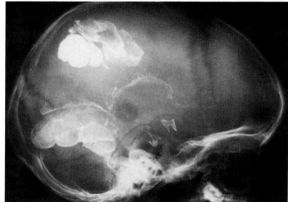

Fig. 13-51. Multiple abscesses. A and B, Early and late phases of a carotid angiogram show marked displacement of the peripheral middle cerebral and posterior cerebral arteries. There also is evidence of transtentorial herniation (arrow). The cerebrogram phase (B) reveals a posterior parietal and a temporo-occipital area of lucency. Note the very slow flow through the peripheral arteries in this phase. C, Barium in the two abscesses, one in the posterior parietal and the other in the temporo-occipital region, correlates with their identification in the cerebrogram phase.

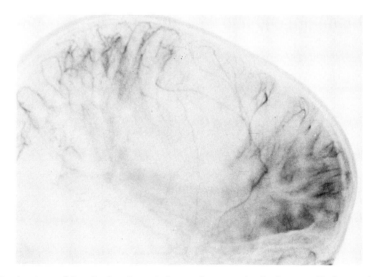

Fig. 13-52. Angiographic ripple sign. A large frontoparietal abscess displaces the cerebrogram effect of the gyri in a concentric ripplelike fashion.

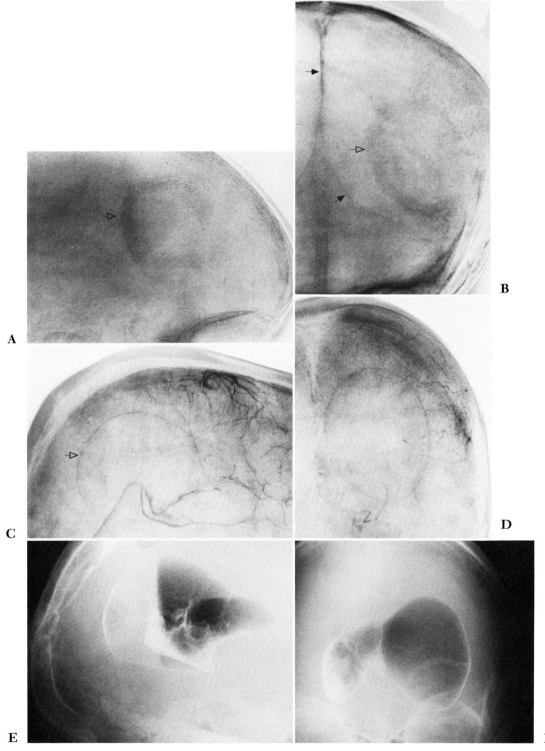

Fig. 13-53. Capsule vascularity. A and **B,** A thick well-defined capsule in a chronic frontal abscess (open arrows). Seen 5 minutes after a carotid angiogram. Note the contrast within the falx and tentorium (solid arrows). This child had sickle cell anemia. **C** to **F,** A very thin capsule around an aseptic chronic abscess (arrow) which has extended across the midline as seen by the instillation of barium and air (**E** and **F**). This vascular ring persisted for 30 minutes after the angiogram.

mass—either forward and above or backward and below—but are not usually stretched over the dome of the mass (Fig. 13-51). Due to the increased pressure, veins tend to fill very slowly and follow a similar sort of displacement as the arteries. The examiner must be aware of bizarre vessel displacements that do not follow a centrifugal pattern, for this discrepancy may indicate *multiple abscesses* (Fig. 13-51).

PERIFOCAL EDEMA ("RIPPLE" SIGN). Heinz and Cooper (1968) described a concentric displacement of edematous gyri rippling away from the center of the mass effect (Figs. 13-43 and 13-52). This may be visualized on lateral angiograms by opacification of compressed vessels within the sulci, through which the blood flow rate is diminished because of local increased cerebral pressure. Since there is an associated edema of the involved gyri between the sulci, the sulci are not compressed together as much as one would expect from the centrifugal pressure.

This ripple effect is commonly seen with abscesses and focal inflammatory brain swelling; however, it may also be seen with cerebral hematoma, focal brain edema due to cerebral trauma, and some tumors (but rarely if ever in a benign cyst).

Heinz and Cooper (1968), quoting Taveras, stated that the ripple effect is not commonly seen in temporal abscesses, the reason being that relatively few sulci are seen in the lateral view of the temporal lobe.

Vascular abnormalities

ALTERATION IN VESSEL CALIBER. Arteries displaced by a mass effect may be compressed (Figs. 13-1 and 13-51); but areas of segmental narrowing may also occur, particularly in the early cerebritis stage (Figs. 13-10, 13-11, and 13-29) (Davis and Taveras, 1966), and may be due to spasm or segmental vessel wall edema. This is probably caused by a concomitant local meningitis. More common, however, are dilated arteries in the area contiguous with the inflamed brain, again being more common in the cerebritis phase than in an organized abscess (Fig. 13-50). Loss of vessel tone, similar to that seen in a contused brain due to trauma, probably accounts for the dilatation.

LOCAL VASCULAR STASIS. Passage of contrast through the artery-capillary-vein pathways in the vicinity of a mass effect is slowed by increased pressure (Fig. 13-50), spasm (Fig. 13-29), or occlusion (Fig. 13-3, A). Slowing of contrast may be evident in the major vessels themselves or in the capillary phase within the sulci (Fig. 13-4), as just described.

CAPSULE VASCULARITY. A prolonged ringlike persistence of contrast medium within fine vessels (Fig. 13-53), together with a relatively avascular center, is sometimes seen around the site of an abscess.

This is due to two phenomena: (1) compressed normal capillaries in the brain tissue immediately surrounding the inflammatory focus, which at angiography provide an ill-defined circular shadow in acutely expanding abscesses, and (2) vascular proliferation within the capsule of a mature abscess (Wickbom, 1948; Chou et al., 1966).

The chronic abscess cavity is enclosed by a layer of granulation tissue that merges with a hyperemic fibrous capsule in the peripheral zone of a gliosis (Blackwood et al., 1966). The vessels in these layers, together with the vascular stasis, can probably be identified at angiography—appearing during the capillary and early venous phases and often persisting from a few seconds to 30 minutes (Fig. 13-53, C to F) after contrast has disappeared from the deep veins.

This capsule is *not* commonly seen on angiograms of children with an abscess, having occurred in only 15% of the children in the HSC series. Capsuled abscesses tend to be chronic and large, and often there is no positive culture; most children with such an abscess had been on antibiotic therapy elsewhere prior to being admitted. Contrariwise, the compressed brain stain or capillary blush (Figs. 13-3, B, and 13-49) was commonly seen in children with acute cerebritis or a rapidly growing abscess. It was also frequently a concomitant of the ripple sign.

The low incidence of capsule vascularity in our series agrees with the 20% incidence reported by Davis and Taveras (1966) but is far less than the 48% reported by Lecuire and co-workers (1966). Chou and co-workers (1966) found this capsule during angiography in six children—all of whom had associated cyanotic CHD and whose abscesses, presenting late in the disease, were large and in the frontoparietal region.

ARTERIAL OCCLUSIONS. Jordan and co-workers (1972) believe that the infarcts so formed (Fig. 13-8) do not create the mass effect observed in abscesses. These occlusions are not commonly seen among children (Fig. 13-3, A); but if they do occur in the absence of congenital heart disease, they are probably related to an associated meningitis or to bona fide cerebral artery thrombosis.

EARLY-FILLING VEINS. Ferris and co-workers (1968) and Segall and co-workers (1973) reported the early appearance of regional cerebral veins concomitant with an associated avascular mass in an abscess. This phenomenon is uncommon among children and adults (Davis and Taveras, 1966); but when it occurs, it often is not associated with any other abnormal circulation in the arterial tree.

VENOUS OR SINUS THROMBOSIS OR BOTH. Small cortical venous thromboses are often associated with abscesses in children. Identification of these occlusions necessitates good angiographic subtraction and magnification (Fig. 3-20) as well as meticulous scrutiny, since the occlusions frequently occur in very small veins. The affected veins are often tortuous and are similar to veins under the capsule of a chronic subdural hematoma.

If the thrombosis is not caused directly by middle ear disease, a sinus thrombosis may be associated with the infected cerebral site itself or be secondary to the accompanying toxemia and dehydration.

Pneumoencephalography and ventriculography. Under no circumstance should pneumoencephalography be performed on a child who has raised intra-cranial pressure and in whom an abscess is suspected. We have found a small chronic encapsulated abscess sometimes leads to local neurological signs without raised intracranial pressure; on such children we perform pneumoencephalography. This has occurred particularly with small abscesses located deep in the area of the basal ganglia. There was also a child who had no clinical evidence of acute raised intracranial pressure but who did have a slowly enlarging head and in whom a mild EVOH was suspected; at pneumoencephalography we found, to our surprise and obvious consternation, a large supratentorial mass that was shown at subsequent surgery to be a

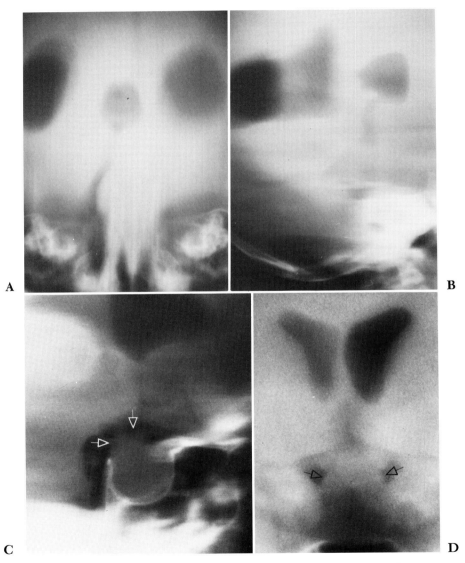

Fig. 13-54. Pneumoencephalography and ventriculography in abscesses. A and **B,** A ventriculogram demonstrates kinking of the aqueduct and elevation and displacement of the fourth ventricle to the right due to a large left cerebellar abscess. **C** and **D,** An enlarged sella contains a mass lesion that projects into the chiasmatic cistern (arrows). At operation, the mass was found to be a staphylococcal abscess.

chronic abscess. Paradoxically, such a large mass provided only a few clinical signs.

Ventriculography has demonstrated a posterior fossa abscess (Fig. 13-54, *A* and *B*) which simulated a neoplasm, and pneumoencephalography outlined a rare pituitary abscess (Fig. 13-54, *C* and *D*).

Similarly, large abscesses have been found in infants at The Hospital for Sick Children, Toronto, who were relatively well clinically but who presented with progressively enlarging heads (Hoffman et al., 1970). At the attempted ventriculography in some, the needle entered not a large ventricle but a huge and often multiloculated abscess (Fig. 13-55).

To reiterate, therefore, we shall merely state that CT and angiography are the diagnostic procedures of choice in the investigation of postinflammatory sequelae, particularly in children who have raised intracranial pressure.

Brain cystography with barium. We insert a suspension of sterile micropaque (barium sulfate) into a drained abscess cavity. This radiopaque marker provides, by means of standard radiographs, an estimation of the site and size of the cavity and evidence of the subsequent course of the abscess (Fig. 13-56). We have used the technique in sixty-five of the 135 children with cranial abscesses. Thorotrast was used until 1960. In no surviving patient has any untoward development of local malignancy occurred that could be ascribed to the latter marker (Dahlgren, 1961; Kyle et al., 1963; Horta et al., 1965).

Micropaque barium sulfate was first used in 1962 by Clarke and co-workers, and further experience was detailed by Allen and Meacham in 1969. Blinderman (1964) reported the reaction of the ependyma and arachnoid to micropaque in monkeys (i.e., macrophage ingestion of barium and resultant nonspecific acute inflammation). We have found, however, that when barium ruptures into the ventricles and subarachnoid space cells in the ependyma and arachnoid phagocytose it; the ingested barium does *not* cause any untoward effect on cerebrospinal fluid passage in the subarachnoid and ventricular systems (Fig. 13-57). Even inadvertent direct instillation of barium into a ventricle did not cause any obstructive reaction.

Even in the aqueduct, micropaque barium sulfate does not produce obstructive arachnoiditis or ependy-

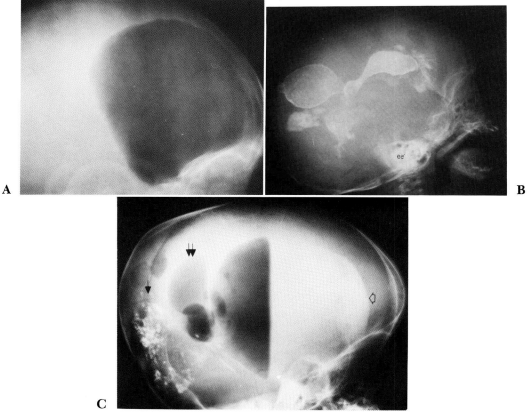

Fig. 13-55. Infantile abscesses. A, Large frontal, filled with air after tapping in a 3-week-old child. **B,** Extensive loculated hemispheric, lined by barium in an infant. **C,** Initial large occipital, filled with barium (solid arrow). Another frontoparietal abscess contains barium and air (open arrow). The dilated occipital horns are also filled with air (double arrow).

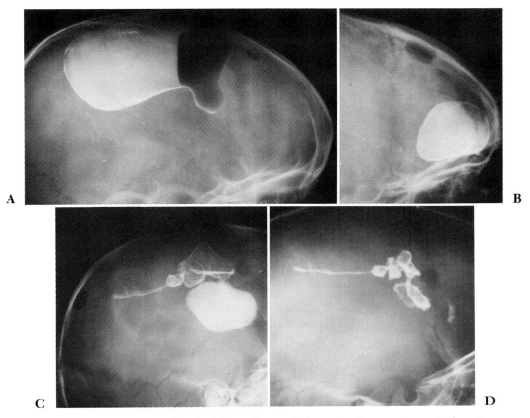

Fig. 13-56. Barium cystography. A, A large elongated abscess in the anterior cerebral territory. Note the uptake of barium by the lining of the abscess. B, A well-defined frontal abscess due to sinusitis. C, A large anterior parietal loculated abscess. D, One year later it has satisfactorily shrunk. The patient remains without symptoms.

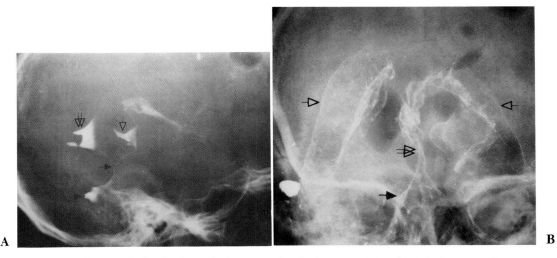

Fig. 13-57. Ventricular barium. A, Rupture of a barium-containing frontal abscess outlines the posterior third ventricle (open arrow), occipital horn (double arrow), and aqueduct and fourth ventricle (solid arrows). B, Barium within the entire ventricular system due to a similar occurrence. Again the lateral ventricles (open arrows), aqueduct (double arrow), and fourth ventricle (solid arrow) are particularly well seen. This patient has been followed for seven years, and the ventricles have not increased in size.

mitis. This lack of significant clinical sequelae is even more remarkable in view of the fact that the barium is intimately mixed with the unsavory contents of the abscess itself, contents which should cause considerable inflammatory reaction in the cerebrospinal fluid pathways. Reddy and co-workers (1967) did report one child with a cerebellar abscess and posterior fossa subdural empyema in whom a distant spinal subdural granuloma may have resulted from barium in the subdural space.

Parasites

Parasitic infection of the brain is generally confined to endemic areas of the world, rarely presenting at our hospital except in unusual cases from among the immigrant population. The infection presents with the mass effect of a large cyst, with calcification (Chapter 2), or with occlusion of the ventricular or subarachnoid pathways by intraventricular or subarachnoidal cysts giving rise to hydrocephalus (Proctor, 1964). Some of the more common parasites that infect the brain are *Cysticercus cellulosae, Coenurus cerebralis, Echinococcus granulosus* (hydatid), *Paragonimus westermani* (lung fluke), *Trichinella spiralis, Plasmodium falciparum, Schistosoma japonicum,* and *Trypanosoma cruzi* (Chagas' disease). *Toxoplasma gondii* is discussed in Chapter 2.

Cysticercosis

A complete dissertation on the subject of parasitosis of the brain is given by Arana-Iñiguez and López-Fernández (1966). The pathology of *Cysticercus* may be obtained from any standard textbook on pathology or from reports by Cárdenas Y Cárdenas (1962), Olivé and Angulo-Rivero (1962), and Arana-Iñiguez and López-Fernández (1966) from Mexico; and by Proctor (1964) from South Africa.

Radiological identification of this disease relies on the sites of infection and on the presence of calcification (Fig. 13-58, A). The commonest site is the meninges (56%), then the meninges with associated fourth ventricular and parenchymal cysts (20%), then the ventricles (16%) (Fig. 13-58, B), and finally the parenchyma (8%) (Dorfsman, 1963). Calcifications may be found in the scolex or in the wall of the dead cysticerci and occur in 15% to 50% of cases (Dorfsman, 1963; Santín and Vargas, 1966). These calcifications may be single or multiple and may either be small and round (1 to 5 mm in diameter) and centered in the scolex or have a partially or totally calcified spherical wall (7 to 12 mm in diameter) which was the body of the cystic larva.

Paragonimiasis

The lung fluke, *Paragonimus westermani,* travels from the lungs to the brain by hematogenous spread via the arteries or via loose connective tissue around the jugular vein to the head (Higashi et al., 1971). The occipital and temporal lobes are commonly infected. Radiological recognition of this brain infestation is by the mass effect and the dramatic calcification that occurs in 50% to 70% of cases, "an aggregated round or oval cystic calcification with an increased peripheral density" (Higashi et al., 1971). Six of the ten cases reported by Higashi and his co-workers were in children.

Hydatidosis of the nervous system

Hydatidosis, infection with *Echinococcus,* affects primarily the cerebral tissue and rarely the cerebro-

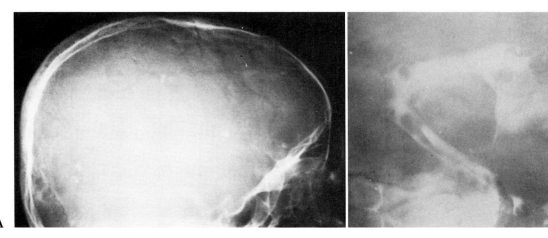

A   B

Fig. 13-58. Cysticercosis. A, Multiple dense calcifications throughout the cranium. B, Intraventricular, demonstrated by a Conray ventriculogram. (Courtesy F. Rueda-Franco, M.D., Mexico City.)

spinal fluid pathways de novo (Carrea and Murphy, 1964). Cerebral involvement occurs in 1% to 4% of cases and is manifested by generalized hydatid infestation (Orman and Le Roux, 1968). In endemic areas the presentation is mainly during childhood, between the ages of 6 and 18 years (Samiy and Zadeh, 1965), with increased intracranial pressure usually being the first manifestation in children. The cysts may be large but do not provoke a reaction from neighboring nervous tissue.

If a hydatid cyst ruptures into the ventricles or into the subarachnoid space, either spontaneously or by ill-advised tapping for cisternography, the larvae within it will contaminate the cerebrospinal fluid and cause subsequent satellite cysts to develop.

Abnormalities seen on standard skull radiographs may be one or more of the following: *split sutures, calvarial thinning* at the site of the cyst, and *calcifications*, linear (which is rare) or circumscribed (Fig. 13-59) (i.e., an outline of the cyst with fine and stippled foci or a dense conglomeration indicating a chronic partially collapsed cyst).

Angiography reveals a nonspecific mass typical of any cyst, with no characteristic changes in the vessels. Ventriculography (or pneumoencephalography in the absence of raised intracranial pressure) also reveals a nonspecific mass effect.

Involvement of the extradural space and the cranial vault itself has rarely been described. As Samiy and Zadeh (1965) state, 2% of hydatid cysts occur in the skeleton, with only 3.4% of these in the skull: an incidence rare indeed!

Miscellaneous parasitic infections

Through its infection of the fetus, *Toxoplasma* causes a devastating postinflammatory brain destruction that leads to subsequent brain atrophy in neo-

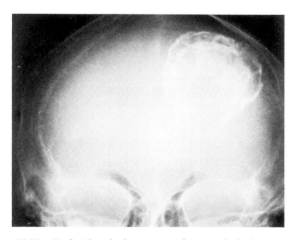

Fig. 13-59. Hydatid calcification. A large calcified cyst was found in the left cerebral hemisphere. (Courtesy M. Reeder, M.D., Washington, D.C.)

nates and calcification in numerous cerebral granulomas (Chapter 2).

Schistosomiasis, trypanosomiasis, cerebral malaria, and trichinosis are very uncommon. The reader is referred to the excellent discussion of these infections by Arana-Iñiguez and López-Fernández (1966).

Granulomas

Except in those instances when the neoplasm is caused by the protozoan *Toxoplasma gondii*, a granuloma is rarely found in a child's brain. This infection, acquired in utero, leads to typical cerebral calcifications (Chapter 2). Both intracranial sarcoidosis and intracranial histiocytosis are extremely uncommon in children. In the last ten years, we have identified neuroradiologically only two cases of intracranial histiocytosis at this hospital (Chapter 2).

Tuberculosis

Although in our experience intracranial tuberculosis is uncommon, its unusual neuroradiological manifestations deserve mention. A complete clinical description of tuberculosis in the central nervous system is given by Mathai and Chandy (1966). The following description is based on their report.

Tuberculous meningitis. Onset and progression in children with raised intracranial pressure are rapid.

Tuberculous arachnoiditis. Multiple cranial nerve palsies not associated with meningeal irritation are present, as well as raised intracranial pressure due to hydrocephalus.

Tuberculous meningoencephalitis (pseudotumor syndrome). This has a slower onset than tuberculous meningitis alone. It may present with signs and symptoms similar to those of a cerebral tumor, but neuroradiological procedures do not often show a focal mass effect.

Mixed meningitis, arachnoiditis, and meningoencephalitis. A combination of any of these signs may present in a child.

Tuberculoma. This is a common cause of space-occupying brain lesions in many tropical countries—particularly in India, where 20% of space-occupying lesions in children are attributed to tuberculoma (Mathai and Chandy, 1966). In children, cerebellar rather than cerebral sites are more common. An avascular mass is seen at angiography. Both calcification (Fig. 13-60) and abscess formation are rare. Calcifications within the basal cisterns have been demonstrated after recovery from childhood tuberculous meningitis (Segall et al., 1973).

Tuberculous cerebral vasculitis. Characteristic stenoses of the intradural part of the carotid siphon and its branches occur (Fig. 13-61) (Greitz, 1964; Ferris et al., 1968). These stenoses may be focal or

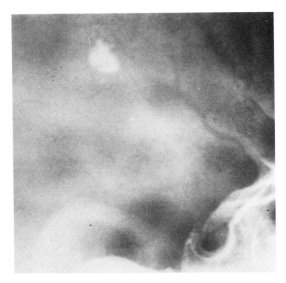

Fig. 13-60. Tuberculoma. This densely calcified mass is in the posterior frontal lobe.

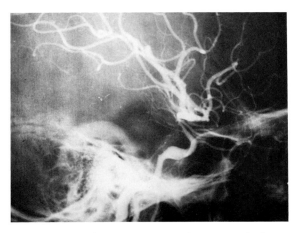

Fig. 13-61. Tuberculous meningitis. There is marked stenosis of the supraclinoid internal carotid artery in a child with chronic tuberculous meningitis. (Courtesy C. Suwanwela, M.D., Bangkok.)

may involve a considerable portion of an intracerebral artery; vasculitis, together with surrounding basilar arachnoiditis due to the tuberculous granulomatous tissue, causes them. Smaller vessels may be totally occluded as part of the vasculitis. A diffuse collateral arterial pattern in the midbrain may result from bilateral intracranial internal carotid stenosis (Mathew et al., 1970).

Fungal infections

Fungal infections of the nervous system are caused by saprophytes that primarily involve the lung (Utz, 1966). The saprophytes spread to the brain hematogenously, causing granulomatous reactions in the meninges. Seldom does a brain abscess result.

Although this type of infection is rare, commoner agents are *Cryptococcus neoformans, Histoplasma capsulatum, Coccidioides immitis, Blastomyces,* and *Candida albicans* (Utz, 1966). *Aspergillus* and *Nocardia asteroides* are uncommon etiological agents that have been implicated in pulmonary infections.

REFERENCES

Allen, J. H., and Meacham, W. F.: Colloidal barium sulfate as radiographic marker in surgical treatment of cavitary brain lesions; report on three years experience, Acta Radiol. [Diagn.] **9**:15, 1969.

Andrews, J. M.: Giant-cell ("temporal") arteritis; a disease with variable clinical manifestations, Neurology **16**:963, 1966.

Arana-Iñiguez, R., and López-Fernández, J. R.: Parasitosis of the nervous system, with special reference to echinococcosis, Clin. Neurosurg. **14**:123, 1966.

Arseni, C., Horvath, L., and Dumitrescu, L.: Cerebral abscesses in children, Acta Neurochir. **14**:197, 1966.

Askenasy, H. M., and Kosary, I. Z.: Brain abscess in cyanotic congenital heart disease, J. Neurosurg. **17**:851, 1960.

Benson, P., Nyhan, W. L., and Shimizu, H.: The prognosis of subdural effusions complicating pyogenic meningitis, J. Pediatr. **57**:670, 1960.

Berman, P. H., and Banker, B. Q.: Neonatal meningitis; a clinical and pathological study of 29 cases, Pediatrics **38**:6, 1966.

Bickerstaff, E. R.: Aetiology of acute hemiplegia in childhood, Br. Med. J. **2**:82, 1964.

Bigelow, N. H.: Multiple intracranial arterial aneurysms—an analysis of their significance, Arch. Neurol. Psychiatry **73**:76, 1955.

Birnbaum, G., Lynch, J. I., Margileth, A. M., Onergan, W. M., and Sever, J. L.: Cytomegalovirus infections in newborn infants, J. Pediatr. **75**:789, 1969.

Blackwood, W., McMenemy, W. H., Meyer, A., Norman, R. M., and Russell, D. S.: Greenfield's pathology, ed. 2, Baltimore, 1966, The Williams & Wilkins Co.

Blinderman, E. E.: An evaluation of micropaque barium sulphate as a radiographic marker for cerebral abscess, J. Neurosurg. **21**:867, 1964.

Bolton, C. F., and Ashenhurst, E. M.: Actinomycosis of the brain; case report and review of the literature, Can. Med. Assoc. J. **90**:922, 1964.

Byers, R. K., and Hass, G. M.: Thrombosis of the dural venous sinuses in infancy and in childhood, Am. J. Dis. Child. **45**:1161, 1933.

Cantu, R. C., LeMay, M., and Wilkinson, H. A.: The importance of repeated angiography in the treatment of mycotic-embolic intracranial aneurysms, J. Neurosurg. **25**:189, 1966.

Cárdenas Y Cárdenas, J.: Cysticercosis of the nervous system. II. Pathologic and radiologic findings, J. Neurosurg. **19**:635, 1962.

Carrea, R., and Murphy, G.: Primary hydatid cyst of the spinal cord, Acta Neurol. Lat. Am. **10**:309, 1964.

Charrier, A., and Ferradou, M.: Sur les abcès métastatiques du cerveau et du cervelet au cours des suppurations bronchopulmonaires, Rev. Chir. Orthop. **74**:642, 1936.

Chou, S. N., Story, J. L., French, L. A., and Peterson, H. O.: Some angiographic features of brain abscess, J. Neurosurg. **24**:693, 1966.

Clark, D. B.: Brain abscess and congenital heart disease, Clin. Neurosurg. **14**:247, 1966.

Clark, D. B., and Clarke, E. S.: Brain abscess as a complication of congenital cardiac malformation, Trans. Am. Neurol. Assoc. 77:73, 1952.

Clarke, P. R., Langmaid, C., and Wray, S.: The use of micropaque barium sulphate in the treatment of abscesses of the brain, Neurochirurgie 4:211, 1962.

Conen, P. E., Walker, G. R., Turner, J. A., and Field, P.: Invasive primary aspergillosis of the lung with cerebral metastasis and complete recovery, Dis. Chest 42:88, 1962.

Courville, C. B.: Subdural empyema secondary to purulent frontal sinusitis; clinicopathologic study of 42 cases verified at autopsy, Arch. Otolaryngol. 39:211, 1944.

Cussen, L. J., and Ryan, G. B.: Hemorrhagic cerebral necrosis in neonatal infants with enterobacterial meningitis, J. Pediatr. 71:771, 1967.

Dahlgren, S.: Thorotrast tumours; a review of the literature and report of 2 cases, Acta Pathol. Microbiol. Scand. 53: 147, 1961.

Davis, D. O., DiLenge, D., and Schlaepfer, W.: Arterial dilatation in purulent meningitis; case report, J. Neurosurg. 32: 112, 1970.

Davis, D. O., and Taveras, J. M.: Radiological aspects of inflammatory conditions affecting the central nervous system, Clin. Neurosurg. 14:192, 1966.

Dodge, P. R., and Swartz, M. N.: Bacterial meningitis—a review of selected aspects. II. Special neurologic problems, postmeningitic complications and clinicopathological correlations, N. Engl. J. Med. 272:954, 1965.

Doll, R., and Vessey, M. P.: Relation between use of oral contraceptives and thromboembolic disease, Br. Med. J. 2: 199, 1968.

Dorfsman, J.: The radiologic aspects of cerebral cysticercosis, Acta Radiol. [Diagn.] 1:836, 1963.

Eberhard, S. J.: Diagnosis of brain abscess in infants and children; a retrospective study of twenty-six cases, North Carolina Med. J. 30:301, 363, 1969.

Evans, W.: Pathology and aetiology of brain abscess, Lancet 1:1231, 1931.

Farmer, T. W., and Wise, G. R.: Subdural empyema in infants, children and adults, Neurology 23:254, 1973.

Ferris, E. J., and Ciembroniewicz, J.: Subdural empyema—report of a case demonstrating the unusual angiographic triad, Am. J. Roentgenol. Radium Ther. Nucl. Med. 92:838, 1964.

Ferris, E. J., and Levine, H. L.: Cerebral arteritis: classification, Radiology 109:327, 1973.

Ferris, E. J., Rudikoff, J. C., and Shapiro, J. H.: Cerebral angiography of bacterial infection, Radiology 90:727, 1968.

Gabrielsen, T. O., and Heinz, E. R.: Spontaneous aseptic thrombosis of the superior sagittal sinus and cerebral veins, Am. J. Roentgenol. Radium Ther. Nucl. Med. 107:579, 1969.

Garfield, J.: Management of supratentorial intracranial abscess: a review of 200 cases, Br. Med. J. 2:7, 1969.

Goodman, J. M., and Mealey, J., Jr.: Postmeningitic subdural effusions: the syndrome and its management, J. Neurosurg. 30:658, 1969.

Greitz, T.: Angiography in tuberculous meningitis, Acta Radiol. [Diagn.] 2:369, 1964.

Greitz, T., and Link, H.: Aseptic thrombosis of intracranial sinuses, Radiol. Clin. Biol. 35:111, 1966.

Gross, S. W., 1866. In Gurdjian, E. S., 1969.

Gross, S. W., 1873. In Gurdjian, E. S., 1969.

Gurdjian, E. S., editor: Cranial and intracranial suppuration, Springfield, Ill., 1969, Charles C Thomas, Publisher.

Hannesson, B., and Sachs, E., Jr.: Mycotic aneurysms following purulent meningitis; report of a case with recovery and review of the literature, Acta Neurochir. 24:305, 1971.

Harwood-Nash, D. C., McDonald, P., and Argent, W.: Cerebral arterial disease in children; an angiographic study of 40 cases, Am. J. Roentgenol. Radium Ther. Nucl. Med. 111: 672, 1971.

Harwood-Nash, D. C., Reilly, B. J., and Turnbull, I.: Massive calcification of the brain in a newborn infant, Am. J. Roentgenol. Radium Ther. Nucl. Med. 108:528, 1970.

Heinz, E. R., and Cooper, R. D.: Several early angiographic findings in brain abscess including the "ripple sign," Radiology 90:735, 1968.

Heinz, E. R., Geeter, D., and Gabrielsen, T. O.: Cortical vein thrombosis in the dog with a review of aseptic intracranial venous thrombosis in man, Acta Radiol. [Diagn.] 13:105, 1972.

Higashi, K., Aoki, H., Tatebayashi, K., Morioka, H., and Sakata, Y.: Cerebral paragonimiasis, J. Neurosurg. 34:515, 1971.

Hilal, S. K., Solomon, G. E., Gold, A. P., and Carter, S.: Primary cerebral arterial occlusive disease in children. I. Acute acquired hemiplegia, Radiology 99:71, 1971.

Hoffman, H. J., Hendrick, E. B., and Hiscox, J. L.: Cerebral abscesses in early infancy, J. Neurosurg. 33:172, 1970.

Holt, L. E., 1898. In Hoffman, H. J., 1970.

Horta, J. S., da Motta, L. C., Abbatt, J. D., and Roriz, M. L.: Malignancy and other late effects following administration of thorotrast, Lancet 2:201, 1965.

Isler, W.: Acute hemiplegias and hemisyndromes in childhood, Clin. Dev. Med., vol. 41/42, 1971.

Johnson, R. T., and Johnson, K. P.: Hydrocephalus following viral infection: The pathology of aqueductal stenosis developing after experimental mumps virus infection, J. Neuropathol. Exp. Neurol. 27:591, 1968.

Jordan, C. E., James, A. E., Jr., and Hodges, F. J., III: Comparison of the cerebral angiogram and the brain radionuclide image in brain abscess, Radiology 104:327, 1972.

Kalbag, R. M., and Woolf, A. L.: Cerebral venous thrombosis, London, 1967, Oxford University Press.

Krayenbühl, H. A.: Abscess of the brain, Clin. Neurosurg. 14: 25, 1966a.

Krayenbühl, H. A.: Cerebral venous and sinus thrombosis, Clin. Neurosurg. 14:1, 1966b.

Kyle, R. H., Oler, A., Lasser, E. C., and Rosomoff, H. L.: Meningioma induced by thorium dioxide, N. Engl. J. Med. 268:80, 1963.

Lebert, H., 1856. In Gurdjian, E. S., 1969.

Lecuire, J., Buffard, P., Goutelle, A., Thierry, A., Dechaume, J. P., and Kofman, J.: Considérations sur les aspects angiographiques des abcès du cerveau, Acta Radiol. [Diagn.] 5:315, 1966.

Lehrer, H., Larson, P. F., and McGarry, P. A.: Cryptococcal meningoencephalitis; two new radiologic signs, Radiology 88:531, 1967.

Lorber, J., and Pickering, D.: Incidence and treatment of post-meningitic hydrocephalus in the newborn, Arch. Dis. Child. 41:44, 1966.

Lyons, E. L., and Leeds, N. E.: The angiographic demonstration of arterial vascular disease in purulent meningitis; report of a case, Radiology 88:935, 1967.

MacEwen, W., 1893. In Gurdjian, E. S., 1969.

Macpherson, R. I., and Dunbar, J. S.: The radiology of mastoid disease in infants and children, J. Can. Assoc. Radiol. 16:40, 1965.

Margolis, M. T., Glickman, M. G., and Hoff, J.: Focal encephalitis simulating neoplasm, Neuroradiology 4:3, 1972.

Mathai, K. V., and Chandy, J.: Tuberculous infections of the nervous system, Clin. Neurosurg. 14:145, 1966.

Mathew, N. T., Abraham, J., and Chandy, J.: Cerebral angiographic features in tuberculous meningitis, Neurology 20:1015, 1970.

Matson, D. D.: Intracranial arterial aneurysms in childhood, J. Neurosurg. 23:578, 1965.

McDonald, C. A., and Korb, M.: Intracranial aneurysms, Arch. Neurol. 42:298, 1939.

McGreal, D. A.: Brain abscess in children, Can. Med. Assoc. J. 86:261, 1962.

Morgan, H., Wood, M. W., and Murphey, F.: Experience with 88 consecutive cases of brain abscess, J. Neurosurg. 38:698, 1973.

Morgagni, J. B., 1761. In Byers, R. K., and Hass, G. M., 1933.

Morriss, F. H., Jr., and Spock, A.: Intracranial aneurysm secondary to mycotic orbital and sinus infection; report of a case implicating Penicillium as an opportunistic fungus, Am. J. Dis. Child. 119:357, 1970.

Nager, G. T.: Mastoid and paranasal sinus infections and their relation to the central nervous system, Clin. Neurosurg. 14:288, 1966.

Nelson, D. A., Holloway, W. J., Kara-Eneff, S. C., and Goldenberg, H. I.: Neurological syndromes produced by sphenoid sinus abscess; with neuroradiologic review of pituitary abscess, Neurology 17:981, 1967.

Nestadt, A., Lowry, R. B., and Turner, E.: Diagnosis of brain abscess in infants and children, Lancet 2:449, 1960.

Newton, E. J.: Haematogenous brain abscess in cyanotic congenital heart disease, Q. J. Med. 25:201, 1956.

Norrell, H., and Howieson, J.: Gas-containing brain abscesses, Am. J. Roentgenol. Radium. Ther. Nucl. Med. 109:273, 1970.

Ojemann, R. G., New, P. F. J., and Fleming, T. C.: Intracranial aneurysms associated with bacterial meningitis, Neurology 16:1222, 1966.

Olivé, J. I., and Angulo-Rivero, P.: Cysticercosis of the nervous system. I. Introduction and general aspects, J. Neurosurg. 19:632, 1962.

Orman, D. N., and Le Roux, P. A. T.: Cerebral hydatid disease. A radiological review, S. Afr. Med. J. 42:1048, 1968.

Overall, J. C.: Neonatal bacterial meningitis: analysis of predisposing factors and outcome compared with matched control subjects, J. Pediatr. 76:499, 1970.

Peison, B., and Padleckas, R.: Granulomatous angiitis of the central nervous system, Ill. Med. J. 126:330, 1964.

Peters, E. R., and Davis, R. L.: Congenital rubella syndrome: cerebral mineralizations and subperiosteal new bone formation as expressions of this disorder, Clin. Pediatr. 5:743, 1966.

Proctor, N. S. F.: Tapeworm cyst infestation of the central nervous system; some observations, Med. Proc. 10:168, 1964.

Radcliffe, W. B., Guinto, F. C., Jr., Adcock, D. F., and Krigman, M. R.: Herpes simplex encephalitis; a radiologic-pathologic study of 4 cases, Am. J. Roentgenol. Radium Ther. Nucl. Med. 112:263, 1971.

Radcliffe, W. B., Guinto, F. C., Jr., Adcock, D. F., and Krigman, M. R.: Early localization of herpes simplex encephalitis by radionucleide imaging and carotid angiography, Radiology 105:603, 1972.

Raimondi, A. J.: Pediatric neuroradiology, Philadelphia, 1972, W. B. Saunders Co.

Raimondi, A. J., Matsumoto, S., and Miller, R. A.: Brain abscess in children with congenital heart disease, J. Neurosurg. 23:588, 1965.

Reddy, G. N. N., Harris, P., and Gordon, A.: Spinal subdural granuloma caused by micropulvarized barium sulphate; case report, J. Neurosurg. 26:425, 1967.

Roach, M. R., and Drake, C. G.: Ruptured cerebral aneurysms caused by micro-organisms, N. Engl. J. Med. 273:240, 1965.

Rowen, M., Singer, M. I., and Morgan, E. T.: Intracranial calcification in the congenital rubella syndrome, Am. J. Roentgenol. Radium Ther. Nucl. Med. 115:86, 1972.

Samiy, E., and Zadeh, F. A.: Cranial and intracranial hydatidosis; with special reference to roentgen-ray diagnosis, J. Neurosurg. 22:425, 1965.

Sanford, H. N., 1928. In Hoffman, H. J., et al., 1970.

Santin, G., and Vargas, J. S.: Roentgen study of cysticercosis of central nervous system, Radiology 86:520, 1966.

Schaffer, A. J.: Diseases of the newborn. Philadelphia, 1966, W. B. Saunders Co.

Schultz, P., and Leeds, N. E.: Intraventricular septations complicating neonatal meningitis, J. Neurosurg. 38:620, 1973.

Segall, H. D., Rumbaugh, C. L., Bergeron, R. T., Teal, J. S., and Gwinn, J. L.: Brain and meningeal infections in children; radiological considerations, Neuroradiology 6:8, 1973.

Shillito, J., Jr.: Carotid arteritis: a cause of hemiplegia in childhood, J. Neurosurg. 21:540, 1964.

Sievers, K., Nissila, M., and Sievers, U. M.: Cerebral vasculitis visualized by angiography in juvenile rheumatoid arthritis simulating brain tumour, Acta Rheumatol. Scand. 14:222, 1968.

Suwanwela, C., Suwanwela, N., Charuchinda, S., and Hongsaprabhas, C.: Intracranial mycotic aneurysms of extravascular origin, J. Neurosurg. 36:552, 1972.

Swischuk, L. E.: Radiology of the newborn and young infant, Baltimore, 1973, The Williams & Wilkins Co.

Taveras, J. M.: Caldwell lecture, 1968. Multiple progressive intracranial arterial occlusions: a syndrome of children and young adults, Am. J. Roentgenol. Radium Ther. Nucl. Med. 106:235, 1969.

Thompson, J. R., Harwood-Nash, D. C., and Fitz, C. R.: Cerebral aneurysms in children, Am. J. Roentgenol. Radium Ther. Nucl. Med. 118:163, 1973.

Tolosa, E.: Periarteritic lesions of the carotid siphon with the clinical features of acarotid infraclinoid aneurysm, J. Neurol. Neurosurg. Psychiatry 17:300, 1954.

Turner, E., and Whitby, J. L.: Nocardial cerebral abscess with systemic involvement successfully treated by aspiration and sulphonamides; case report, J. Neurosurg. 31:227, 1969.

Utz, J. P.: Fungal infections of the central nervous system, Clin. Neurosurg. 14:86, 1966.

Vines, F. S., and Davis, D. O.: Clinical-radiological correlation in cerebral venous occlusive disease, Radiology 98:9, 1971.

Wagenvoort, C. A., Harris, L. E., Brown, A. L., and Veeneklass, G. M. H.: Giant-cell arteritis with aneurysm formation in children, Pediatrics 32:861, 1963.

Wickbom, I.: Angiography of the carotid artery, Acta Radiol., supp. 72, 1948.

Wilkins, R. H., and Goree, J. A.: Interhemispheric subdural empyema: Angiographic appearance, J. Neurosurg. 32:459, 1970.

Wintrobe, M. M., Thorn, G. W., Adams, R. D., Bennett, I. L., Jr., Braunwald, E., Isselbacher, K. J., and Petersdorf, R. G., editors: Harrison's principles of internal medicine, ed. 6, New York, 1970, McGraw-Hill Book Co.

Wise, B. L., Mathis, J. L., and Jawetz, E.: Infections of the central nervous system due to Pseudomonas aeruginosa, J. Neurosurg. 31:432, 1969.

Woodhall, B.: Osteomyelitis and epi-, extra-, and subdural abscesses, Clin. Neurosurg. 14:239, 1966.

Wright, R. L., and Ballantine, H. T., Jr.: Management of brain abscesses in children and adolescents, Am. J. Dis. Child 114:113, 1967.

Wyss, 1871. In Eberhard, S. J., 1969.

Yaşargil, M. G., and Damur, M.: Thrombosis of the cerebral veins and dural sinuses. In Newton, T. H., and Potts, D. G., editors: Radiology of the skull and brain. Vol. 2, book 4, Angiography, St. Louis, 1974, The C. V. Mosby Co.

CHAPTER 14

Abnormalities of the cerebral arteries

The advent of safe and expert percutaneous catheter selective cerebral angiography in infants and children has encouraged an aggressive neuroradiological approach to the diagnosis of vascular disease in children. Though neuroradiological abnormalities peculiar to the cerebral vessels alone are rare in children, secondary vascular changes may be common sequelae of cerebral infection, trauma, and neoplasia.

Spontaneous subarachnoid hemorrhage does not occur often in children, nor do aneurysms or arteriovenous malformations. Except in the hospital referral practice, acute hemiplegia of infancy and childhood is also rare. These vascular disorders, however, require aggressive and intensive angiographic study and etiological speculation; and the understanding of their morphology and characteristics not infrequently relies solely on cerebral angiograms.

• • •

In infants and children, many arterial afflictions are not fatal. Catastrophic spontaneous intracranial hemorrhages are uncommon. Vascular occlusions are counteracted by a remarkably quick development of existing and potential collateral channels, with an equally remarkable adaptability of cerebral function to insult. Consequently, the devastating disturbance

of these functions that occurs in adults does not usually occur in children. Repeated vascular accidents and loss of consciousness and motor function are not morbid features in the young.

Thus the neuroradiological themes of this discussion are the study in the child of spontaneous intracranial hemorrhage (be it in the brain or subarachnoid or both), cerebral aneurysms and arteriovenous malformations, acute onset of hemiplegia from an obvious or unexplained source, and vascular abnormalities or angiodysplasias secondary to general systemic or local intracranial diseases. Serendipitous detection of intracranial vascular disease during angiography is extremely rare.

It is our general conviction that some types of arterial disease which occur in adults occur in children but the character of the disease is quite different; hence the early presentation in children. Some so-called congenital lesions, however (e.g., small but latent berry aneurysms), are not found "in evolution" in children; what is destined to present in adults *originates in adults*. The reader is reminded that arteriovenous malformations in the adult can develop into a larger and more significant edition of the childhood anlagen.

SPONTANEOUS BLEEDING

Intracerebral bleeding from any cause is usually associated with a subarachnoid hemorrhage; but the subarachnoid hemorrhage does not necessarily occur alone. The causes of each are often common to both; and therefore it is valid to consider them together.

Subarachnoid hemorrhage

The paediatric neuroradiologist is charged with the detection of the cause and site of frank blood in the CSF as seen on lumbar puncture or indicated clinically.

Sharpe and Maclaire (1925a,b) stated that 14% of newborn infants have a subarachnoid hemorrhage within 24 hours of birth and that 9% do within the first two days of birth. In spite of the normal trauma to intracranial contents during the delivery process, Alpers (1949) and Potter (1961) believe that most subarachnoid hemorrhages in neonates are due to anoxia which leads to venous congestion and increased venous and CSF pressures with subsequent rupture of small vessels. Also blood may escape into the CSF from vessels lying within the subarachnoid itself (cortical and basal vessels, choroid plexus) and join brain parenchymal hemorrhage or subdural blood through an arachnoid defect. Laitinen (1964) reported an incidence of spontaneous subarachnoid hemorrhage in 3% of 1,175 patients under 15 years of age. An aneurysm was identified in only nine of these children.

Causes of subarachnoid hemorrhage in infants and children may be listed as follows:

Aneurysm
Arterial or venous occlusive disease
Arteriovenous malformation
Birth process—trauma and anoxia
Bleeding in an intracranial neoplasm
Blood dyscrasia
Hypersensitivity vasculopathy
Infection
Postnatal trauma
Primary cerebral hemorrhage
Unknown

In a large series of patients of all ages with subarachnoid hemorrhage, Locksley (1966) stated that 51% of the hemorrhages were due to a ruptured

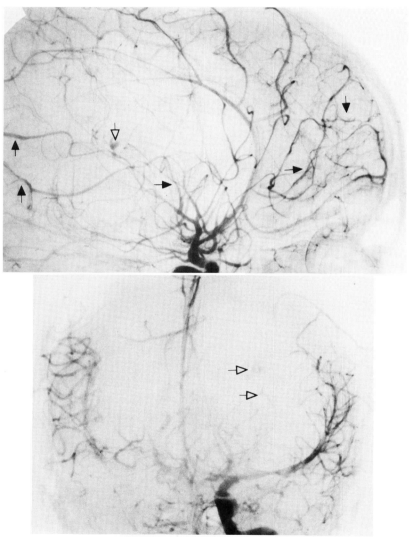

Fig. 14-1. Subarachnoid and intracerebral hemorrhage in leukemia. A deep cerebral hemorrhage and extravasation of contrast (open arrows), together with intraventricular hemorrhage, caused hydrocephalus and subarachnoid hemorrhage with diffuse stenoses and dilatation of the peripheral vessels (solid arrows).

aneurysm, 15% were associated with primary intracerebral hemorrhage, 6% were associated with a bleeding arteriovenous malformation, and 6% were of miscellaneous causes. The cause of 22% was unknown.

Aneurysms and *arteriovenous malformations* are lesions that rarely present in childhood; but when they do, their common presentation is hemorrhage into either the cerebral tissue or the subarachnoid space. Rupture of spinal arteriovenous malformations, rare in children, may present with subarachnoid hemorrhage. One or another of these lesions must therefore be thought of as a cause of spontaneous subarachnoid hemorrhage in the postneonatal age group.

A more common cause of subarachnoid hemorrhage in the infant is a hemorrhagic infarction due to either venous thrombosis (Chapter 13) or, less likely, arterial occlusion (Bailey and Hass, 1937a,b; Szancer, 1955; Kalbag and Woolf, 1967; Ford, 1973).

Venous thrombosis in the infant is usually of the aseptic type and associated with dehydration. Septicemia is also a significant cause of thrombosis.

Although an *intracerebral infection* does not usually cause subarachnoid hemorrhage, a relationship between the two may exist in cerebral embolic bacterial endocarditis (Starrs, 1949). Acute arteritis from a meningitis seldom bleeds into the subarachnoid space (Walton, 1956). A cerebral abscess rarely leads to bleeding from an involved adjacent artery or vein (Walton, 1956; Locksley et al., 1966). A bacterial cerebral aneurysm can rupture (Russell, 1954).

A *hypersensitivity vasculopathy*, such as polyarteritis nodosa, is rare in children and uncommonly involves the intracranial vessels (Hiller, 1953).

Seldom will spontaneous bleeding within an *intracranial neoplasm* lead to subarachnoid hemorrhage. Of those neoplasms that do bleed, grade 3 and grade 4 astrocytomas are common (De Saussure et al., 1951). The rare metastatic melanoma usually presents with a subarachnoid hemorrhage (Madonick and Savitsky, 1951). A hemorrhaged intraspinal neoplasm will infrequently lead to a subarachnoid hemorrhage (Nassar and Correll, 1968).

A *blood dyscrasia* such as leukemia (Fig. 14-1) (Moore et al., 1960), sickle cell anemia (Ballard and Bondar, 1957), or thrombocytopenia (Simpson and Robson, 1960) can lead to subarachnoid hemorrhage together with intracerebral hemorrhage. Adequate modern management of hemophiliacs avoids the previously common complication of intracranial bleeding (Kerr, 1964).

Frequently in adults, there is no detectable cause for the subarachnoid hemorrhage (22%) (Locksley, 1966); but this is not true in children. If total cerebral angiography fails to determine the cause of sub-arachnoid hemorrhage in a child, a myelogram must follow. The myelogram will detect possible spinal malformations or neoplasms, rare though they may be as causes of subarachnoid hemorrhage in children. The CSF must be clear of blood, however, before Pantopaque myelography is performed. If the myelogram reveals a possible spinal arteriovenous malformation, spinal selective angiography is indicated. The neuroradiology of subarachnoid hemorrhage is primarily total cerebral angiography, including both distal vertebral arteries and the origins of the PICAs.

Finally, it is important to remember that *hemorrhagic meningitis*, a frequent post–subarachnoid hemorrhage reaction within the subarachnoid space (Iwanowski and Olszewski, 1960), can induce a fibrotic arachnoiditis with occlusion of the subarachnoid space either by encroachment into the CSF pathway or by occlusion of the action of the arachnoid granulations (Ellington and Margolis, 1969). This leads to posthemorrhagic hydrocephalus, usually of the extraventricular obstructive type (Babson, 1944; Foltz and Ward, 1956).

Intracerebral hemorrhage

Relatively more common in adults, primary cerebral hemorrhage rarely occurs in children. Most infantile and childhood cerebral hemorrhages can be attributed to trauma or to one of the abnormalities listed as the causes of subarachnoid hemorrhage. The neuroradiology of such hemorrhages is concerned with detecting the mass effect (Fig. 14-2, A and B) and possibly the cause (e.g., an arteriovenous malformation) (Fig. 14-2, C) of the hemorrhage. Iatrogenic hemorrhage may also occur in the cerebral tissue or the ventricles, or both, and usually results from ventricular tapping.

The neuroradiological investigation of suspect intracerebral hemorrhage and its cause is done by computed tomography (CT) and angiography. Huckman and Davis (1974) describe in detail the angiographic nuances of the various sites of intracranial hemorrhage occurring in adults, most of which can also be applied to children. Though hemorrhage in the ventricles may be visible only by CT or ventriculography (Fig. 14-3), the neuroradiologist should use ventriculography only after other resorts have been exhausted (Murtagh and Baird, 1961). *CT* (Chapter 8) is now an essential preliminary investigation to angiography and will reveal the presence and location of clotted blood with great precision (Scott et al., 1973; Berger et al., 1976).

In the investigation of a suspect cerebral brain hemorrhage, we recommend that, in addition to a carotid angiogram, a vertebral angiogram be obtained so good filling of the posterior cerebral arteries will

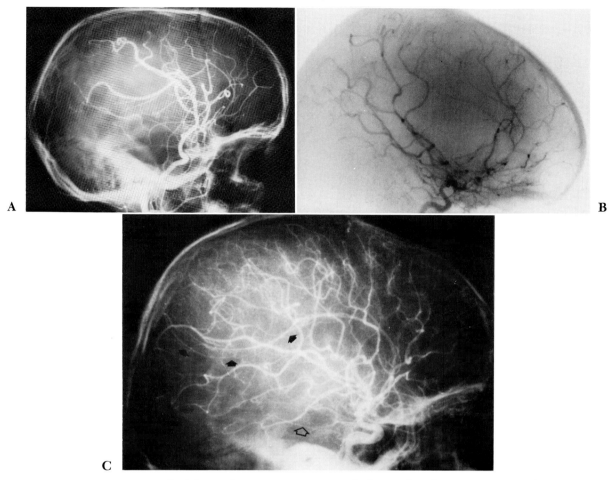

Fig. 14-2. Intracerebral hemorrhages. A, Large parietal, due to thrombocytopenia. Note the paradoxical dilatation of cortical vessels over the hemorrhage due to loss of autoregulation. B, Large superficial frontoparietal, spreading the cortical vessels apart. C, Large deep parieto-occipital, with downward displacement and stretching of the distal anterior cerebral arteries (solid arrows) and a hypertrophied tentorial artery (open arrow). An underlying AVM was confirmed at surgery.

enable the neuroradiologist to best evaluate the occipital lobes and visualize the posterior choroidal arteries and deep perforating arteries of the basal ganglia. Furthermore, the vertebral angiogram will show possible cerebellar or brain stem hemorrhage (Fig. 14-4). Thus not only can deep basal ganglionic cortical or posterior fossa hemorrhages be localized but possible causes of intracerebral hemorrhage (i.e., arteriovenous malformations, aneurysms, arteriopathies) can be identified.

Magnification subtraction selective cerebral angiog-

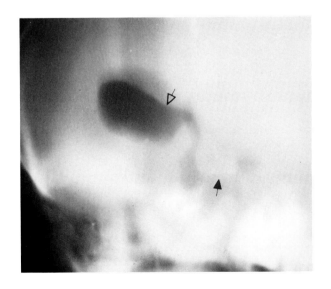

Fig. 14-3. Intraventricular hemorrhage. A newborn infant had a large hemorrhage (open arrow) in the lateral ventricle extending into the third ventricle (solid arrow) as seen on this midline tomogram and during ventriculography. (The nose is to the left.)

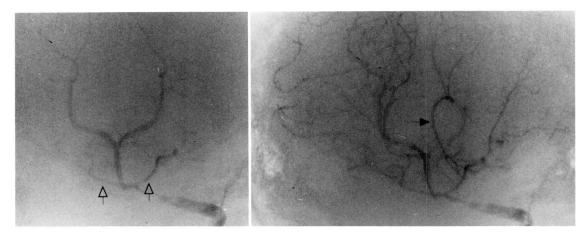

Fig. 14-4. Spontaneous brain stem and cerebellar hemorrhage. Sequential radiographs demonstrate stretching and displacement of both PICAs (open arrows) around an enlarged brain stem as well as medial and upward displacement of the distal left PICA (solid arrow) in the later phase and poor blood flow to the left cerebellar hemisphere. At operation a hemorrhage of the brain stem and left cerebellar hemisphere was present.

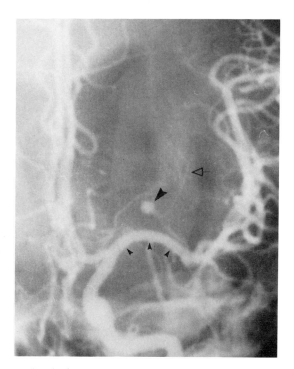

Fig. 14-5. Basal ganglionic hemorrhage. A spontaneous deep cerebral hemorrhage, probably from a hamartoma with a local pseudoaneurysm (large arrowhead) or a true aneurysm, displaces the lenticulostriate arteries laterally (open arrow) and extends in the subarachnoid space beneath the proximal middle cerebral artery (small arrowheads). (From Thompson, J. R., et al.: Am. J. Roentgenol. Radium Ther. Nucl. Med. **118**:163, 1973.)

raphy is also essential for accurately visualizing the character and displacements of the small deep perforating and lenticulostriate arteries (Krayenbühl and Yaşargil, 1968). The angiographic identification of the rare primary hemorrhage of the internal capsule (Fig. 14-5) and basal ganglia is by discrete displacement of the lenticulostriate vessels themselves. There may be a concomitant contralateral displacement of the internal cerebral vein, together with a downward displacement of the basal vein of Rosenthal or an upward displacement of the thalamostriate vein (Andersen, 1963). Forward extension of the hemorrhage into the sylvian fissure will elevate the horizontal portion of the middle cerebral artery (Fig. 14-5) and depress the anterior choroidal artery. Differentiating by angiography alone between an intracranial hemorrhage and edema from an infarct is difficult unless extravasation of contrast is visualized with the mass effect (Figs. 14-1 and 14-5). A computed tomogram will best identify extravasated blood.

A sudden loss of consciousness in an infant or child together with a large cerebral mass lesion detected in the posterior occipital region must be presumed to be a large hematoma prior to computed tomographic or surgical confirmation of angiographic changes. Intraventricular hemorrhage is best identified by CT or a ventriculogram. Angiography will reveal only the size and shape of the ventricles, not the intraventricular mass itself.

ANEURYSMS

An aneurysm is a localized and persistent dilatation of an artery and is comprised of components of the vessel wall. Aneurysms of the cerebral arterial system in infants are rare and are associated with local structural change (Stehbens, 1972). A false aneurysm is formed by an arterial wall rupture with an organized hematoma enclosing a lumen connected with that of the vessel. Local arterial ectasia, an arterial or venous varix, or an arteriovenous malformation is not an aneurysm. A *dissecting* aneurysm is correctly an extravasation of circulating blood within and along the substance of a vessel wall.

Carmichael (1950) suggested that the formation of a cerebral arterial aneurysm depends on two factors: (1) a defect in the media, or some congenital anomaly, and (2) a superimposed lesion of the internal elastic lamina, which in adults is probably due to early atheroma (Crawford, 1959). In a careful and extensive analysis, du Boulay (1965) compared the etiology and natural history of cerebral aneurysms from angiographic studies in man with dissection studies in animals and concluded that there is indeed an association between atherosclerosis and aneurysms. Close study of his report is recommended, as is scrutiny of the cooperative study of intracranial aneurysms in subarachnoid hemorrhage by Locksley (1966) and Sahs (1969).

The statistics and complications of adult cerebral aneurysms are beyond the scope of this chapter. A few generalities, however, are pertinent and apply to all ages:

1. At least twenty-five instances of *familial occurrence* of cerebral aneurysms have been reported (Brisman and Abbassioun, 1971), particularly between a mother and a son or daughter or between two brothers or two sisters.

2. *No specific pattern* to support a mendelian inheritance has been found. In a review of the literature, Bigelow (1953) reported that twenty-one of 360 patients (5.9%) with a congenital intracranial aneurysm had polycystic kidneys. Conversely, he reported that 10% of 499 patients with polycystic kidneys had a subarachnoid hemorrhage. Dalgaard (1957) studied 284 patients with bilateral polycystic kidneys and estimated the incidence of cerebral aneurysm to be 16%.

3. *Coarctation of the aorta* has uncommonly been described associated with a cerebral aneurysm. In at least thirty-two instances, Schwartz and Baronofsky (1960) found this concomitance; and Patel and Richardson (1971) reported that nine of fifty-eight children under 20 years of age with a cerebral aneurysm had been found to have a coarctation.

4. Other lesions reported to occur with cerebral aneurysm vary from *multiple angiomas* to *neurofibromatosis* (Bergouignan and Arne, 1951). Cronqvist and Troupp (1966) found that 9% of cerebral aneurysms also had a cerebral arteriovenous mal-

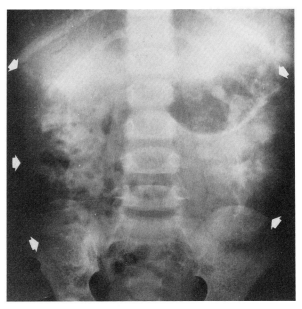

Fig. 14-6. Aneurysms and polycystic kidneys. This child had large polycystic kidneys (arrows) and congenital intracranial aneurysms. (From Thompson, J. R., et al.: Am. J. Roentgenol. Radium Ther. Nucl. Med. 118:163, 1973.)

formation. Two children with intracranial congenital aneurysms had enlarged bilaterally polycystic kidneys (Fig. 14-6). The Ehlers-Danlos syndrome has also been connected with cerebral aneurysm (Rubinstein and Cohen, 1964).

5. George and co-workers (1971b) described the association of *intracranial aneurysm* with a *persistent trigeminal artery* and reported a collected incidence of 13.8% in 232 cases. The aneurysm is commonly found at the carotid origin of the persistent trigeminal artery, and rarely at the basilar connection (Wolpert, 1966).

As far as we are aware, no clinically latent cerebral aneurysms have been discovered at angiography or serendipitously at autopsy in infants and children (Housepian and Pool, 1958; Harwood-Nash and Fitz, 1974; Raimondi, 1975). The incidence of aneurysms in adults at autopsy varies from 0.6% to 7.6% (Stehbens, 1972). The conclusion therefore is that most aneurysms presenting in childhood are due to some often unknown superimposed defect of the arterial wall other than atherosclerosis. Furthermore, it is obvious that aneurysms presenting in adults develop in adults and do not begin to form in infancy or childhood. Apparently the inherent medial wall weakness, particularly at the bifurcation, exists at any age; but the superadded intimal changes or medial damage in children differ as to origin from the usual atherosclerotic changes in adults.

Matson (1965), however, described two children

(one a 4-year-old) with atherosclerotic plaques at the neck of the aneurysm; and Patel and Richardson (1971) reported the presence of atherosclerosis in the coronary arteries and aorta of three children with intracerebral and intracranial aneurysms.

The types of aneurysm that we recognize neuroradiologically in children are congenital, inflammatory (bacterial and fungal), and traumatic. In our experience, there have been some aneurysms that were not typical in site or characteristics of any of the foregoing; these, by default, we consider to be congenital aneurysms.

Cerebral aneurysms in infants and children

The ensuing descriptions of aneurysms in infants and children should be compared and contrasted with the extensive neuroradiological data concerning adult aneurysms presented by Allcock (1974).

Matson (1969) reported thirteen children under 17 years of age with cerebral aneurysms. Patel and Richardson (1971) reported fifty-eight children under the age of 20 with aneurysms presumed to be congenital. Our own experience now totals twenty-six children each with an intracranial aneurysm from any cause (Table 14-1). (Four more children with intracranial aneurysms have been seen since our initial report of twenty-two children [Thompson et al., 1973].) In the preantibiotic era, McDonald and Korb (1939) found a 34% incidence of mycotic etiology in forty-four children with intracranial aneurysms.

Age and sex. Aneurysms presenting before 1 year of age are quite rare. In our series, one posterior cerebral aneurysm in a 9-month-old girl and one aneurysm of the anterior cerebral in a 4-month-old boy occurred. In a collective series of eleven aneurysms presenting before the age of 1 (Thompson and Pribram, 1969; Valpalahti et al., 1969; Shucart and Wolpert, 1973), the youngest patient was 2 days old. We combined our two patients with the eleven in the total series and found four of the thirteen aneurysms to have occurred in the middle cerebral artery, three in the posterior cerebral artery, two in the internal carotid artery, two in the basilar artery, and two in the anterior cerebral artery. In both Matson's (1969) and our series, approximately half and two thirds respectively of the aneurysms presented before the age of 10 (Table 14-1).

Many of the patients (72%) in the series of Patel and Richardson (1971) were in their late teens, between 15 and 19 years of age. Thus this series is heavily weighted toward the older age group and the figures are not exactly comparable with figures in the other two series. Twelve of the thirteen children in Matson's series were boys. In our series, however, there were more girls (sixteen, 62%) than boys (ten,

Table 14-1. Cerebral aneurysms in infants and children

	Matson (1969)	Patel and Richardson (1971)	Hospital for Sick Children (1976)
Number	13	58	26
Possible cause			
Congenital	12 (92%)	58	20 (77%)
Mycotic	1 (8%)	–	3 (11%)
Traumatic	–	–	3 (11%)
Age (yr)			
0-7	4 (30%)	0	7 (27%)
8-10	2 (15%)	4 (7%)	10 (38%)
11-14	6 (46%)	12 (21%)	7 (27%)
15+	1 (8%)	42 (72%)	2 (8%)
Site			
Supraclinoid internal carotid	3 ⎱ 4	– ⎱ 26	2 ⎱ 8
Internal carotid bifurcation	1 ⎰	26 ⎰	6 ⎰
Middle cerebral	2	3	6
Proximal	–	–	4
Distal	–	–	2
Anterior cerebral	5	23	5
Proximal	5	–	2
Distal	0	–	3
Posterior cerebral	–	–	2
Posterior communicating	–	–	1
Basilar tip	1	3	4
PICA	1	–	1
Multiple	–	3	1

38%) and twelve of the twenty congenital aneurysms occurred in girls. Thirty-two patients (55%) of the series of Patel and Richardson were boys and twenty-six (45%) were girls. No clear sex incidence therefore seems to be apparent.

Size and site. There was no real predilection for any site other than the supraclinoid portion of the internal carotid artery (Table 14-1). Four children in our series had basilar tip aneurysms (Table 14-1). Locksley (1966) reported in adults a 41% incidence of internal carotid aneurysms, a 34% incidence of middle cerebral aneurysms, a 20% incidence of anterior cerebral aneurysms, and only a 3% incidence of basilar aneurysms.

Only one child in our series had multiple aneurysms, and these were mycotic and involved the basilar and middle cerebral systems. A large aneurysm was a common occurrence. As measured by angiography or by direct visualization at autopsy or operation, thirteen (50%) were larger than 1 cm in diameter (Fig. 14-7). This figure actually may be greater since, in some children, angiography filled only the lumen of the aneurysm. The largest congenital aneurysm was 3.5 cm in diameter, and at least half the congenital aneurysms were larger than

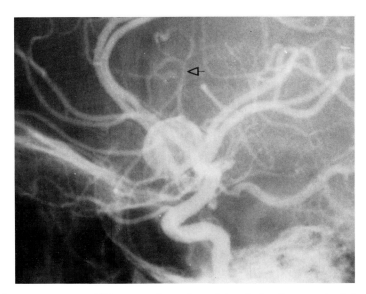

Fig. 14-7. **Large aneurysm.** This arose from the origin of the frontoparietal branch of the middle cerebral artery with associated spasm of the distal artery (arrow).

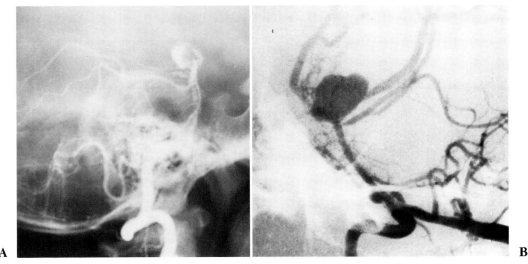

Fig. 14-8. **Mycotic aneurysms. A,** Large basilar, partially filled by a clot and with an associated spasm of the distal artery. **B,** Large lobulated basilar tip, with general spasm of the artery and of the superior cerebellar as seen on an oblique view. This aneurysm had an associated small aneurysm of an angular branch of the middle cerebral artery.

1 cm. Large aneurysms are rare in adults (Morley and Barr, 1969).

Cause. In our series, twenty aneurysms (77%) were judged to be *congenital* because no other cause could be identified. Three aneurysms were *mycotic* and secondary to congenital heart disease with septic emboli. Two of these three were associated with a meningitis; two of the three also were at the basilar tip (Fig. 14-8) (one with an additional aneurysm of the distal middle cerebral artery); one was in a branch of the anterior cerebral. Aneu-

rysms resulting from cavernous sinus thrombophlebitis (Chapter 13), osteomyelitis of the skull, and meningitis have been described by Suwanwela and co-workers (1972). Three aneurysms were *traumatic.* Two of these were in the anterior cerebral artery (Fig. 14-9)—one along the pericallosal branch and the other at the genu. In the third child the aneurysm arose from the supraclinoid portion of the internal carotid artery; this aneurysm thrombosed and calcified. The anterior cerebral aneurysm that arose from the genu was due to direct penetrating injury and con-

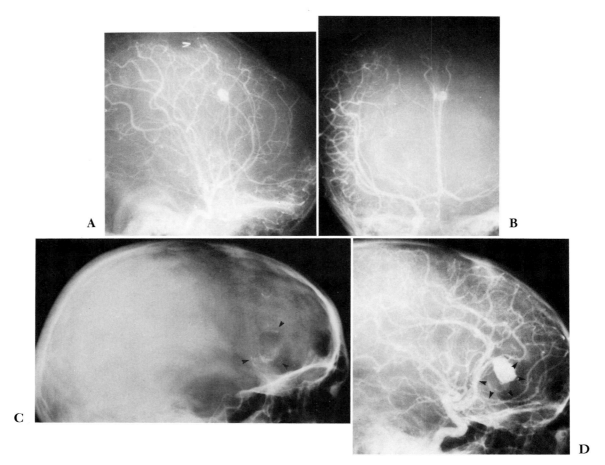

Fig. 14-9. Traumatic aneurysms. A and **B**, Large, of the pericallosal branch of the anterior cerebral artery in an infant with a severe head injury. The artery impinges on the falx at this site. **C** and **D**, Off the genu of the anterior cerebral, due to a penetrating injury six years prior to the angiogram. The thick wall (arrowheads) is calcified and creates a smaller irregular lumen. (**C** and **D** from Thompson, J. R., et al.: Am. J. Roentgenol. Radium Ther. Nucl. Med. **118**:163, 1973.)

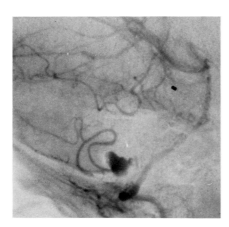

Fig. 14-10. Cerebellar artery aneurysm. This large lobulated aneurysm off the PICA was presumably congenital and is best seen by subtraction. (Courtesy D. Hardman, M.D., Hartford, Conn.)

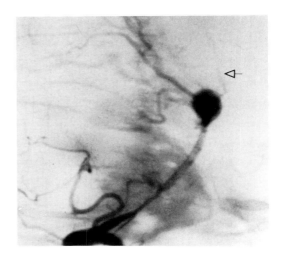

Fig. 14-11. Angiotomography and aneurysms. Large perforating vessels (arrow) can be seen arising from the fundus of a basilar tip aneurysm.

tained calcium in a thick wall (Fig. 14-9, C). The other two were due to severe head injury.

In a summary of the literature, Benoit and Wortzman (1973) stated that traumatic aneurysms are rare and may occur in the large basal arteries or peripherally, especially the middle cerebral artery. In one of our cases, that of a 4-month-old boy, the pericallosal artery must have been torn for it presumably pressed against the sharp edge of the falx during severe head injury (Fig. 14-9, A and B).

Aneurysms of the external carotid arteries. Without a traumatic cause, an aneurysm of the middle meningeal artery is rare; and we have not seen one in a child (New, 1963; Holland and Thomson, 1965). A small spontaneous aneurysm of the superficial temporal artery did occur in a 10-year-old girl; but this type also is rare (Wilson, 1969). A kink or loop in the upper internal carotid artery of an infant is commonly seen and is quite normal, but it is sometimes mistaken for an aneurysm (Sarkari et al., 1970).

Neuroradiology

In the investigation of subarachnoid hemorrhage in children, we customarily perform as complete a cerebral angiography as is necessary. This usually entails studying all four vessels by selective catheter angiography with magnification and subtraction. To locate a possible blood clot either within the aneurysm (Chapter 8) or within the adjacent brain tissue, we precede the angiography by computed tomography. Magnified, subtracted, and often oblique angiograms are necessary in the investigation of basilar or proximal anterior cerebral lesions and cerebellar artery aneurysms (which are rare in children) (Fig. 14-10). Angiotomograms will aid in the detection of small basal perforating arteries that may emerge from the apex of a basilar aneurysm (Fig. 14-11). Because of the common large size of the aneurysm, however, a well-defined neck will not commonly be identified in children (Fig. 14-12).

Except that aneurysms of the supraclinoid internal

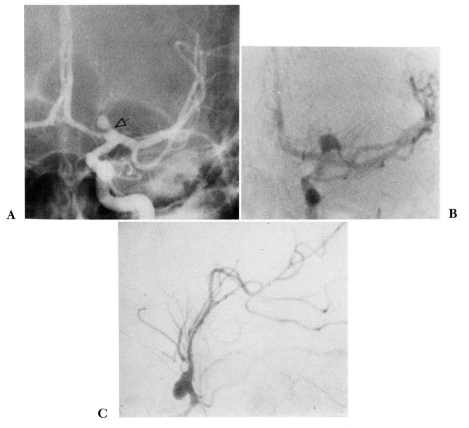

Fig. 14-12. Neck of the aneurysm. A, Well-defined (arrow), in a bifurcation internal carotid aneurysm. **B,** Without clear definition, in a large lobulated aneurysm of the same site. **C,** Large sessile middle cerebral aneurysm. Note the massive swelling of the temporal lobe and spasm of the anterior middle cerebral branches. A temporal subdural hematoma was also present.

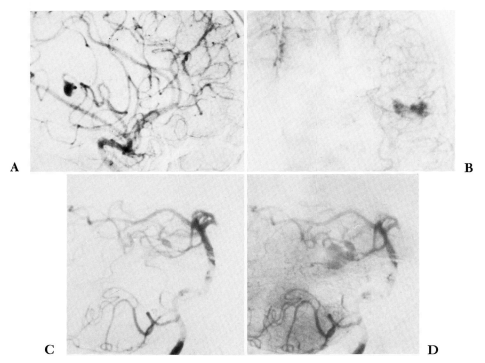

Fig. 14-13. Mycotic aneurysms and changing size. A, A lateral carotid angiogram shows a left distal middle cerebral artery aneurysm. B, A repeat anteroposterior carotid angiogram shows that the aneurysm increased markedly in size and became lobulated. C, A lateral vertebral angiogram in the same child shows a small superior cerebellar artery aneurysm. D, A repeat lateral vertebral angiogram shows that the aneurysm enlarged and became lobulated. (Courtesy B. Annis, M.D., La Crosse, Wis.)

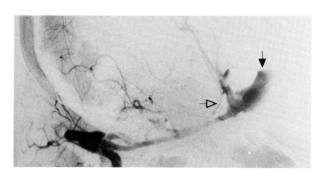

Fig. 14-14. Giant basilar aneurysm. This aneurysm had a lumen that at autopsy was two thirds filled with clot and one third filled with liquid blood (solid arrow). The child also had a primitive accessory basilar artery (open arrow) from which the superior cerebellar arteries arose.

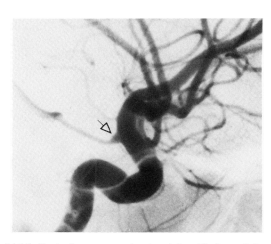

Fig. 14-15. Posterior communicating infundibulum. Infundibular dilatation of the origin of the posterior communicating artery (arrow) is rare in children and should not be mistaken for an aneurysm.

carotid artery are likely to be congenital, we have found few reliable specific angiographic features in children to differentiate mycotic, congenital, and traumatic aneurysms.

The *mycotic* type is often multiple and may change in size (Fig. 14-13). An associated *congenital* vascular anomaly may be identified—e.g., a primitive double basilar artery from one of whose lumina the superior cerebellar artery arises and from the other a large basilar aneurysm (Fig. 14-14). Contrast may fill a lumen within an intra-aneurysmal clot and the aneurysm may be so large as to occlude part of the CSF pathway, in particular the aqueduct, and produce a hydrocephalus (Pribram et al., 1969; Ekbom and Greitz, 1971). A ventriculogram may reveal an extra-axial mass, and subsequent angiography will demonstrate its true character. We have not identified a persistent trigeminal artery in any of our cases (George et al., 1971a).

Spasm of the parent or other artery in children, similar to that occurring in adults and due to subarachnoid hemorrhage, can take place. A concomitant bleeding into the cerebral tissue can occur and may create a large hematoma. The bleeding may be localized within the CSF space surrounding the aneurysm, such as in the sylvian fissure. If the intracranial source of a subarachnoid hemorrhage is not determined, a myelogram should be obtained to identify a possible spinal angioma. We have not found aneurysms associated with intracranial arteriovenous malformations, but there is a 7% incidence of this association in adults (Perret and Nishioka, 1966).

Cerebral angiograms may identify increasing size or lobulation of the aneurysm (Figs. 14-8, *A*, and 14-13) or even diminished size of the intra-aneurysmal lumen due to a progressive luminal thrombosis (Figs. 14-8, *B*, and 14-14). A subdural hematoma with a bleeding aneurysm is an uncommon association in children (Fig. 14-12, *C*) but is stated to occur in 5% to 20% of ruptured intracranial aneurysms in adults (Stehbens, 1972). Infundibular dilatation of the posterior communicating artery, often mistaken for an aneurysm, is common in adults but rare in children (Fig. 14-15).

ARTERIOVENOUS MALFORMATIONS

The generic term arteriovenous malformation is used to describe a number of vascular anomalies occurring within the brain, some of which in fact are not arteriovenous but are venous only; indeed, some are comprised of arteries and venules but no abnormal shunting is present. We shall consider those vascular anomalies that are commonly demonstrated by cerebral angiography to be arteriovenous malformations and merely mention the rare venous angiomas and small hemangiomas or telangiectasias of the brain.

Stehbens (1972) classifies the vascular anomalies as follows:

1. *Telangiectasias*—rare small solitary anomalies of capillary-like channels often found in 0.4% of adult autopsies. These usually occur in the pons and rarely bleed.

2. *Cavernous hemangiomas*—sometimes presenting with epilepsy or hemorrhage. These occur even less frequently (0.02%), are found at autopsy, and may be single or multiple and scattered throughout the brain. They are large vascular spaces tightly packed by and contained within endothelium and collagen, and they may calcify. Their size varies from a few millimeters to 3 or 4 cm in diameter.

3. *Arteriovenous malformations*—constituting the majority of vascular malformations in children. These are widespread throughout the cerebrum, particularly but less commonly in the posterior fossa; there may be scattered multiple foci. They are made up of a focal tangle of arteries and veins ranging in size from small cryptic malformations to large complexes 4 or 5 cm across. The arteries may shunt directly, or via a network of tortuous capillaries, into veins; the arterial and venous walls may be segmentally hyalinized or fibrosed. Vascular ectasia, thrombosis, and calcification may occur within the malformation.

4. *Venous angiomas*—single or several tortuous veins with normal or calcified walls and no arterial component. These may occur anywhere throughout the brain substance but will often be found in a pia-based cone. They rarely bleed, may cause seizures, and are usually situated within the middle cerebral territory. Stehbens (1972) considers the venous varix component of an arteriovenous shunt to be a venous angioma; but we, like McCormick (1966), prefer to consider venous angiomas as part of an arteriovenous malformation per se.

AVMs are the most common vascular anomalies of the central nervous system. Stehbens (1972) considers them to be "vascular hamartomas in which there is an arteriovenous shunt of variable degree." Padget (1956) described the development of arteries as preceding that of veins, the veins developing in subjacent tissue usually at right angles to the path of the arteries. A persistent fistula between these two primitive endothelial vessels at their crossing could explain the development of an AVM. Vessels of the choroid plexus have a similar juxtaposition but rarely develop into AVMs. The anomalous connection therefore is the malformation and not the secondary dramatic dilatation of abnormal veins. Kaplan and co-workers (1961) stated that AVMs originate as congenital maldevelopments in the primitive AV communications of the early embryo, these shunts being normally replaced by an intervening capillary network; thus an AVM may be a defect in capillary development.

The malformations often have a wedge-shaped configuration, the base being the pial surface. This follows the pattern of the developing transcerebral veins proposed by Padget (1956). The malformations therefore are present at birth and grow and develop symptoms due to hemorrhage and AV shunting; they may also thrombose. The majority are fed by multiple arterial vessels, commonly by a predominant middle cerebral artery supply often including the deep perforating and thalamic arteries.

Numerous extensive reports are available describing in great detail the pathology, radiology, and treatment of AVMs in adults; and the reader is referred to those by Poppen and Avman (1960), Perret and Nishioka (1966), Gomes and Bernatz (1970), Stehbens (1972), Houser and co-workers (1973), and in particular the exhaustive neuroradiological data compiled by Newton and Troost (1974). Except for the spectacular infantile AVMs involving the galenic system, there is little reference other than by Matson (1969) to AVMs occurring in children.

Arteriovenous malformations in infants and children

Matson (1969) reported thirty-four infants and children with AVMs of the brain (excluding galenic venous varices). We have encountered fifty infants and children with intracranial AVMs (Table 14-2). This includes twelve AVMs with aneurysmal dilatation of the vein of Galen. We identified these AVMs by angiography. Rarely did we discover small asymptomatic pial telangiectasias, and *never serendipitously* a large AVM without clinical symptoms. Thus, like paediatric cerebral aneurysms, these AVMs present in children because they are different in some way from those that continue to present in adults.

Age and sex. Eleven infants in our series were under 6 months of age, and eight had a large varix of the vein of Galen. In six of these eight children, the AVM presented within the first few weeks of life. Only two children were seen at 6 months to 2 years of age, whereas eleven children were seen between and including the ages of 2 and 5 years. Ten children were ages 6 to 10 years inclusive, and sixteen were over 11 years of age (Table 14-2). AVMs other than those central types with galenic varices, which commonly present in infancy, tend to present at an older age.

Twenty-eight children (56%) were boys, and twenty-two (44%) were girls. These figures are nearly identical with the figures in a collected series of patients of all ages by Stehbens (1972) (54% and 46% respectively) and in Matson's series of thirty-four children (53% and 47% respectively).

Size and site. Forty children (80%) had a supratentorial AVM (lesions of the posterior cerebral artery at the tentorial hiatus are considered to be supratentorial), and eight (16%) an infratentorial AVM. In two children the lesion was confined to the dura of the vault (Table 14-3). In collected series of patients of all ages with AVMs, supratentorial outnumber infratentorial 82% to 18%—the range being 7% to 93% for supratentorial and 32% to 68% for infratentorial (Perret and Nishioka, 1966; Stehbens, 1972; Houser et al., 1973). In adults, cerebellar AVMs outnumber brain stem AVMs 2 to 1; in children, the opposite is true (Perret and Nishioka, 1966).

Table 14-2. Age and arteriovenous malformations in children

Age	Total HSC series	Large galenic varix	Other AVMs	Total Matson series*
0-6 mo	11	8	3	1
6 mo-1 yr	2	–	2	2
2-5 yr	11	3	8	5
6-10 yr	10	1	9	14
11 yr+	16	–	16	12
Total	50	12	38	34

*Excluding AVMs with large galenic varices.

Table 14-3. Site of fifty arteriovenous malformations in children

	Number	Percent
Supratentorial	40	80
Midline (with large galenic varix)	12	
Cerebral hemispheric	28	
Superficial (± deep)	25 }	
Deep thalamic only	3 }	
Unilateral single	20 }	
Unilateral multiple	4 }	
Bilateral	4 }	
Involvement		
Parietal		42
Temporal		25
Occipital		16
Frontal		14
Choroid plexus alone		3
Dural	2	4
Alone	2	
And cerebral (eight, classified with cerebral hemispheric)		
Infratentorial	8	16
Brain stem	6	
Cerebellar	2	

The majority of AVMs located in the cerebral hemispheres were cortical, often with a deep extension. Most (70%) were fed by more than one major pial artery, a few (19%) were fed by only one pial artery, and even fewer (11%) were purely thalamic and fed by perforating vessels. A vascular anomaly of the retina along with a cerebral hemispheric AVM rarely presents in children (Wyburn-Mason, 1943; Newton and Troost, 1974). The AVMs drained into the superficial cerebral veins to the sinuses and/or into the deep venous system and thence into the vein of Galen and straight sinus. Mild dilatation of the vein of Galen may occur. Those children in whom the arteries pass centrally and *directly* into the vein of Galen should be considered separately, however, for the vein then becomes immensely dilated (the so-called aneurysm of the vein of Galen).

Within the cerebral hemisphere alone (twenty-eight children), single unilateral AVMs (71%) were common but multiple unilateral (14%) and bilateral (14%) were less common (Table 14-2). Bilateral AVMs are rare in any series and are reported at approximately 5% (Perret and Nishioka, 1966). Midline AVMs, such as those with large galenic varices, are often fed by both carotid vessel branches but are not considered to be bilateral.

The parietal lobe is involved more often than the temporal lobe (42% to 25%) (Table 14-3). In children, as in adults, AVMs tend to occur at the watershed blood supply areas between major cerebral arteries (Houser et al., 1973). The choroid plexus of the lateral ventricles is seldom involved alone (in only one child of our series). Dural AVMs more commonly present in adults, usually in the posterior venous sinuses (Newton and Cronqvist, 1969; Houser et al., 1972). Pure dural AVMs rarely present in children; but malformations of the cerebrum and posterior fossa frequently receive part of their blood supply by external carotid vessels, tentorial arteries, or meningeal vessels of the vertebrobasilar arterial tree. Dural AVMs in our series tended to be fed by external carotid, vertebrobasilar meningeal, and tentorial arteries. A rare meningeal artery from a posterior cerebral artery occurred in one child with a dural AVM similar to that reported by Newton and Troost (1974).

Infratentorial arteriovenous malformations, uncommon in our series (eight children, 16%), involved the brain stem commonly (six) and the cerebellum alone rarely (two). AVMs of the brain stem may encroach on the fourth ventricle or involve small portions of contiguous cerebellum (McCormick et al., 1968).

When the AVM complex first presents in children, it is usually large, its area of involvement is considerable, and its feeding and draining vessels are wide (Henderson and Gomez, 1967). Houser and co-workers (1972) have reported the size of AVMs to be inversely proportional to the propensity for bleeding. We have not found this to be true, however, in our experience with children. The AVMs that presented with bleeding were very large. At angiography, a few children had relatively small remnants of an AVM that had partially destroyed itself. In three children not in our series, large hematomas of the brain contained microscopic remnants of an AVM—so-called "cryptic" vascular malformations (Russell, 1954; McCormick and Nofzinger, 1966; Matson, 1969).

Clinical presentation. In all the AVMs of infancy and childhood, common presenting signs and symptoms were focal headache (35%), hemiplegia, aplasia, and cranial nerve palsies (35%), and subarachnoid hemorrhage (35%).

Severe headaches, always a difficult symptom to evaluate in children, are uncommon. They should never be disregarded clinically, however, since in our experience they were often the only symptom in older children with a cerebral AVM.

Seizures were uncommon (19%)—as either the sole presentation or a concomitant of intracranial hemorrhage. AVMs rarely presented in children with epilepsy alone. In the majority of children in whom an AVM was thought to be the cause of seizures, additional clinical or radiological evidence of an AVM was usually present.

Nineteen percent of the children were comatose when we saw them. Cardiac failure was present in only those infants and children with cerebral galenic AVMs, occurring in seven of these infants. Cronqvist and co-workers (1972), however, described two infants with congestive cardiac failure and a peripheral AVM of the cerebral hemisphere. Hydrocephalus was a presenting sign in ten children (20%), five of whom had a central AVM with a galenic varix. Intraventricular bleeding and a subarachnoid hemorrhage also contributed to the hydrocephalus. A large cranial bruit may not be present or may be of varying intensity from one examination to the next; but a soft intracranial bruit is quite common in both normal and hydrocephalic children. Infants with a postnatal galenic AVM were often investigated initially by the cardiac unit for their congestive cardiac failure. The appearance of early filling of the jugular vein and a high jugular venous oxygen content indicated an intracranial AVM.

Infratentorial AVMs often presented with a focal brain stem or cerebellar neurological defect or ataxia. Subarachnoid hemorrhage and headache or an altered sensorium were less commonly seen. Rebleeding may occur in untreated cases and is more common after subarachnoid hemorrhage (but only if an intracerebral hemorrhage was not previously present).

Neuroradiology

Central arteriovenous malformation with a large galenic varix. Separate and specific descriptions of these fascinating anomalies are essential. Amacher and Shillito (1973) presented a detailed review of thirty-seven cases from the literature and added five of their own. The neuroradiological course is often predicated on the clinical presentation (Gold et al., 1964b). At our hospital approximately three infants per year with this lesion are seen, and not all survive long enough to be investigated neuroradiologically.

From the clinical point of view, the *first group* includes those children with cardiac failure who are seen soon after birth or in early infancy (Gomez et al.,

1963; Holden et al., 1972). Failure to detect a preangiogram cranial bruit leads to cardiac rather than to cerebral vascular catheterization in the infant. The high jugular venous oxygen content and the early return of contrast down the superior vena cava are foundation for immediate neuroradiological consultation and investigation. These children are in a fast–shunt flow situation.

The *second group* includes children with hydrocephalus due to compression and occlusion of the posterior third ventricle and aqueduct (Fig. 14-16) who are seen between 6 months and 3 years of age. They may have mild heart failure and rarely convulsions with subarachnoid hemorrhage. They may or

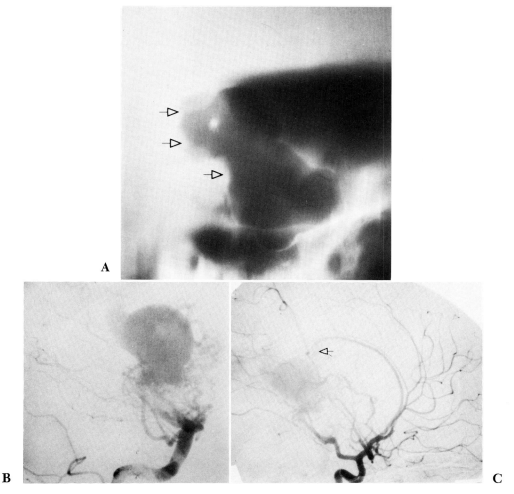

Fig. 14-16. Central galenic arteriovenous malformation and hydrocephalus. A, A two-year-old child had hydrocephalus and no cranial bruit. A ventriculogram demonstrates an irregularly surfaced mass in the posterior third ventricle (arrows) occluding the aqueduct. **B** and **C,** Internal carotid and vertebral angiograms show a large galenic varix fed by the posterior cerebral artery and numerous posterior perforating arteries (**B**). Both the feeders and the varix have produced occlusion and an irregular posterior surface of the third ventricle. Note the hydrocephalic sweep of the anterior cerebellar artery which provides some small posterior callosal feeders (**C,** arrow).

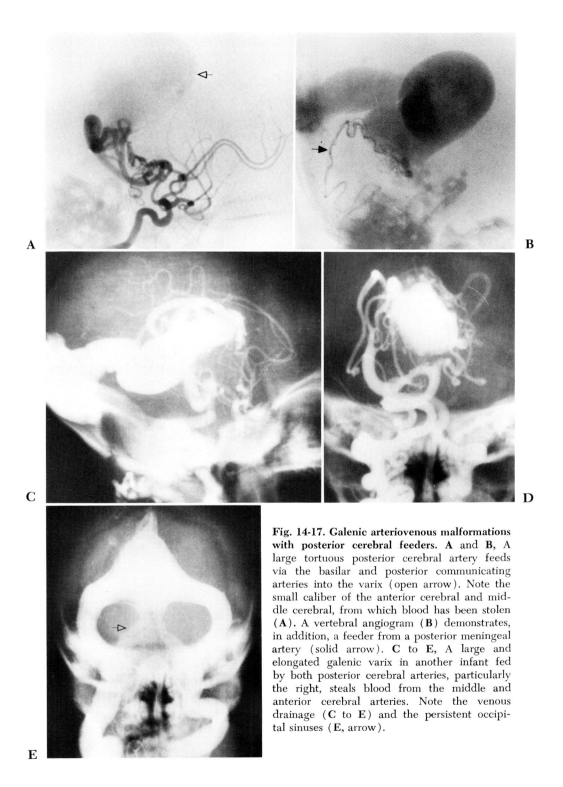

Fig. 14-17. Galenic arteriovenous malformations with posterior cerebral feeders. A and **B,** A large tortuous posterior cerebral artery feeds via the basilar and posterior communicating arteries into the varix (open arrow). Note the small caliber of the anterior cerebral and middle cerebral, from which blood has been stolen (**A**). A vertebral angiogram (**B**) demonstrates, in addition, a feeder from a posterior meningeal artery (solid arrow). **C** to **E,** A large and elongated galenic varix in another infant fed by both posterior cerebral arteries, particularly the right, steals blood from the middle and anterior cerebral arteries. Note the venous drainage (**C** to **E**) and the persistent occipital sinuses (**E,** arrow).

may not have a bruit. In this group the shunt is of a relatively slow-flow type.

The *third group* is the most uncommon and is comprised of older children and adults—who are in a very slow–shunt flow type of situation, often without spectacular enlargement of the venous varix. Since these children often have associated intrinsic cerebral hemispheric AVMs, we tend to include them with children having cerebral AVMs that involve the galenic system rather than with children having central AVMs.

Skull radiography in children with a central AVM and large galenic varix either is normal (e.g., the first group) or reveals a chronic hydrocephalus (the second group). Enlarged dural inner table markings around the torcular may also be seen. Rarely will the varix calcify (Ozonoff and Burrows, 1971). We have not seen such calcification.

A radionuclide brain scan will show on both immediate and delayed images a large central area of increased uptake (Chapter 9). Computed tomography will show a large image centrally with an absorption coefficient of 18 to 20 EMI units, the same as that of flowing blood (Chapter 8). To identify every feeding artery, selective angiography of both internal carotids and one vertebral is the minimum essential examination. A totally successful method of treating AVMs with numerous feeding vessels is still not at hand.

An essential component of these galenic varices is a direct connection between one or more major feeding arteries into the varix. Litvak and co-workers

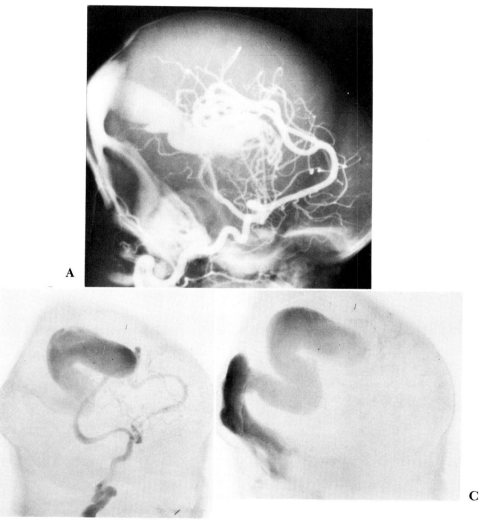

Fig. 14-18. Dominant anterior cerebral feeder. A, To a galenic AVM, together with relatively minor supply from the posterior cerebral artery. **B,** A single large anterior cerebral and a single large posterior cerebral feeder. Note the small remaining anterior cerebral and middle cerebral arteries. **C,** This venous varix is a highly placed venous drainage system.

(1960) defined the "true aneurysm of the vein of Galen" as a gross dilatation of the vein being fed directly by a large anomalous vessel or vessels off the carotid or basilar circulation. We have adopted this concept; and we relegate all other AVMs with indirect drainage into the deep venous system—some with relatively large tubular-like dilatations of the vein of Galen—to the group that includes cerebral AVMs involving the galenic system (O'Brien and Schechter, 1970).

The posterior cerebral artery and its branches, especially the posterior choroidal and posterior perforating arteries, are commonly involved (90%) (Fig. 14-17) in central AVMs. We have found that the anterior cerebral artery also feeds the aneurysm in 40% of our cases (Fig. 14-18), a much higher incidence than the 13% reported by Amacher and Shillito (1973). Both the anterior and the posterior cerebral arteries were dominant feeders in a majority of these infants. The middle cerebral artery did not feed even one AVM in our series, and only 5% of those discussed by Amacher and Shillito. Much of the blood flow from this vessel actually is diverted through the shunt and a small-caliber middle cerebral artery results (Fig. 14-18, C).

Thus only one or two large feeders may be present and create a filling jet effect (Fig. 14-19), or a myriad of small arteries may feed directly into the varix (Fig. 14-16, C). We industriously counted forty-seven such feeders in one infant! Single feeders are eminently treatable, whereas multiples are not. Catheter embolization may have a preoperative benefit, but often the feeders are so large that huge artificial emboli would be needed. In any case, embolic treatment of infantile AVMs necessitates that the emboli be inserted by a large catheter placed in the carotid or vertebral artery rather than by a subcutaneous catheter (Hilal, 1974).

The galenic varix may be so large and its walls so thick that it contains its own vasa vasorum; and the vasa vasorum, in turn, may be dilated and tortuous and exist as part of the vascular malformation complex itself (Fig. 14-20). The huge galenic varix may drain down an equally large straight sinus or may have a clublike appearance; it may be large and spherical with a small draining sinus; or it may drain directy upward toward the central sinus through a persistent primitive venous pathway (Figs. 14-18, C, and 14-21), so clearly described by Padget (1956).

The confluence of the straight and sagittal sinuses (at the torcular) often produces another varix through which contrast-opacified blood from the anomaly and unopacified blood via the sagittal sinus create artistic swirls and vortices (Fig. 14-20). The varix will rarely thrombose spontaneously (Heinz et al., 1968).

If a ventriculogram is inadvertently obtained, it will reveal a large smooth (Fig. 14-19) or gently irregular (Fig. 14-16, A) mass behind the third ventricle obstructing the aqueduct and creating an IVOH. In these (older) children, heart failure or a bruit may not be present. Angiography is essential; and the correct diagnosis may be suspected by the results of the radionuclide scan and computed axial tomography,

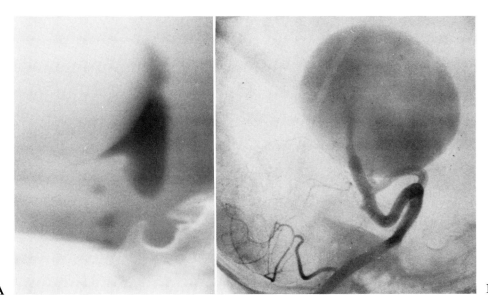

A   **B**

Fig. 14-19. Arterial jet effect. A, A ventriculogram reveals a smooth indentation into the posterior third ventricle in an infant with hydrocephalus and a faint cranial bruit. B, An angiogram shows the sole feeder from the right posterior cerebral artery creating a remarkable jet effect into the galenic varix.

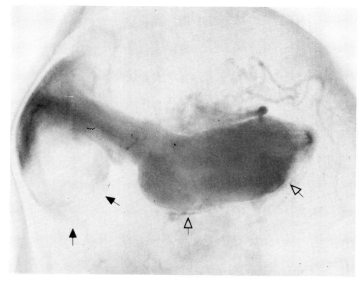

Fig. 14-20. Varix and its vasa vasorum. Note the swirling eddy effect in a slow-flowing varix at the torcular (solid arrows). This malformation was fed by the anterior and posterior cerebral arteries. Its walls contain their own vasa vasorum (open arrows).

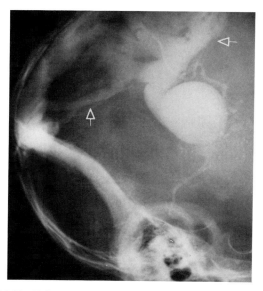

Fig. 14-21. Galenic arteriovenous malformation and primitive venous drainage. A large galenic varix drains superiorly through a fanlike falcine system of veins (arrows) similar to those seen in early embryonic life.

which will show a highly vascular mass. In the absence of angiography, an atypical pineal teratoma may be mistakenly diagnosed on a ventriculogram—particularly if calcification is present within the varix (Wilson and Roy, 1964).

Supratentorial arteriovenous malformation

Skull radiographs. In our series of twenty-eight children with a supratentorial AVM other than a large galenic varix, skull radiographs were entirely

normal in 51%. Abnormalities were due to either direct or indirect effects of the arteriovenous malformation (Lindblom, 1936; Rumbaugh and Potts, 1966).

DIRECT ABNORMALITIES

CALCIFICATION. Calcification of the AVM varix occurred in 20% of the children in our series and was most common in older children. It developed within the venous or sinus varix (Fig. 14-22, A) and was rounded or crescentic, often with an irregular coarse border, suggesting that a mural hematoma might also be calcified. Large cavernous angiomas rarely calcify (Runnels et al., 1969).

Calcification was seen in 30% of the sixty-one patients of all ages reported by Rumbaugh and Potts (1966). These patients demonstrated marked prominence of vascular markings on or in the vault and foramina (Fig. 14-23), especially along the course of the meningeal arteries and the venous sinuses or dural veins (particularly the sphenoparietal) (Fig. 14-23, C).

VASCULAR MARKINGS. If the meningeal arteries are involved, large meningeal grooves will be seen. Vascular markings occurred in eight children (16%). All these children had superficial cerebral AVMs with or without dural involvement. Perforating channels from the external vessels into the cerebrum may create small round lucent areas. Large occipital emissary veins may also be seen in AVMs of this area.

A superficial cortical venous varix may produce a large well-corticated scalloped erosion of the inner table (Fig. 14-24). Enlarged vascular foramina commonly occur in children. The carotid canal may be

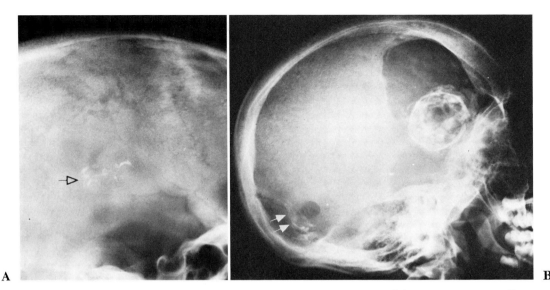

Fig. 14-22. **Calcification and arteriovenous malformation. A,** Fine flakes (arrow) in small venous varices within the main complex of the AVM. **B,** Gross calcifications in large varices, both within the AVM anteriorly and in a large varix in the transverse sinus posteriorly (arrows).

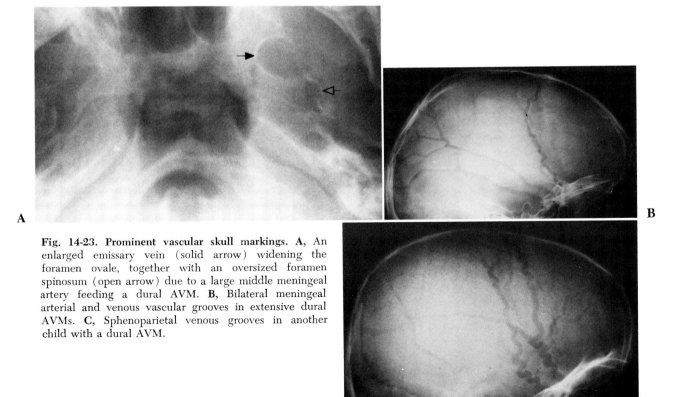

Fig. 14-23. **Prominent vascular skull markings. A,** An enlarged emissary vein (solid arrow) widening the foramen ovale, together with an oversized foramen spinosum (open arrow) due to a large middle meningeal artery feeding a dural AVM. **B,** Bilateral meningeal arterial and venous vascular grooves in extensive dural AVMs. **C,** Sphenoparietal venous grooves in another child with a dural AVM.

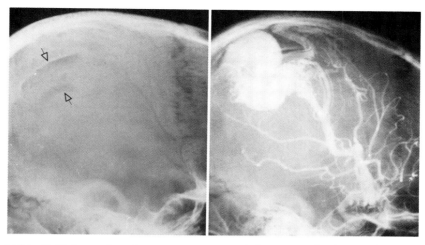

Fig. 14-24. Skull impression due to venous varix. A large superficial cortical parietal AVM with a large varix produces scalloping on the inner table of the vault (arrows).

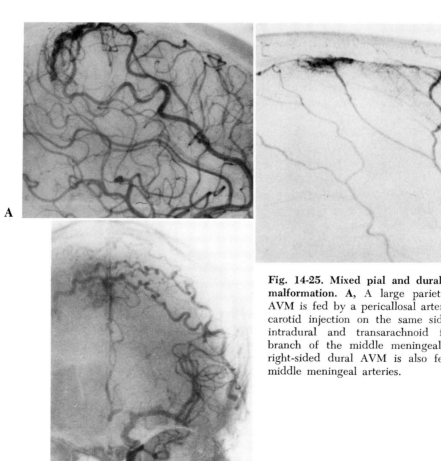

Fig. 14-25. Mixed pial and dural arteriovenous malformation. A, A large parietal parasagittal AVM is fed by a pericallosal artery. B, External carotid injection on the same side reveals tiny intradural and transarachnoid feeders off a branch of the middle meningeal artery. C, A right-sided dural AVM is also fed by the left middle meningeal arteries.

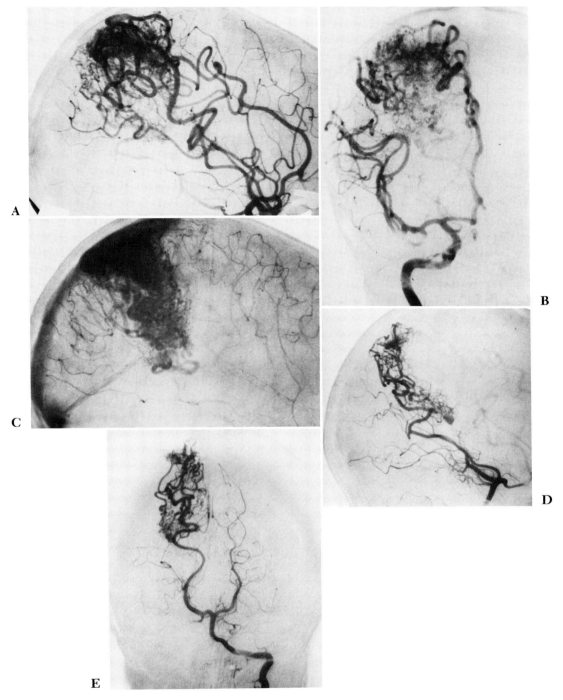

Fig. 14-26. Cortical arteriovenous malformation with numerous feeders and pyramidal form.
A and B, Right carotid injection shows a posterior parietal and occipital AVM fed by the
anterior cerebral and middle cerebral arteries. C, Characteristic broad-based periphery—
pyramidal shape with the apex centrally. D and E, Additional feeding vessels via the right
posterior cerebral artery.

quite enlarged, but anteroposterior and lateral tomograms will usually identify a bony carotid canal precisely. Similarly, the foramen transversarium of the vertebral artery in the C2 vertebra or the jugular foramen may be enlarged (Rumbaugh and Potts, 1966). If its meningeal artery is involved (Fig. 14-23), the foramen spinosum will enlarge and emissary venous foramina connecting the dural venous sinuses to the cranial or facial venous plexus may also enlarge (e.g., around the foramen ovale) (Fig. 14-23).

INDIRECT ABNORMALITIES

RAISED INTRACRANIAL PRESSURE. Split sutures and macrocrania due to variceal obstruction of the CSF pathway constitute evidence of increased intracranial pressure. Subarachnoid hemorrhage and hematoma may also obstruct the CSF pathway or the subarachnoid space system and create an EVOH. The mass effect of an intracranial hematoma due to acute bleeding from an arteriovenous malformation may produce acute raised intracranial pressure with splitting of the sutures.

THICKENING OF THE VAULT. In older children, vault thickening rarely may be local at the site of the arteriovenous malformation and may result from loss of cerebral tissue as part of the local cerebral atrophy or indeed some diploic hypertrophy due to the ex-

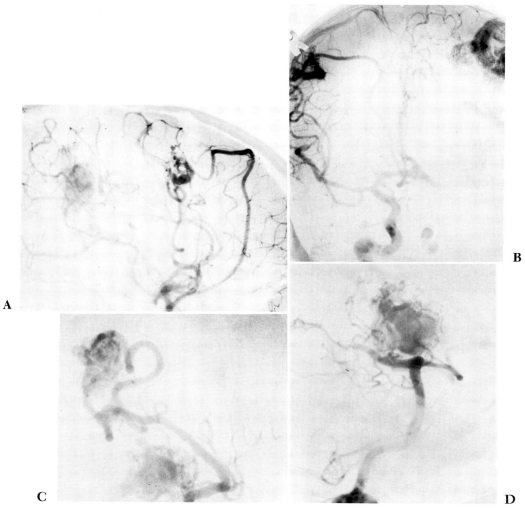

Fig. 14-27. Multiple and bilateral cerebral arteriovenous malformation. A and **B,** A right carotid arteriogram shows filling of a right anterior parietal AVM fed by the middle cerebral and anterior cerebral arteries. There is also cross filling of a large left posterior parietal AVM fed by the same arteries on the left side. **C,** A left carotid arteriogram shows filling of a deep thalamic AVM, including the parietal AVM. **D,** A vertebral arterial angiogram reveals the deep thalamic AVM via posterior perforators.

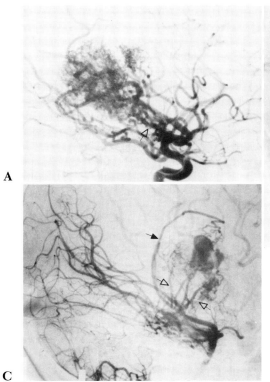

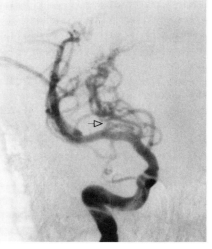

Fig. 14-28. Deep basal ganglia arteriovenous malformations. A and B, A large deep basal ganglionic AVM is fed by the lenticulostriate arteries (arrows). C, A large thalamic AVM is fed by posterior thalamoperforating arteries (open arrows) and a posterior choroidal artery (solid arrow) and contains a venous varix.

uberant blood flow (Rumbaugh and Potts, 1966). Pneumoencephalography will reveal local cerebral atrophy if present (McRae and Valentino, 1958).

Computed tomograms. Particularly if enhanced by contrast media, CT will detect large blood-containing varices or collections of dilated arteriovenous capillaries as a blood-containing mass (Chapter 8). It will also detect the presence of associated intracerebral hemorrhage or calcification.

Angiograms. Our practice is to perform selective bilateral internal and external carotid angiography and unilateral vertebral angiography. If no reflux into the other vertebral artery occurs, this latter artery is selectively studied. Hyperventilation angiography is helpful in the better visualization of implicated small arteries, particularly those of the thalamic and lenticulostriate groups.

The external carotid injection demonstrates transarachnoid or intradural feeding vessels (Fig. 14-25), which may be small and few or large and made up of mixed pial and dural anomalies (Fig. 14-25) (Newton and Cronqvist, 1969; Houser et al., 1972). External carotid vessels sometimes cross at the midline and feed an AVM on the opposite side (Fig. 14-25, C).

One, two, or many arterial feeders can pass into a tangle of enlarged capillaries, often broad based at the cortex with an apex pointing centrally (Fig.

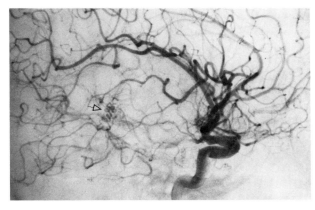

Fig. 14-29. Spontaneous bleeding of an arteriovenous malformation and a hematoma. Due to spontaneous bleeding of an AVM, whose remnants can be still seen (arrow), a posterior temporal mass elevates the middle cerebral artery.

14-26). In addition to these pial feeders, both a dural and a deep perforating arterial supply may be present. AVMs are sometimes multiple and in a combination of sites, sometimes peripheral and deep (Fig. 14-27), sometimes cerebral and in the posterior fossa. Deep thalamic AVMs are usually fed by posterior perforating and posterior choroidal arteries (Fig. 14-28). Demonstration of the precise geography of these complex anomalies is essential prior to successful surgical treatment. Each feeding vessel must be identified. To this end, we believe that selective hyperventilated magnified subtraction angiography is invaluable. Oblique and even basal views also frequently are helpful.

An AVM does not produce a mass effect unless (1) it has bled and created a hematoma, together with the attendant cerebral edema (Fig. 14-29), or (2) a large venous varix has formed. A hemorrhage may partially or completely destroy an AVM (Krayenbühl and Siebenmann, 1964). If the AVM is completely destroyed, remnants of it may appear in the clot and be identified only by pathological examination; the angiogram will merely show the ravages of the cerebral hematoma. If it is only partially destroyed, differentiating its remnants from the mass effect and abnormal vasculature of a cerebral neoplasm (particularly a grade 3 or 4 astrocytoma) may be quite difficult (Goree and Dukes, 1963).

The venous drainage of an AVM may be through large cortical veins (Fig. 14-30, A) or into the deep venous system of the internal cerebral and galenic veins (Fig. 14-30, B); or it may be via dural and diploic veins or a combination of these latter channels. Regardless of how extensive, involvement of the galenic system by draining veins from a deep cerebral AVM (Fig. 14-30, B) (O'Brien and Schechter, 1970) should not be equated with the previously described direct AV fistulae of the so-called vein of Galen aneurysm in infants.

The internal cerebral and galenic veins may be extremely varicosed, and the pial veins may form an aneurysmal dilatation (Fig. 14-30, A). In older children, calcification may occur in these large varices and often be crescentic. Involved dural veins and sinuses (Fig. 14-22) are always large and may be tortuous; they also may calcify.

In a bleeding AVM, angiographic contrast may pool in a large hematoma cavity; or if intraventricular hemorrhage has occurred, contrast may pool in one or the other occipital horn (the patient being in a brow-up position) (Fig. 14-31).

In our series an AVM localized in the choroid

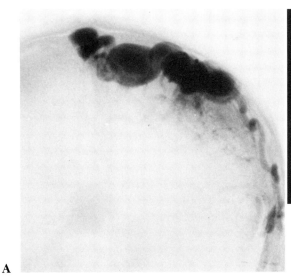
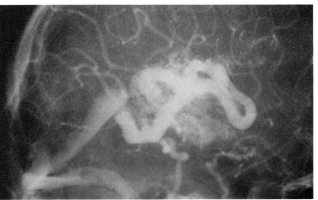

Fig. 14-30. Large draining veins. A, Cortical, draining into the sagittal sinus from a parietal AVM. **B,** Thalamostriate, draining into the internal cerebral and galenic veins and into the straight sinus.

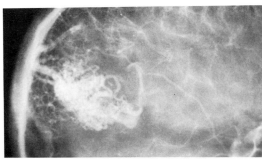
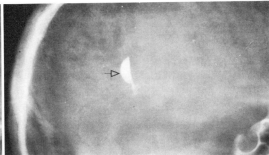

Fig. 14-31. Arteriovenous malformation bleeding into a lateral ventricle. At angiography, contrast pooled in the occipital horn (arrow).

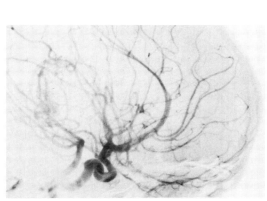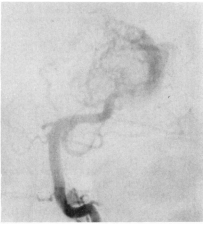

Fig. 14-32. Arteriovenous malformation of the choroid plexus of the lateral ventricle. This blocked the foramen of Monro anteriorly and caused hydrocephalus. It was fed by the posterior choroidal arteries alone, as demonstrated by a lateral carotid (left) and an antero-posterior vertebral (right) angiogram.

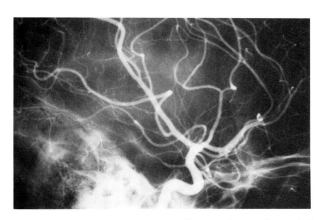

Fig. 14-33. Venous angioma. Stretching and spreading of the middle cerebral branches resulted from a large venous angioma within the sylvian triangle. No arterial feeders or vascularization of the venous angioma were seen, and the diagnosis was made at operation.

plexus of the lateral ventricle was fed by both anterior and posterior choroidal vessels and caused occlusion of one foramen of Monro (Fig. 14-32). The tela choroidea was not involved; hence we were able to demonstrate a segmental isolated blood supply to the third and lateral ventricular choroid plexuses respectively.

A venous angioma (McCormick, 1969; Stehbens, 1972) occurred in one child and presented as a mass lesion in the region of the sylvian triangle (Fig. 14-33). No abnormal arteries were seen, however, and the angioma did not fill with contrast. Surgical exploration revealed a flabby lake of venous blood within thin-walled venous sacs. Such angiomas rarely calcify (Runnels et al., 1969).

We perform postoperative angiography after each direct surgical procedure or before a repeat attempt at occlusion of the arterial feeders or total excision of the anomaly. Transfemoral catheter embolization of the intracranial and dural AVMs is increasingly being safely used (Luessenhop et al., 1965; Hilal et al., 1970; Kricheff et al., 1972). It is a difficult procedure in small children, however, due to the small size of the femoral catheter. Direct exposure of a carotid and vertebral artery must be employed (Hilal, 1974). A larger catheter will then permit emboli to be injected.

Infratentorial arteriovenous malformation. Abnormalities of skull radiography that may suggest an AVM of the posterior fossa are increased vascular markings of the occipital bone, enlargement of a foramen tranversarium of the upper cervical vertebra, and enlargement of a jugular foramen (Hoare, 1953).

In our experience, patients with infratentorial AVMs have frequently manifested focal brain stem neurological abnormalities without subarachnoid hemorrhage (Lessell et al., 1971). The first investigation is usually by pneumoencephalography or ventriculography, depending on whether or not hydrocephalus is present. As a result, in three cases a local mass arising from the floor of the fourth ventricle was detected and a subsequent abnormal tangle of vessels identified on angiography—suggesting a localized brain stem AVM (Fig. 14-34).

Patients with sudden severe loss of consciousness and/or acute hydrocephalus had large AVMs and cerebellar hematomas, whereas patients with ataxia were found to have AVMs of the cerebellum and/or brain stem without an associated hematoma. Hemorrhage usually resulted in an acute IVOH. In three

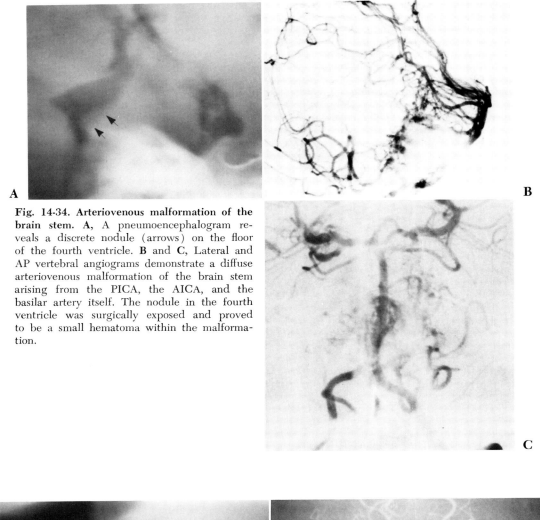

Fig. 14-34. Arteriovenous malformation of the brain stem. A, A pneumoencephalogram reveals a discrete nodule (arrows) on the floor of the fourth ventricle. B and C, Lateral and AP vertebral angiograms demonstrate a diffuse arteriovenous malformation of the brain stem arising from the PICA, the AICA, and the basilar artery itself. The nodule in the fourth ventricle was surgically exposed and proved to be a small hematoma within the malformation.

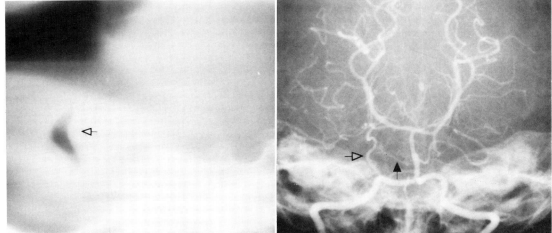

Fig. 14-35. Cryptic arteriovenous malformation of the brain stem and hematoma. A, A ventriculogram reveals a posteriorly displaced fourth ventricle (arrow) with a posteriorly convex floor. B, An AP vertebral angiogram demonstrates lateral displacement of the right PICA (open arrow), stretching of the right AICA (solid arrow), and spasm of the distal basilar artery and the origins of the SCA and posterior cerebral arteries. At operation a large brain stem hematoma was found. Histology of the hematoma revealed evidence of an underlying AVM.

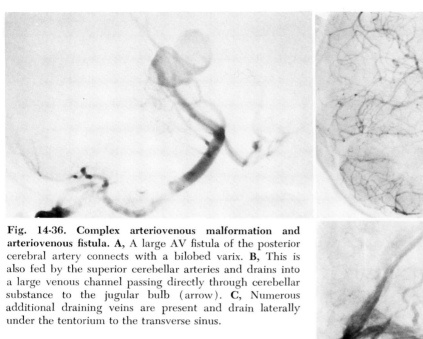

Fig. 14-36. Complex arteriovenous malformation and arteriovenous fistula. A, A large AV fistula of the posterior cerebral artery connects with a bilobed varix. **B,** This is also fed by the superior cerebellar arteries and drains into a large venous channel passing directly through cerebellar substance to the jugular bulb (arrow). **C,** Numerous additional draining veins are present and drain laterally under the tentorium to the transverse sinus.

children, however, each with a small brain stem hematoma and an AVM of the floor of the fourth ventricle (the youngest being 9 months old), no hydrocephalus ensued. Scott and co-workers (1973) described surgical evacuation of a pontine hematoma due to a "cryptic" vascular malformation (Fig. 14-35) and quoted six previous surgically evacuated pontine hematomas. Successful surgery was performed on two of the three children in our series.

In one arteriovenous malformation the feeding arteries were off the posterior cerebral and superior cerebellar arteries of the cerebellum, and a large varix drained through the cerebellum itself (Fig. 14-36); in another, the feeders were off the AICA and PICA; however, in arteriovenous malformations of the brain stem, vessels arose from the AICA and the PICA and directly from the basilar trunk (Fig. 14-34).

AVMs of the cerebellum or brain stem with meningeal involvement (Newton et al., 1968) were uncommon in our series. Veins in posterior fossa AVMs were less often varicosed (Fig. 14-37) than in supratentorial AVMs. Cerebellar veins and the basal vein of Rosenthal were commonly involved (Fig. 14-37).

Associated vascular abnormalities. Subarachnoid hemorrhage and associated arterial spasm due to a ruptured AVM are common and may be segmental locally or at a distance from the malformation. Angiography may demonstrate thrombosis in venous varices (Weir et al., 1968) or even in afferent arteries (Rodda and Calvert, 1969). A subdural hematoma associated with a bleeding AVM is rare in children (Teabeaut, 1951; Paterson and McKissock, 1956).

An associated cerebral aneurysm and an AVM did not occur in our series, but this has been reported in as many as 7% of AVMs in a cooperative study (Perret and Nishioka, 1966). An AVM of the cerebrum and another of the cord occurred together in one child (Fig. 14-38). A coarctation of the aorta was also present in a child with a cerebral AVM.

ACUTE HEMIPLEGIA OF CHILDHOOD

Children with hemiplegias have been mentioned throughout religious and historical writings. They have been painted by the Masters (Ribera, The Louvre) and have been the subject of academic study by at least two great physicians, Osler (1889) and Freud (1897). The much abused term *cerebral palsy* includes childhood hemiplegia as one of the many clinical entities making up this ill-defined spectrum (Bax, 1961). Whether "congenital" or acquired, hemi-

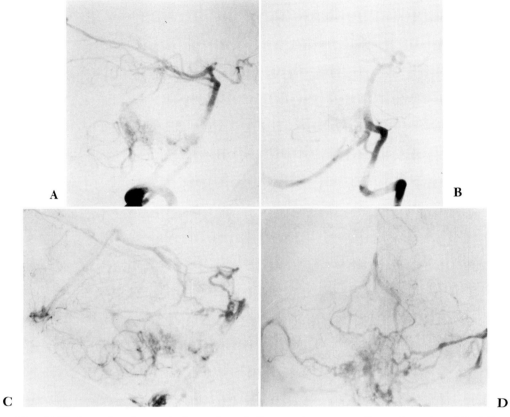

Fig. 14-37. Intra–fourth ventricular and cerebellar arteriovenous malformations. A and B, Off the PICA and AICA, passing through the brain stem into the fourth ventricle and cerebellar hemispheres in the midline. **C and D,** Numerous and extensive draining veins upward to the mesencephalic vein, basal vein of Rosenthal, and lateral cerebellar veins.

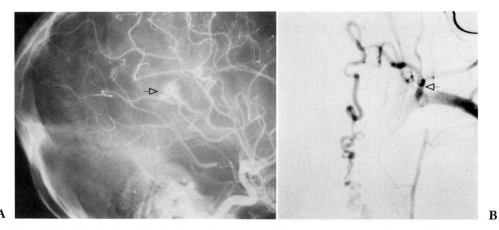

Fig. 14-38. Cerebral and spinal arteriovenous malformations. A, Small cortical posterior temporal (arrow). **B,** Extensive, of the spinal cord and fed from a branch of the thyrocervical trunk on the left (arrow).

plegia accounts for a third of all cases of cerebral palsy; and of these hemiplegics, one quarter acquired hemiplegia postnatally.

In 1927, Ford and Schaffer introduced the term *acute infantile acquired hemiplegia* and described those cases due to acute infectious diseases; but they also described cases occurring in apparently healthy children. Since that time the literature has become replete with descriptions of the causes, syndromes, radiological characteristics, and pathology of the syndrome—including extensive monographs on the subject (Bax and Mitchell, 1962; Isler, 1971). Acute hemiplegia in childhood is not a disease but a symptom. Neuroradiology alone often provides evidence of the specific intracranial vascular abnormalities that must be related to any clinical sign or symptom present, enabling investigators to suggest a cause. In many cases, however, no direct cause is apparent.

Etiology

There are myriad causes of acute hemiplegia in a child (Carter and Gold, 1967); but basically either a primary occlusion of some part of the cerebral vasculature leads to cerebral damage (Banker, 1961; Gold et al., 1964a) or there are abnormalities of the cerebral tissue per se—traumatic brain destruction, postictal states, hemorrhage, cerebral edema, encephalopathies, neoplasms.

These diverse causes may be identifiable with a specific type of intracranial disease, accounting for the respective pathogenesis of the vascular abnormality, or not be identifiable. To have a practical and relatively simple neuroradiological approach, it is necessary to subdivide the lesions and their causes that lead to acute childhood hemiplegia into four broad groups: (1) specific vascular abnormalities with a known cause, (2) general cerebral vascular abnormalities with a known cause, (3) specific vascular abnormalities with no known cause, and (4) no detectable abnormality or cause. The following subdivisions deal with the causes of detectable vascular angiographic abnormalities. Many of the causes are rare, and many do not necessarily produce acute hemiplegia even in the face of angiographically demonstrable abnormalities.

Specific vascular abnormalities with known cause
　Arterial emboli from extracranial source
　　Congenital heart disease
　　Endocarditis
　　Fat
　　Air
　　Iatrogenic (neuroradiology, cardiac surgery)
　　Carotid thrombosis
　　Pulmonary sepsis
　Thrombosis
　　Arterial thrombosis
　　　Polycythemia
　　　Sickle cell anemia
　　　Atherosclerosis
　　　Inflammatory
　　　Traumatic
　　　Iatrogenic
　　Venous thrombosis
　　　Dehydration in infants
　　　Sepsis
　　　Meningitis and encephalitis
　　　Infiltrations (leukemia, neuroblastoma)
　Abnormalities of the vascular wall
　　Meningitic
　　Traumatic
　　Neurocutaneous syndromes
　　Atherosclerosis
　　Dissecting aneurysms
　　Neoplasia
　　Radiation
　　Spasm (traumatic, subarachnoid hemorrhage, iatrogenic)
　　Lupus erythematosus
　　Periarteritis nodosa
　　Migraine
General cerebral vascular abnormalities with known cause
　Postictal edema
　Traumatic cerebral destruction
　Nontraumatic hemorrhage into brain
　　"Spontaneous" aneurysm
　　Arteriovenous malformation
　　Hematological abnormality
　Dural hematoma
　Encephalopathies
　　Meningoencephalitis (herpes, *Haemophilus influenzae*, postvaccinal exanthema)
　Brain abscess (intact or ruptured)
　Brain tumor (with hemorrhage, edema)
　Transcompartmental cerebral shifts
Specific vascular abnormalities with no known cause
　(acute idiopathic hemiplegia of infancy and childhood)
　Carotid stenosis with intracranial arterial obstructions (thromboses, emboli, stenoses)
　Intracranial arterial obstructions
　　Narrowing
　　　General (smooth or irregular)
　　　Local (webs or stenoses)
　　Occlusion (proximal, distal, single, multiple, bilateral)

Neuroradiology

Specific vascular abnormalities with known cause
Extracranial arterial emboli. These include endocarditis due to congenital heart disease (Tyler and Clark, 1957; Banker, 1961), rheumatic fever, prolapsed mitral valve, and the rare myxoma of the left atrium (Joynt et al., 1965; New, 1970). The emboli may be infected (Morgan and Bland, 1959) or sterile (Barron et al., 1960). Perinatal middle cerebral artery occlusions can be of embolic origin; Cocker and co-workers (1965) suggested that the emboli may arise from fetal placental veins.

Fat emboli can arise from severe limb trauma (Bergentz, 1961; Fuchsig et al., 1967; Drummond et al., 1969). Fat emboli, however, are rarely large

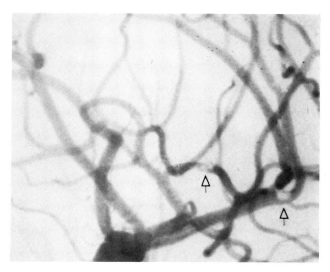

Fig. 14-39. Iatrogenic catheter emboli. Residing within the anterior cerebral and middle cerebral branches, these emboli (arrows) were presumably due to faulty catheter technique. The patient suffered no untoward sequelae.

enough to cause obstruction of major intracerebral arteries and tend to lodge in the small arterioles. Their effect may be detected only by magnification subtraction angiography.

Cerebral arterial emboli may occur with pulmonary sepsis (Banker, 1961). Air emboli may rarely result from open heart surgery or be caused by extreme carelessness during a carotid or aortic arch angiogram injection.

Other angiographic *iatrogenic* emboli are catheter thrombi, broken catheters (rare) or fractured guide wire tips, and finally glove powder or cotton fibers. The last two produce occlusions of the very small arterioles that are not usually seen on angiograms. Similar small occlusions can occur after open heart surgery from platelet emboli originating in the bypass pump (Aguilar et al., 1971). We have had experience with six children (in over 3,000 cerebral angiograms) in whom we judged emboli within one or another major intracerebral artery (Fig. 14-39) to

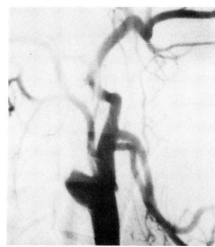

Fig. 14-40. Cervical internal carotid artery thrombosis. A, Abrupt idiopathic, at the origin of the artery. **B,** An irregular thrombosis and stenosis (large and small arrowheads) resulted when a child fell with a pencil in his mouth. The pharyngeal wall was pierced. **C,** A left carotid *(LC)* angiogram, oblique projection, in this child shows cross filling of the right middle cerebral artery *(Rmc)* with numerous intraluminal emboli (arrowheads).

A

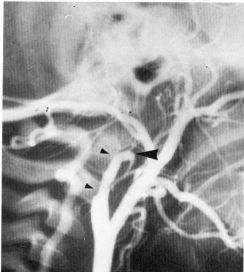

B

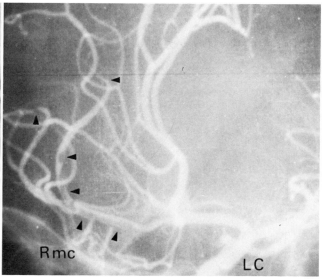

C

have followed poor catheter technique (Harwood-Nash and Fitz, 1974b). These children experienced no postangiographic sequelae, much to our relief. A rapid dissolution of the embolus occurred as visualized on immediate or late repeat angiograms.

Thrombosis. Distal emboli and hemiplegia can result from thrombosis of the cervical carotid artery or intimal irregularities. Thromboses and irregularities due to known cause include falls with a pointed object in the mouth (Fig. 14-40) (Braudo, 1956; Pitner, 1966; Harwood-Nash et al., 1971) and closed trauma to the neck with possible impaction of the carotid on the transverse process of a cervical vertebra or the arch of the atlas (Clarke et al., 1955; Boldrey et al.,

1956; Duman and Stephens, 1963). Infected cervical nodes (Pouyanne et al., 1957) or nasopharyngeal infections or tonsillectomy (Bickerstaff, 1964; Shillito, 1964; Harwood-Nash et al., 1971) have also been implicated. A total cervical carotid occlusion (Fig. 14-40, *A*) does not necessarily lead to hemiplegia but may if distal emboli are present (Fig. 14-40, *B* and *C*).

Intracranial arterial and venous thromboses can occur in hematological diseases such as polycythemia (Chapter 13) (Johnson and Chalgren, 1951) and sickle cell disease (Fig. 14-41) (Hilal et al., 1971a; Stockman et al., 1972).

Inflammatory arterial thromboses occur in men-

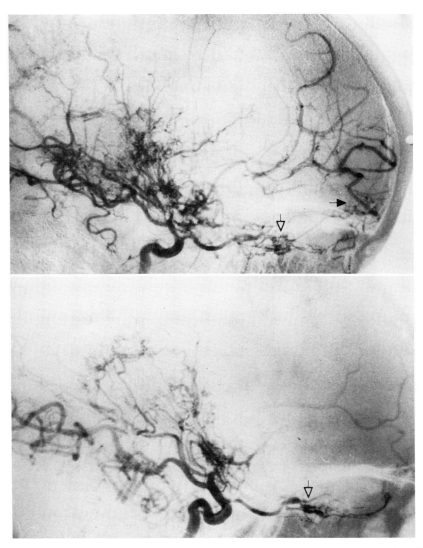

Fig. 14-41. Arterial occlusion and sickle cell anemia. Bilateral internal carotid occlusions distal to the origins of the anterior choroidals resulted in profuse basal collaterals. Faint filling of both anterior cerebral arteries can be seen. Note also the collaterals from the ethmoidal branches of each ophthalmic artery (open arrows) and the transdural anastomoses by the anterior meningeal arteries (solid arrow) on one side.

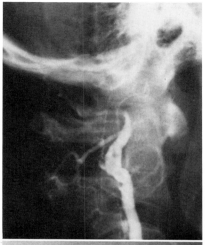

Fig. 14-42. Vertebral and basilar artery occlusion. A, Marked distal vertebral thrombosis of unknown origin on the right; however, the patient had had cervical trauma five years previously. B, The left vertebral (LV) is patent, but the distal basilar (arrowhead) is occluded just proximal to the origin of the superior cerebellar artery. C, A carotid arteriogram demonstrates reflux down a thin basilar artery to the same occlusion site (arrow) as in B.

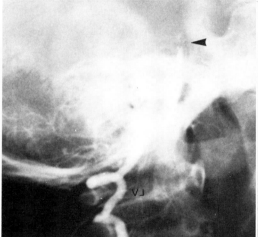

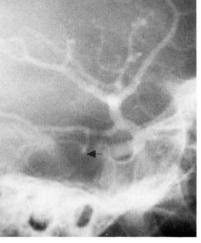

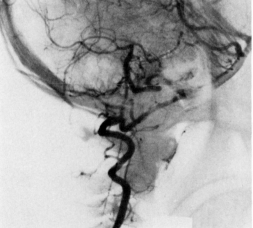

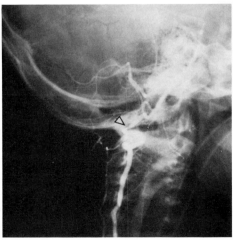

Fig. 14-43. Occlusion of the vertebral artery with neck turning. A, The right vertebral angiogram in the sagittal position with a patent distal artery. B, Turning of the head to the left virtually occludes the artery (arrow), with resultant poor flow through the basilar artery.

ingitides (Perlstein and Hood, 1964) and extracerebral abscesses or osteitis of the skull and mastoids (Chapter 13). Encephalotrigeminal angiomatosis (Sturge-Weber syndrome) may be associated with an arterial thrombosis (Hilal et al., 1971b).

Traumatic arterial thrombosis, either at the base of the skull or in the peripheral vessels, is relatively uncommon in children (Chapter 12). Occlusion of the basilar artery is very rare (Dooley and Smith, 1968) and occurred in only two children of our series (Fig. 14-42); another child had a thrombosis of the proximal vertebral artery, presumably due to trauma. Stenosis of the distal vertebral artery between C1 and the occiput can result from simple neck turning (Fig. 14-43) but rarely will produce symptoms and is probably due to kinking on the ligamentous structures.

Venous thromboses of either the cortical veins or the cortical sinuses (Chapter 13) occur from many causes. They are common in infants and can lead to acute hemiplegia. A venous thrombosis is more frequently seen in this age group than is an arterial thrombosis (Gold et al., 1964a).

Abnormalities of the vascular wall. In association with lesions of the brain and its coverings, intracranial vascular wall abnormalities can lead to focal or widespread stenoses or occlusion. A thrombosis may or may not be a concomitant. Tuberculous and pneumococcal meningitis (Chapter 13), traumatic incarceration in fractures, direct trauma with spasm (Chapter 12), or intramural hemorrhage or rupture are common causes in children.

Severe purulent sphenoidal sinusitis may produce an acute narrowing of the cavernous portion of the internal carotid artery (Fig. 14-44)—a stenosis that usually disappears after successful treatment of the infection.

Neurocutaneous syndromes such as neurofibromatosis and tuberous sclerosis, together with tortuosity and segmental ectasia and stenosis (Hilal et al., 1971b) may be associated with distal branch arterial occlusions.

Atherosclerosis or atheroma in the cerebral arteries of children is rare; and if present, it may be associated with idiopathic hyperlipemia or primary hypercholesterolemia (Hsia, 1959).

Another rare disease is homocystinuria, which may produce irregular stenoses of both carotid and intracerebral vessels (Presley et al., 1968). Irradiation will cause marked irregularities of cerebral arteries in the area surrounding the neoplasm requiring such treatment (Fig. 14-45) (Harwood-Nash et al., 1971). This is relatively uncommon, however (Ferris and Levine, 1973).

Dissecting aneurysms of the branches of the internal carotid arteries in children are rare and are discribed from the clinical and pathological viewpoints by Wisoff and Rothballer (1961), Jacob and co-workers (1970), and Stehbens (1972). We have confirmed one such case in an 8-year-old child (Chang et al., 1975) with bilateral dissecting subintimal aneurysms of both proximal middle cerebral arteries and proximal portions of the anterior cerebral arteries (Fig. 14-46). Autopsy showed the medial dissections, but there was no cause for these dissections and the

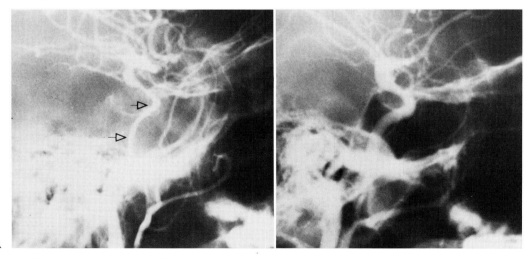

A   **B**

Fig. 14-44. Internal carotid artery stenosis and sphenoidal sinusitis. An acute sphenoidal sinusitis with an opaque sphenoid produces severe stenosis of the suprapetrosal and intracavernous portions of the internal carotid artery (arrows). Successful treatment with reaeration of the sphenoidal sinus resulted in a normal-looking internal carotid artery (**B**). (Courtesy E. Afshani, M.D., Buffalo.)

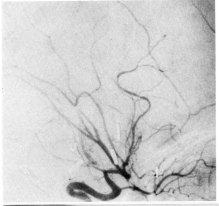

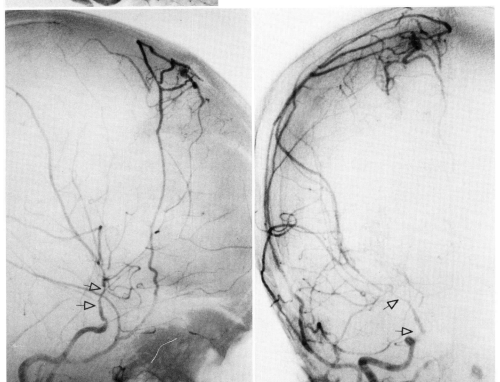

Fig. 14-45. Postradiation arterial occlusions. A, Marked narrowing of the supraclinoid portion of the internal carotid artery with occlusion of the origin of the anterior cerebral and segmental narrowing of the branches of the middle cerebral. Note the increased basal collaterals of the anterior choroidal artery. This patient had a parietal grade 2 astrocytoma that was irradiated. **B** and **C,** Another child, having been administered radiation to a hypothalamic glioma, showed a markedly irregular stenosis of the internal carotid and proximal middle cerebral arteries (arrows). Note the extensive meningeal collaterals.

remainder of the intracranial vessels were normal. No systemic disease was present.

Cerebral neoplasms, particularly grade 3 and grade 4 astrocytomas, may wrap and involve intracerebral arteries—producing irregular stenoses and, less commonly, occlusions (Leeds and Rosenblatt, 1972).

Arterial spasm, frequently associated with subarachnoid hemorrhage or cerebral trauma, may itself produce hemiplegia. Both oral and intravenous amphetamines and other drugs (Margolis et al., 1971; Rumbaugh et al., 1971) may produce alternating areas of dilatation and narrowing in the anterior and middle cerebral arteries. Intrinsic disease of the arteries such as lupus erythematosus and periarteritis nodosa (Ford, 1973) will involve cerebral vessels and

produce an acute hemiplegia, but such occurrences are rare in children.

Strange carotid and cerebral artery ectasia has occurred in children, the most dramatic being in a 12-year-old child with an immunological defense defect against candidiasis. The internal carotids and basilar artery all showed general dilatation, and there were multiple sausage-shaped areas of ectasia throughout the cerebral vascular system (Fig. 14-47). Mucocutaneous candidiasis was rampant, but blood and CSF cultures for *Candida* were negative.

General cerebral vascular abnormalities with known cause. The neuroradiology of such lesions does not directly implicate the vessels since its main purpose is to demonstrate mass lesions, edema, or loss of

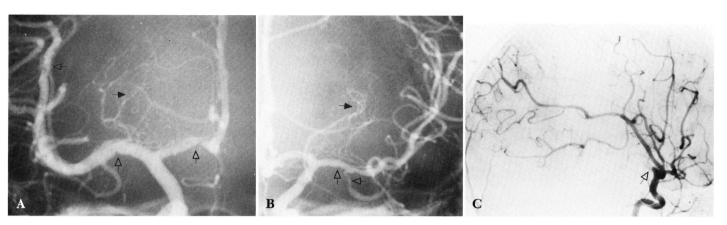

Fig. 14-46. Bilateral cerebral arterial dissecting aneurysms. A and **B,** Right and left carotid angiograms reveal extensive mural and luminal irregularities in the proximal anterior cerebral and middle cerebral arteries bilaterally and of the origin of their branches (open arrows). Numerous irregularities are seen in the lenticulostriate arteries (solid arrows). **C,** A lateral left carotid angiogram demonstrates complete occlusion of the origin of the posterior parietal artery (arrow) and numerous pial collaterals.

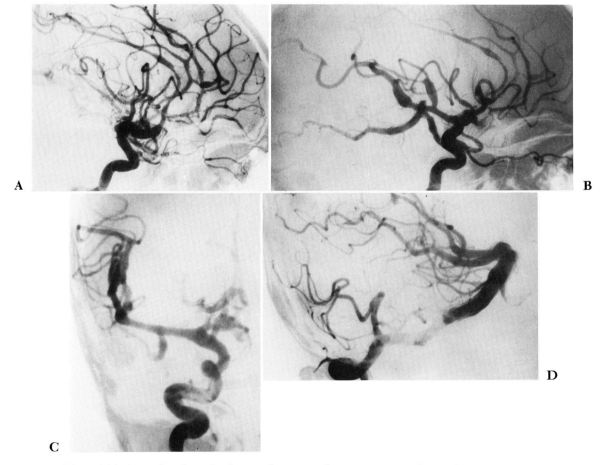

Fig. 14-47. Carotid and cerebral arterial ectasia. There is an extraordinary dilatation of both internal carotid arteries (**A** to **C**) and the basilar artery (**D**), together with general and local areas of ectasia throughout the cerebellar and cerebral arteries, in this stroke patient. The cause is unknown. The patient had mucocutaneous candidiasis but negative blood and CSF cultures.

cerebral substance. These lesions affect brain function more than they affect arterial morphology. Postictal hemiparesis or hemiplegia is usually temporary (Todd's paralysis), probably due to local cerebral dysfunction and edema. Mass lesions like traumatic edema and hemorrhage, dural hematomas from trauma, and intracranial hemorrhage from aneurysms, AVMs, or hematological abnormalities will cause an acute hemiplegia.

Some encephalitides present with acute hemiplegias and a mass effect from edema due to the cerebritis. Herpes encephalitis, in particular, produces a focal cerebral lesion (Chapter 13). An acute or chronic cerebral abscess may present with sudden hemiplegia from rupture of the abscess into the subarachnoid space or ventricles or from sudden cerebral edema around the abscess (Chapter 13).

The abnormality may be of obscure cause, but frequently postictal. Angiography then will show a small area of edema, with stretching of the cortical arteries and veins and often with an early-filling vein, and a prolonged intense gyral cerebrogram effect (Harwood-Nash, 1972). The arteries themselves are normal. Hemorrhage or proximal edema within or around a cerebral neoplasm may precipitate clinical presentation of the neoplasm by acute hemiplegia.

Sudden transcompartmental brain shifts as occur in acute occlusion of some part of the intraventricular CSF pathway leading to an acute hydrocephalus or, contrariwise, a sudden decompression of hydrocephalus by shunting may lead to sudden hemiplegia.

Specific vascular abnormalities with no known cause. A sudden unexplained onset of hemiplegia in an infant or child, usually not associated with a seizure, will commonly reveal on angiography an abnormality of the intracranial arteries (Harwood-Nash et al., 1971; Hilal et al., 1971a).

Possible etiologies. The paediatric stroke, usually not fatal, is nearly always unexplained. The angiographic abnormalities are often the only evidence of the site and characteristics of the arterial lesion. These children have no history or evidence of trauma, neoplasia, infection, hematological or cardiac abnormalities, or generalized diseases. In fact, they are usually perfectly normal prior to the episode (Ford, 1973).

Shillito (1964) reviewed the sparse pathological reports of cerebral arterial lesions in these children and added three cases of his own. He ascertained that an arteritis was indeed present, possibly originating from an inflammation of the internal carotid artery at the base of the skull and either spreading to involve the intracranial arteries or by subsequent thrombosis providing an origin for distal emboli. We support this view. Picard and co-workers (1974) have reported two autopsy studies in which the internal elastic lamina was destroyed but intimal hypoplasia and nonspecific evidence of mild inflammation were present.

Apart from the foregoing studies, the basis for any theory as to the pathogenesis of these arterial lesions remains only with the angiographic abnormality. Afflicted children rarely die, and thus there is no possibility of pathological examination of the many bizarre angiographic abnormalities that appear. Our own sparse studies indicate that a nonspecific postinflammatory fibrosis of the media with intraluminal thrombi occurs.

Bickerstaff (1964), Shillito (1964), and later we suggested a strong relationship between severe nasopharyngeal or tonsillar infections in children and subsequent stenosis or thrombosis of the intracerebral artery. This occurred in a high percentage (60%) of the children in our series.

The direct pathogenetic correlation is not clear. A periarteritic spreading of infection may ascend by the cervical internal carotid artery and affect only the internal carotid and its branches that are bathed by CSF—whence the artery appears to change its character. These occlusive lesions in the intracranial arteries may have the tapered irregular appearance of thromboses or the sharp abrupt occlusive edge suggestive of an embolus. In one child who died, diffuse bilateral irregularities in the middle or anterior cerebral arteries (Fig. 14-46) was shown to be multiple medial dissections (Normal and Urich, 1957; Wolman, 1959; Chang et al., 1975). Sphenoidal sinusitis may cause a severe reversible stenosis of the infracavernous portion of the internal carotid artery (Fig. 14-44). Inflammatory thrombosis of the cavernous sinus may also cause stenosis of the internal carotid artery (Chapter 13). One child, however, had bilateral severe stenosis of the internal carotid arteries at the foramen lacerum area with multiple local collaterals (Fig. 14-48) and no clinical or historical evidence for a lesion that might have caused this abnormality. We suggest therefore that in some children a peculiar susceptibility or undue sensitivity of the arteries is associated with a local nasopharyngeal infection.

In some of our children there occurred an exanthema or high fever within the months prior to the onset of the hemiplegia. Many of these children were vigorously exercising at the moment the hemiplegia began. A severe acute generalized illness may result in local necrosis in the walls of cerebral arteries and lead to sites of thrombosis or dissection (Humphrey and Newton, 1960). There were two sets of siblings with hemiplegia and vascular occlusions. No other disease process was present that could indicate a familial predisposition. Two children in our series

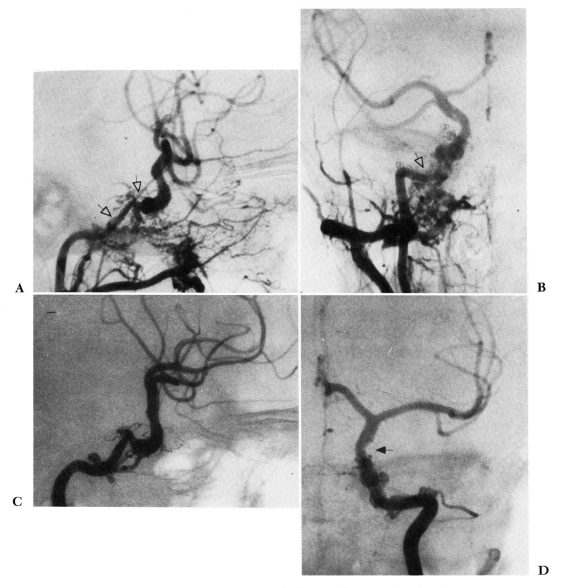

Fig. 14-48. Internal carotid artery stenosis at the foramen lacerum. A and B, Severe stenosis of the transpetrosal portion of the right internal carotid (open arrows). Extensive collaterals about the stenosis are seen between the internal carotid and external carotid arteries. C and D, Similar severe stenosis of the left internal carotid artery with myriad pericarotid collaterals. The supraclinoid portion of the artery is dilated and erect and contains a lateral mural thrombus (solid arrow). The cause of these stenoses is unknown.

had severe hypertension, and one with renal artery stenosis died (Harwood-Nash et al., 1971); no autopsy was obtained. Angiography of the renal arteries in the other child was normal.

Virtually all the children who had demonstrable angiographic abnormalities of the intracranial arteries and hemiplegia (90%) suffered either minor or no seizures in association with the onset of the hemiplegia. Hilal and co-workers (1971a) quoted an incidence of 77%. Our experience also agrees with that of Aicardi and co-workers (1969): most children who

have permanent acute hemiplegia associated with prolonged and severe convulsions have *no detectable intrinsic vascular abnormalities at angiography*. Many of these children had some form of encephalitis, and the only abnormalities at cerebral angiography were mild focal edema usually over the motor strip with slight early filling of veins and a prolonged cerebrogram. In a number of children with "migrainous" hemiplegia, we have performed angiography during or immediately after the headache but have discovered no abnormality.

Table 14-4. Classification of idiopathic cerebral arterial occlusions with hemiplegia

	Number	Percent
Group 1. Extracranial	5	8
Internal carotid	3	
Vertebral and basilar	2	
Group 2. Unilateral intracranial	50	77
a. Internal carotid	30	46
Alone	12	18
Plus distal	18	28
b. Cerebral carotid branch arteries only	20	31
Proximal	14	22
Distal only	6	9
Group 3. Bilateral intracranial	10	15

Table 14-5. Age and sex according to site of arterial occlusion

Group	Age peaks (years)	Sex Female	Male
1	1-4 and 7-10	1.5	: 1
2	1-2 and 7-10	2.1	: 1
2a	7-9	1.5	: 1
2b	1-2 and 7-10	3	: 1
3	2-4	1	: 2.3

George and co-workers (1971b) reported specific occlusion in adults with migraine. Krayenbühl and Yaşargil (1968) warned that occlusive clinical deterioration can occur after angiography in adults with migraine. This has not been the case in our experience with children.

Angiography may be performed for a variety of purposes (e.g., a positive brain scan) in children with headache, visual disturbances, paresthesias, or an abnormal EEG together with headache. We find that iatrogenic catheter emboli fortunately do not lead to any detectable neurological defect in children. This factor tends to suggest to us that in children with an acute onset of hemiplegia, the cerebral arterial lesion is probably a chronic one; and the onset of the lesion probably antedates by some time the onset of the hemiplegia. The acute exacerbation may be caused by the inability of the brain to adapt to additional acute assault or demand on the cerebral vascular system.

Such assaults may be due to additional small peripheral emboli in the cerebral arterioles which further occlude already developed collaterals. High fever, exertion, or mild head trauma may affirm definite but latent arterial disease in these children. In the presence of iatrogenic emboli, the brain and the peripheral cerebral circulation are normal.

We reported a series of 175 children with acute onset of hemiplegia who had previously been quite normal with no evidence of intracranial or systemic disease of any kind (Harwood-Nash et al., 1971). Of the sixty-one children to whom cerebral angiography was administered, forty harbored one or more abnormalities of the cerebral vascular system. Since our report an additional twenty-nine infants and children with such a hemiplegia have been seen. Twenty-two of these twenty-nine children were administered immediate, and seven delayed, angiography—which revealed in all an arterial occlusive lesion of the intra-

cerebral vessels. When we excluded from the original series four children in whom oral trauma produced a cervical internal carotid thrombosis and intracranial occlusive emboli, we found sixty-five children who had had an intracerebral arterial occlusion of unknown cause as identified by angiography. Shillito (1964) reported twenty-one and Hilal and co-workers (1971a) seventeen children with angiographic evidence of such occlusions. Harwood-Nash and co-workers (1971) and Hilal and co-workers (1971a) attempted simultaneously to classify these angiographic occlusions by site and character. The classifications are basically similar (Table 14-4).

Age and sex. Girls (thirty-nine) outnumbered boys (twenty-six) 1.5:1 (Table 14-5). The sixty-five children ranged in age from 4 months to 16 years. Peak age groups were 1 to 4 and 7 to 10 years. In group 2, thirty-four girls outnumbered sixteen boys 2.1:1; in group 2b, fifteen girls and five boys, 3:1. Conversely, in group 3, seven boys outnumbered three girls 2.3:1.

The peak age levels in group 2 were 1 to 2 and 7 to 10 years; in group 2a, 7 to 9; and in group 2b, 1 to 2 and 7 to 10. In group 3 a distinctly increased incidence was observed between 2 and 4 years. Only three of the ten in this group were older than 4 years of age.

These figures are in accordance with the figures of other collected series except those in group 3. In Japanese children, bilateral carotid occlusions were more common in females; in our series they were more common in males. None of the children in our series were Japanese.

Angiographic classification. The following classification of cerebral arterial occlusions with no known cause was chosen quite arbitrarily according to the site or sites of the lesions (Table 14-4). It also groups the children according to certain age and sex parameters.

GROUP 1. EXTRACRANIAL INTERNAL CAROTID OR VERTEBRAL OCCLUSIONS

This group includes nontraumatic stenoses or occlusions of the cervical internal carotid artery without intracranial occlusions (three cases) or vertebral and basilar occlusions (two cases) (Fig. 14-42); it makes up 8% of all idiopathic arterial lesions. We have excluded cases in which intraoral trauma caused the carotid arterial lesion; such a lesion may resemble quite closely nontraumatic stenosis of the vessel. Traumatic cervical internal carotid thrombotic occlusion, however, may give rise to distal intracranial emboli (Fig. 14-40) (Harwood-Nash et al., 1971; Sullivan et al., 1973).

Agenesis of the internal carotid artery is rare (Smith et al., 1972). Infantile supraclinoid internal carotid occlusions will result in a markedly diminished diameter of the internal carotid artery; but true agenesis must have a tomographically absent carotid canal (Davis, 1974). The reader will perceive later in this chapter that some intracranial vascular occlusions do have cervical internal carotid stenoses. Because the intracranial occlusion rather than the cervical occlusion was the dominant lesion, however, we decided to place these children in group 2 rather than in group 1.

The origin of the occlusions in group 1 is not known. Trauma to the neck with hyperextension or hyperflexion that went unnoticed in the patient's history may have caused the lesions (Frantzen et al., 1961; Davie and Coxe, 1967). A localized inflammatory lesion in the neck or nasopharynx previous to the hemiplegia may have led to occlusion (Banker, 1961; Bickerstaff, 1964; Shillito, 1964; Harwood-Nash et al., 1971). Nasopharyngeal infections are so common in children that a statistical correlation may be difficult. Two of the five children in this group had had a nasopharyngeal infection 2 and 3 months previously. We have seen no evidence in these children of concurrent or postinflammatory damage on radiographs of the cervical spine.

Angiography of a suspect extracranial carotid occlusion must be carefully performed. The catheter is initially placed at the orifice of the common carotid, and the hand-injected 4 ml flush is executed under image intensification. If no contrast is seen in the head, the catheter is maintained in this position and common carotid angiography is performed in both planes. The guide wire should not be advanced up the carotid before the possible site of occlusion has been detected. Rarely, however, will the common carotid be occluded if the site of the stenosis is within the internal carotid artery below the base of the skull. With the first common carotid power injection, it is possible to make an angiographic composition of the cervical internal carotid artery and the head on one film.

The occlusion in the neck may be total, or a stenosis of varying length may be present (and is always unilateral). The total occlusion has an abrupt cutoff appearance (Fig. 14-40, A), whereas the stenotic lesion has an irregular orifice and narrows the internal carotid usually just above its origin. The stenosis extends 1 to 2 cm, and this segment of the artery is often curved posteriorly and laterally. With stenotic lesions the distal cervical internal carotid may be quite dilated as compared with the uninvolved side.

Hilal and co-workers (1971a) have shown that the stenotic segment kinks when the head is flexed on the neck, and this suggests rigidity of the segment. The intracranial branches of the affected carotid artery may or may not show a slowed circulation time, and the vessels may or may not have a decreased caliber. The degree of these two phenomena will depend on the degree of the occlusion in the neck.

Total occlusion of the internal carotid artery in the supraclinoid or infracavernous portion may lead to a false occlusion in the proximal portion. The contrast will have a smooth wedge-shaped appearance and will be layered on the posterior wall of the artery within the stagnant column of blood. Opacification of the internal carotid just distal to the occlusion may occur via retrograde filling of the ophthalmic artery.

In our series the vertebral artery was occluded at the atlantoaxial portion in two children. Hyperflexion or hyperextension can be inferred as a possible cause. One such occlusion was associated with a distal basilar artery occlusion, presumably due to an embolus.

A spontaneous basilar occlusion occurred in another child at the midportion of the artery (Fig. 14-49). Associated grossly enlarged cervical internal carotid arteries were present. The etiology in this case was uncertain.

We have no pathological studies of the affected arteries in the neck; and though we think such a phenomenon is unlikely, we cannot entirely dismiss the possibility of fibromuscular hyperplasia of the arteries (Houser and Baker, 1968) from our assessment of these patients. Fibromuscular hyperplasia of the renal arteries has been associated with intracranial aneurysms (Belber and Hoffman, 1968; Handa et al., 1970), but convincing histological proof of intracranial arterial fibromuscular dysplasia is lacking.

Collateral circulation is usually quite adequately maintained via the ophthalmic and anterior communicating arteries (Fig. 14-40) and via posterior communicating and peripheral and cortical leptomeningeal anastomoses. External carotid collaterals to the cavernous portion of the interal carotid are also present (Margolis and Newton, 1969) and were particularly marked in one child with bilateral occlusions of the internal carotid artery at the foramen lacerum (Fig. 14-48). Unless additional intracranial distal

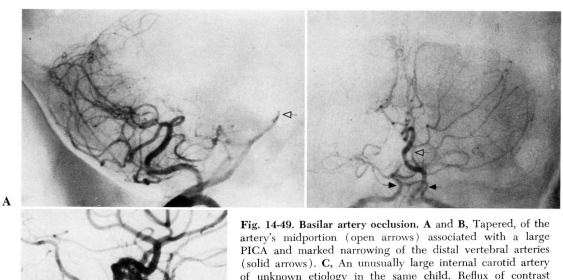

Fig. 14-49. Basilar artery occlusion. A and **B,** Tapered, of the artery's midportion (open arrows) associated with a large PICA and marked narrowing of the distal vertebral arteries (solid arrows). **C,** An unusually large internal carotid artery of unknown etiology in the same child. Reflux of contrast through the posterior communicating artery into the basilar tip with its SCAs can be seen (arrow).

occlusions are present, however, these peripheral leptomeningeal anastomoses are uncommon.

GROUP 2. UNILATERAL INTRACRANIAL INTERNAL CAROTID OCCLUSIONS

This group is the most common and is close to group 1 in Hilal's classification (i.e., basal occlusive disease without telangiectasia). In our series, this group included fifty children (77%). Partial or total occlusions occurred either alone in the internal carotid (18%) or together with distal occlusions in the cerebral vessels (28%). Girls outnumbered boys 2 to 1. The age groups 1 to 2 years and 7 to 10 years were particularly susceptible. The remainder of group 2 (31%) consisted of children with lesions in the branches of the internal carotid artery only; the middle cerebral was far more commonly involved than the anterior cerebral. Proximal occlusions in these branches were common (22%), and most had associated more distal occlusions; however, distal occlusions alone were less common (9%).

The mass effect of a large acute infarction was not observed in these children. The children whom we saw with gross seizures and subsequent hemiplegia thought to be due to focal encephalitis were found not to have arterial occlusions but rather a unilateral cerebral mass effect similar to the findings reported by Aicardi and co-workers (1969).

GROUP 2a. INTRACEREBRAL INTERNAL CAROTID LESIONS

Children with a *major* angiographic occlusion of the internal carotid artery with or without an associated middle anterior cerebral lesion were placed in group 2a. Conversely, children with a major abnormality of the peripheral arteries, often with *minor* narrowing of the internal carotid artery, were placed in group 2b. We reiterate that this is purely an objective angiographic classification. The unilateral nature of the lesions is the important feature, and the subgrouping is arbitrary.

Headache as an accompanying symptom is common, but seizures are very rare. The angiography of this group of lesions is quite bizarre (Fig. 14-50). Occlusions usually occur just distal to the ophthalmic artery origin or distal to the anterior choroidal origin. Occlusions can be complete, with either a tapered or an abrupt character. Weblike projections may occur into the lumen. The internal carotid distal to a stenosis

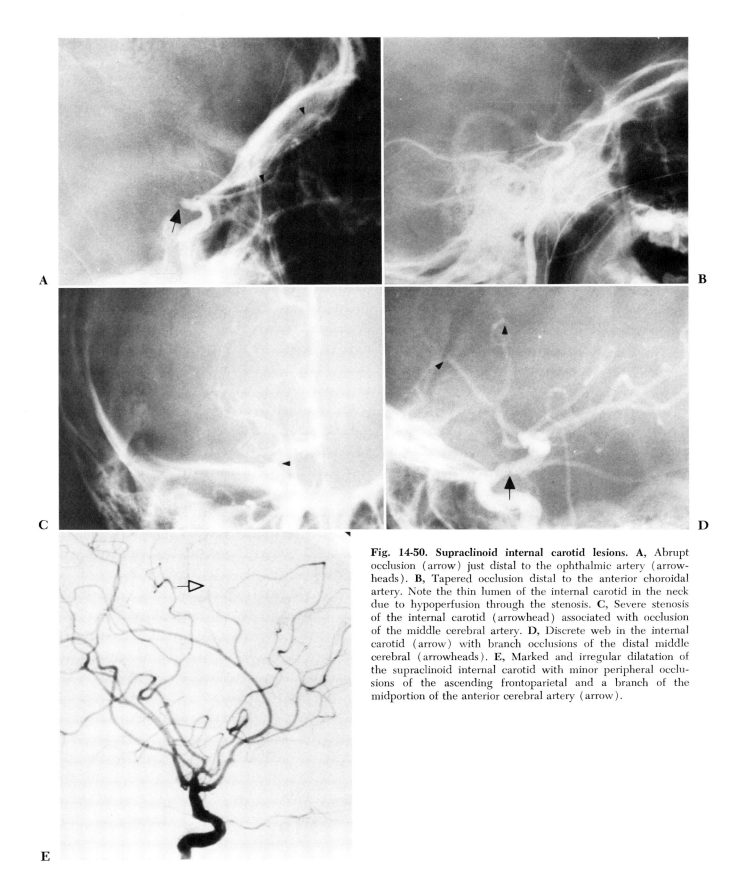

Fig. 14-50. Supraclinoid internal carotid lesions. A, Abrupt occlusion (arrow) just distal to the ophthalmic artery (arrowheads). **B,** Tapered occlusion distal to the anterior choroidal artery. Note the thin lumen of the internal carotid in the neck due to hypoperfusion through the stenosis. **C,** Severe stenosis of the internal carotid (arrowhead) associated with occlusion of the middle cerebral artery. **D,** Discrete web in the internal carotid (arrow) with branch occlusions of the distal middle cerebral (arrowheads). **E,** Marked and irregular dilatation of the supraclinoid internal carotid with minor peripheral occlusions of the ascending frontoparietal and a branch of the midportion of the anterior cerebral artery (arrow).

may be dilated and abnormally erect, or a localized constriction of the supraclinoid portion may occur. The stenosis can have a smooth or an irregular luminal contour. Stenosis or occlusion may be confined to the internal carotid alone or often will be associated with partial or total occlusions of the anterior cerebral or middle cerebral arteries—either contiguously with the internal carotid lesion or segmentally at some distance. The posterior cerebral artery is rarely involved distally, but its origin may be incorporated into the mural abnormality at the internal carotid artery.

A stenosis of the horizontal portions of the anterior cerebral and middle cerebral arteries is usually irregular and often lengthy. Total occlusion of these portions or of branches, either at the origin of the branches or distally, frequently is also present. A discrete intraluminal thrombosis may be identified. The lenticulostriate arteries may be occluded at their origins or can be irregular along their course.

Because the circle of Willis is not occluded elsewhere, basal telangiectasia, a feature of group 3, is not present in this group. We believe the fact that the circle is not obstructed to be the basic reason. Two children did, however, show extensive basal telangiectasias with a unilateral internal carotid arterial stenosis and anterior cerebral occlusion with absent posterior communicating arteries—which could have been a congenital absence or indeed part of the disease. Be that as it may, basal telangiectasia is very rare in unilateral occlusive disease.

Follow-up angiograms often revealed recanalization and better patency of the affected vessels but never a return to normal. This is in no way related to or indicative of possible return of lost motor power.

Due to adaptive narrowing (Fig. 14-50, *B*) (Hilal et al., 1971a) and decreased blood flow, the caliber of the cervical internal carotid artery on one side relative to that on the other is commonly decreased. This is not a developmental hypoplasia but a *secondary* phenomenon. Carotid canals are generally normal. Collateral flow via external carotid arteries through the base of the skull to the supraclinoid internal carotid artery is usually poorly developed, but the anterior choroidal vessels are often large and a lateral ventricular choroidal blush is frequently accentuated. This accentuation of blood flow results in early filling of the internal cerebral vein, similar to the initial phase of the refill phenomenon during hyperventilation angiography (Chapter 7), and should not be misinterpreted as a neoplasm.

Distal retrograde flow from peripheral branches of the middle cerebral arteries is often obtained via peripheral anterior cerebral (Fig. 14-51) and posterior cerebral cortical anastomoses. The posterior choroidal branches may be dilated, as may the meningohypo-

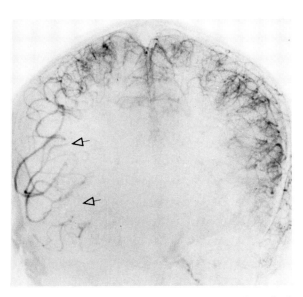

Fig. 14-51. Cortical anastomoses providing collateral flow. The right supraclinoid internal carotid artery is occluded. A left carotid angiogram reveals filling of the right anterior cerebral artery via the anterior communicating artery with filling of the distal right middle cerebral artery branches (arrows) in a retrograde fashion.

physeal arteries. Transarachnoid anastomoses from the external carotid dural and temporal vessels to the pial vessels are not so common as in group 3.

GROUP 2b. CEREBRAL CAROTID BRANCH LESIONS

Partial or complete occlusions of the peripheral arteries with or without associated internal carotid arterial lesions occur frequently. Peripheral arterial occlusions without (or with only minimal) internal carotid artery lesions may occur both proximally and distally (22%) or only distally (9%). Proximal lesions can be associated with intraluminal thrombi and secondary distal embolic spread, or the distal occlusions may be the only evidence of idiopathic arterial disease.

A number of children had a major angiographic abnormality in the middle cerebral artery (Fig. 14-52) with minimal narrowing of the distal internal carotid artery. These children were grouped in 2b. Angiography showed involvement of the middle cerebral artery alone or commonly with some portion of the proximal anterior cerebral artery (Fig. 14-53), but not often was the anterior cerebral artery alone involved. The horizontal proximal portion of the middle cerebral was abnormal for various distances distally. In some patients the stenosis and irregular vessel wall were most marked at the origin of the artery, whereas in others the abnormalities were apparent at the midportion or (rarely) the distal portion. The lenticulostriate arteries were in-

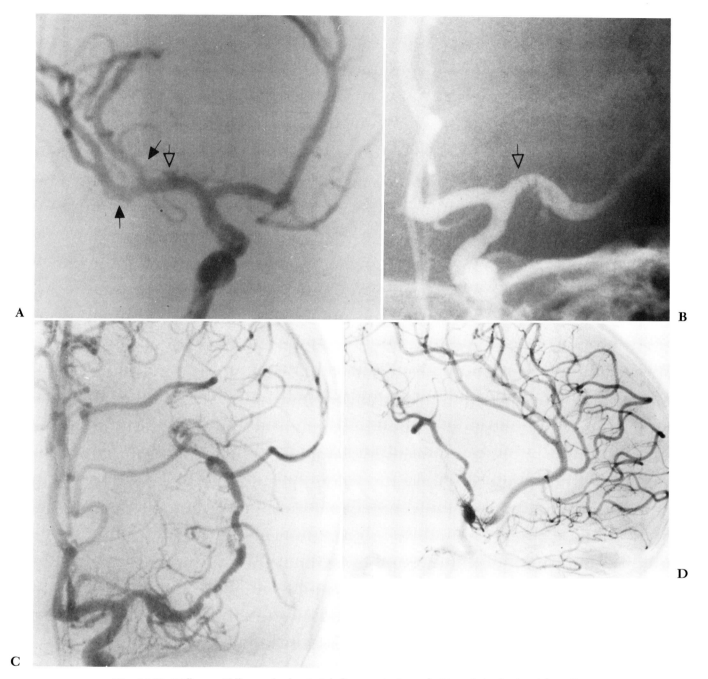

Fig. 14-52. Diffuse middle cerebral arterial disease. A, Irregularities of the horizontal portion of the artery include contrast dissection into the wall of the artery (open arrow) and outpouchings of the proximal branches (solid arrows). B and C, Left AP and, D, lateral carotid angiograms in another child show multiple accordian-like webs proximally (B, arrow), irregular dilatation of the midportion of the artery, and an extraordinary irregularity with stenosis and dilatation of the remainder of what was the posterior parietal artery. Other middle cerebral artery branches are occluded at their origins. (Note the associated mild irregularity of the supraclinoid portion of the internal carotid artery in D.)

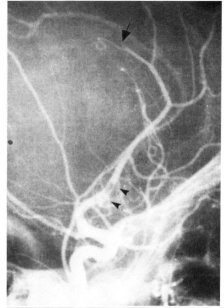

Fig. 14-53. Anterior and middle cerebral arterial occlusions. **A,** Middle, with a discrete thrombus in the proximal anterior cerebral (arrowheads) and a distal occlusion (arrow). **B,** Irregularity of the right middle cerebral (large arrowhead) and occlusion of the origin of the anterior cerebral (small arrowhead). **C,** A left carotid arteriogram in the same child demonstrates the other side of the occlusion (large arrowhead). There is cross filling of the right anterior cerebral with collateral circulation via a persistent recurrent artery of Heubner (small arrowheads).

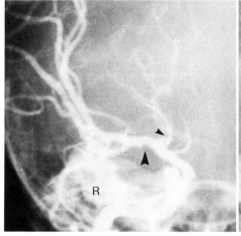

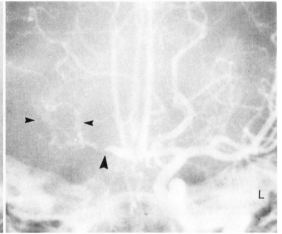

volved either at their origin off the parent vessel or along their course as part of the arterial disease. Our experience as well as the experience of Hilal and co-workers (1971a) has been that dramatic middle cerebral irregularity and stenosis can occur in children *without hemiplegia.*

The angiographic character of these occlusions and irregularities varied from that of simple irregular stenoses of dissimilar lengths to that of an abrupt occlusion suggesting an embolus (Fig. 14-54). Irregular webs into the lumen or clefts into the wall (probably intramural dissections) provided a most distinctive beaded appearance on the horizontal portion of the middle cerebral, particularly the inferior wall (Fig. 14-55), in four chidren similar to that reported by Bickerstaff (1964). This characteristic rarely extended into the sylvian branches by contiguity,

but associated occlusions or discrete stenoses were common distally.

Recanalization or a subsequent widening of the stenotic areas seen on repeat angiograms (the usual course of events) unfortunately is not related to clinical improvement. In our experience, a total occlusion has not often recanalized. Taveras (1969) describes multiple progressive intracranial arterial occlusions and indicates that a few of the children in whom repeat angiograms were obtained did show progressive stenoses, often to occlusion, especially of the supraclinoid internal carotid segment; however, it is very rare for the uninvolved side on the first angiogram to be stenosed on subsequent angiograms. We believe the progressive nature of the stenosis is uncommon; rather the collaterals are what tend to develop dramatically.

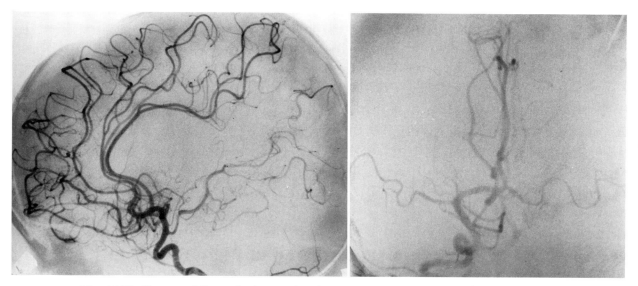

Fig. 14-54. Abrupt middle cerebral arterial occlusion. The right artery is occluded at its origin. Only the anterior frontoparietal branch fills directly from the internal carotid artery.

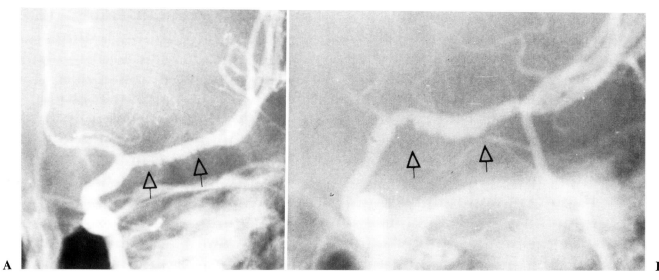

A   B

Fig. 14-55. Stenoses of the middle cerebral artery. A, Numerous circumferential clefts (arrows). **B,** Similar clefts in another child but with inferior pouch formations (arrows). There is also occlusion of the anterior cerebral artery.

A history of severe nasopharyngeal infection, tonsillitis, or tonsillectomy was present in at least 60% of these children. An associated discrete stenosis of the cervical internal carotid artery was noted in five (Fig. 14-56). This abnormality was not due to the catheter technique but was related to the intracranial arterial lesions—by extension of the inflammatory process up the internal carotid artery, resulting in intracranial thrombosis, stenosis, and emboli singly or together—thus providing angiographic evidence to support the thesis that there is indeed a connection

between nasopharyngeal infections and intracranial arteriopathies (Harwood-Nash et al., 1971).

Collateral circulation occurs in proportion to the degree of the occlusion of the middle and anterior cerebral arteries. Central collaterals (group 3) are rare in unilateral lesions unless the circle of Willis is anatomically deficient. Common collateral channels that do occur in this group are ipsilateral interleptomeningeal branches whose flow is retrograde and also choroid plexus vessels. Transdural external carotid–internal carotid anastomoses are uncommon in uni-

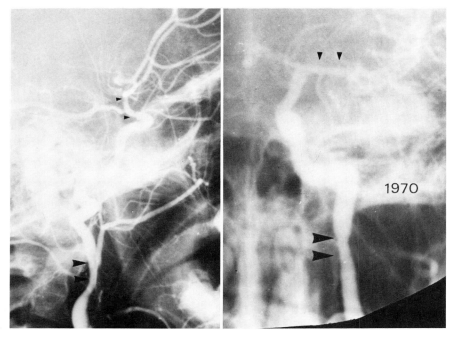

Fig. 14-56. Intracranial arterial disease associated with cervical internal carotid disease. A, Discrete stenosis of the internal carotid artery in the neck (large arrowhead) with irregularity of the supraclinoid internal carotid (small arrowheads) and occlusion of the middle cerebral. **B,** Marked irregularity of the middle cerebral (small arrowheads) in another child. Both patients had a discrete stenosis (large arrowheads) of the upper cervical internal carotid which was directly related to the tonsillar fossa, and both had had previous severe tonsillitis.

lateral disease. Peripheral arterial occlusions of the middle cerebral, posterior cerebral, or anterior cerebral occurring with hemiplegia were uncommon (9%). Distal occlusions were common in the middle cerebral artery and were abrupt, suggesting emboli. Peripheral collateral circulation was via the leptomeningeal pial collaterals.

In some children, pneumoencephalography was performed soon after the onset of the hemiplegia; in others, months or years after the onset. We discovered that atrophic changes were quite marked even at the onset of hemiplegia, indicating that the abnormalities had antedated the onset by a considerable length of time. For fear of disturbing the delicate balance that may be present within confirmed collaterals from the external to the internal carotid system, we do not now consider it wise to perform pneumoencephalography in these children. Air within the subarachnoid space through which the collaterals pass may cause some physical disturbance. CT is preferred.

GROUP 3. BILATERAL INTRACRANIAL OCCLUSIONS

Group 3 is characterized by a distinct form of cerebral vascular disease with occlusion of the circle of Willis at multiple and varying points. Subsequent to these occlusions is the development of a distinctive profuse central and transdural arterial collateral system. Hilal and co-workers (1971a) classified this group as basal occlusions with telangiectasia—group 2.

The bilateral occlusive disease of the supraclinoid internal carotid arteries and their branches in children and young adults was first noted by Kudo in 1956, and reported by him in 1965, and by Takeuchi in 1961 to be associated with a profuse meshlike arterial network at the base of the brain. Initially this was thought to be a malformation and confined to patients of Japanese descent. The first Japanese reports (Nishimoto and Sugiu, 1964; Nishimoto et al., 1965; Handa et al., 1970; Handa and Handa, 1972; Nishimoto and Takeuchi, 1972) were followed by reports of the same disease entity from all over the world. It was called the *moyamoya* syndrome by the Japanese, who likened the fine profuse central collaterals to a puff of smoke (moyamoya) emitting from a volcano. Taveras (1969) termed it multiple progressive intracranial arterial occlusions. The reader is referred to an excellent and extensive review of the subject by multiple authors under the chairmanship of L. Picard (1974a,b). We have had experience with ten children in whom the syndrome occurred.

This group is a syndrome of the young: 70% of the reported cases are in patients under 20 years of age, 50% in patients under 10. The youngest child in our series was 6 months old, and the majority were less than 4. Contrary to the reported findings among Japanese of a 65% incidence in female children, seven boys and three girls made up our series (none of our patients were Japanese).

There again appears to be a distinct relationship between previous nasopharyngeal infections, severe pyrexia, and exanthema and the development of hemiplegia. All these conditions predated the onset by weeks or months. We have found that angiography, often performed within 24 hours of the onset of hemiplegia, revealed an already well-developed central collateral system together with bilateral internal carotid arterial stenoses. We strongly believe that whatever caused the initial bilateral arterial occlusion did

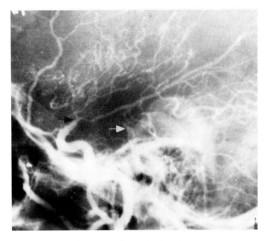

Fig. 14-57. Internal carotid and basilar stenoses. Multiple occlusions in the circle of Willis can cause profuse central collaterals to develop, as in this patient. The internal carotid artery is occluded at the origin of the posterior cerebral (black arrow), and the basilar artery is occluded at its tip (white arrow).

so some time *before* the hemiplegia occurred and that the collaterals developed prior to this onset. The high fever, exanthema, or even intense exertion (in four of our series) precipitated a hemiplegia in an already compromised intracranial vascular circulation. Alternating hemiplegias may occur, as may subarachnoid hemorrhages or subdural hemorrhages due to rupture of one or more transdural collaterals. Both the latter conditions are rare in children (Nishimoto and Takeuchi, 1968).

For the deep arterial collaterals to develop, the circle of Willis must be obstructed in at least two points. Stenosis of both supraclinoid internal carotid arteries is the usual combination, but the basilar and posterior cerebral system will uncommonly be involved (Fig. 14-57).

Angiographic characteristics. Standard radiographs may reveal increased meningeal arterial grooves caused by increased flow to the external carotid–internal carotid anastomoses (Taveras, 1969).

Such grooves are uncommon in children less than 10 years of age. Suzuki and Takaku (1969) suggested an angiographic orientation with six stages of natural history of this disease in group 3. These stages are dependent on the degree of stenosis of the internal carotid arteries and the natural history of the basal and transdural collaterals. We have simplified their classification into three types:

In *type 1* (stage 1 of Suzuki and Takaku) there is bilateral stenosis of the supraclinoid internal carotid arteries (possibly including the basilar artery) with no basal collaterals (Fig. 14-58). This is uncommon.

In *type 2* (stage 2 and stage 3 of Suzuki and Takaku) there are mild basal collaterals at the site of occlusion, increasing to marked basal collaterals from all basal arteries and perforators (Fig. 14-59) (anterior choroidal, posterior communicating, posterior

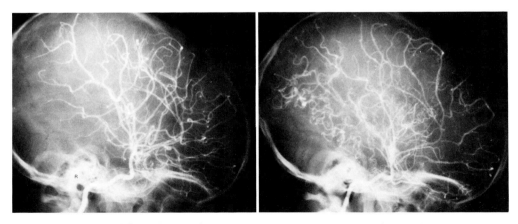

Fig. 14-58. Type 1 bilateral internal carotid arterial stenosis. This includes a mild right internal carotid stenosis and a more severe left internal carotid stenosis in the supraclinoid portions. Except for those between the cortical branches, there are no basal collaterals.

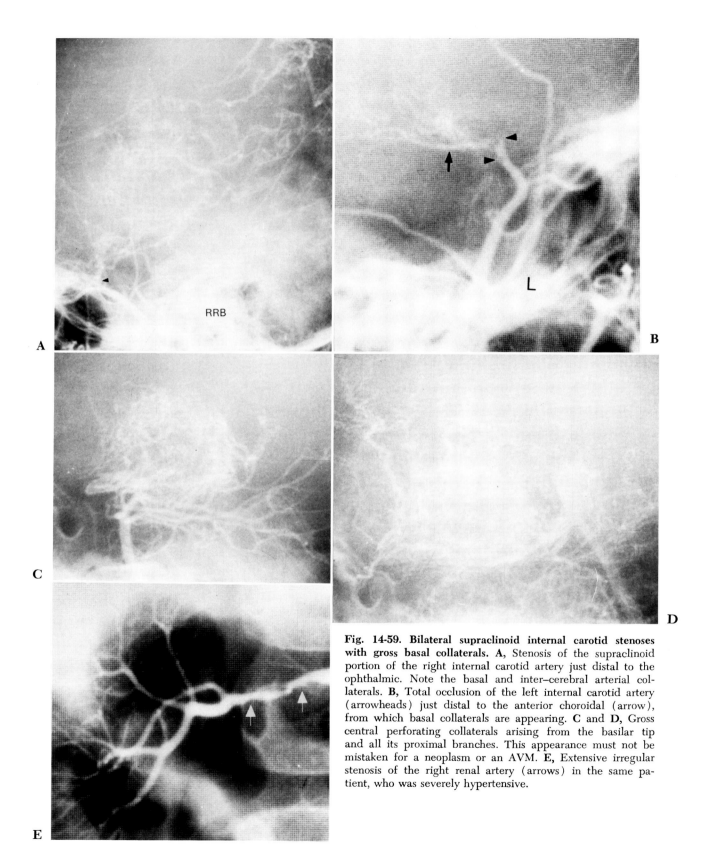

Fig. 14-59. Bilateral supraclinoid internal carotid stenoses with gross basal collaterals. A, Stenosis of the supraclinoid portion of the right internal carotid artery just distal to the ophthalmic. Note the basal and inter–cerebral arterial collaterals. **B,** Total occlusion of the left internal carotid artery (arrowheads) just distal to the anterior choroidal (arrow), from which basal collaterals are appearing. **C** and **D,** Gross central perforating collaterals arising from the basilar tip and all its proximal branches. This appearance must not be mistaken for a neoplasm or an AVM. **E,** Extensive irregular stenosis of the right renal artery (arrows) in the same patient, who was severely hypertensive.

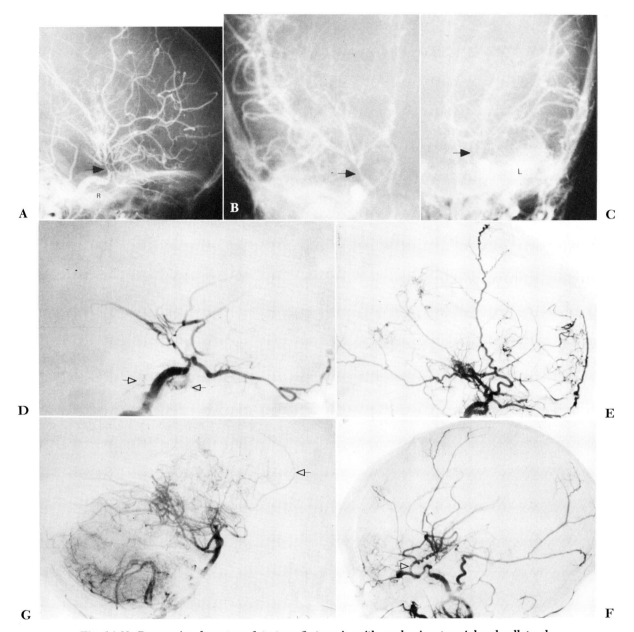

Fig. 14-60. Progression from type 1 to type 3 stenosis, with predominant peripheral collaterals. **A** to **C,** An initial angiogram in an infant with bilateral supraclinoid internal carotid artery stenoses (arrows). Note the developing early central basal collaterals bilaterally. **D,** Three years later, the right internal carotid is completely occluded distal to the origins of the ophthalmic and posterior communicating arteries; and the origins are irregular. There also is a lack of basal collaterals, but note the large meningohypophyseal vessels (arrows). **E,** The right stenosed internal carotid now demonstrates spectacular transdural anastomoses from the anterior meningeal and middle meningeal branches to the middle cerebral and anterior cerebral arteries. **F,** Similar changes are seen on the left side, which has a large middle meningeal artery (arrow) arising from the ophthalmic. **G,** Some large basal collaterals still arise from the posterior communicating artery, the tip of the basilar artery, and the proximal basilar branches. Note the filling of the pericallosal artery (arrow).

cerebral, basilar, lenticulostriate). There may be poor arterial flow with decreased caliber of the cerebral vessels, and total occlusions may replace the stenoses. This type is common in children.

In *type 3* (stages 4, 5, and 6) there are now diminished basal collaterals and only the larger remain (Fig. 14-60). Associated stenoses of the proximal middle cerebral and anterior cerebral occur together with external carotid–internal carotid transdural anastomoses. The peripheral arterial perfusion is markedly delayed. Total occlusion of the internal carotid and of the origins of the middle cerebral and anterior cerebral now develop. Finally, bilateral internal carotid occlusions are seen with transdural collaterals only (rare in young children).

Thus we consider three main types, whose natural history progresses from that of type 1 to that of type 3 with increasing age. Type 1 is usual among infants and young children and consists of bilateral supraclinoid internal carotid arterial stenoses with no basal collaterals. This progresses to type 2, in which there are additional mild or marked basal collaterals. Finally, in type 3, which is more common among older children and young adults, there is occlusion of the supraclinoid internal carotid arteries and origins of the anterior cerebral and middle cerebral arteries with decreasing basal collaterals and increasing transdural collaterals.

The stenosis of the supraclinoid internal carotid arteries is usually distal to the origin of the anterior choroidal or is between the origins of the ophthalmic and anterior choroidal arteries. Complete occlusion of the bifurcation of the internal carotid artery was common, as was severe stenosis of this site with occlusion of the origin of the anterior cerebral and/or middle cerebral arteries. The sites of stenoses or occlusions were not necessarily symmetrical and were different in the majority of the ten cases. Basilar arterial occlusion occurred in two cases, one at the distal tip and the other just proximal to the origins of the superior cerebellar arteries. Stenoses or occlusions of the peripheral middle cerebral and/or anterior cerebral arteries occurred in four children; and these lesions could have been due to either the same disease process or embolization from the proximal arterial abnormalities. If the middle cerebral or anterior cerebral did fill, the caliber of and flow through both vessels were markedly diminished. The mass effect of an acute infarction was *not* seen in children. Subsequent pneumoencephalography, which we now believe is inadvisable, showed the dilated ventricles and sulci of bilateral cerebral atrophy.

In addition to the progression of the stenotic lesions, we tend to think that the collateral circulation varies in degree and site from child to child and also varies with the geography and characteristics of the arterial occlusions. From an angiographic point of view, the degree and distribution of the occlusions and the extent of the collateral pathways, regardless of site, are the important features. More often, however, the degree of collateral circulation rather than the degree of stenosis of the basal arteries progressively increases (Harwood-Nash et al., 1971). Taveras (1969) and Handa and Handa (1972) documented cases of the progression of stenotic arterial lesions alone. We have had experience with two additional cases (Fig. 14-60). Because follow-up angiograms are not usually indicated except for curiosity, many children do not have them.

Collateral circulation

The collateral pathways that develop from the moyamoya disease process involve preexisting rather than new vessels. They are not vascular malformations, nor are they tumor vessels—both common misdiagnoses. No mass effect or rapid vascular flow is present, and the extent of the collaterals has a differing pattern from that of a diffuse neoplasm or an arteriovenous malformation. Arterial occlusions may rarely be seen in infiltrating neoplasms, but not in arteriovenous malformations. Tuberculous meningitis can produce gross and extensive basal cerebral arterial stenoses and occlusions. Trauma can occlude or stenose both the basal and the peripheral arteries. The history, clinical findings, and additional radiological features will differentiate these two entities from group 3 arterial abnormalities. Mishkin and Schreiber (1974) have provided a general discussion of all forms of cranial vascular collateral circulation.

On selective hyperventilated magnified subtracted angiograms in infants, the normal arterioles that dilate in this disease are quite clearly seen (Chapter 7). We believe these enlarged vessels that make up the collateral circulation develop within hours of an acute block.

Basal collaterals

The following vessels are commonly involved in the basal collateral system:

1. Meningohypophyseal vessels off the internal carotid artery (Fig. 14-60, *D*)
2. Anterior perforating arteries to the basal ganglia off the posterior communicating artery (Fig. 14-61, *A*)
3. Perforating arteries off the anterior choroidal artery
4. Hypothalamic vessels off the bifurcation of the internal carotid and proximal anterior cerebral and middle cerebral arteries—including lenticu-

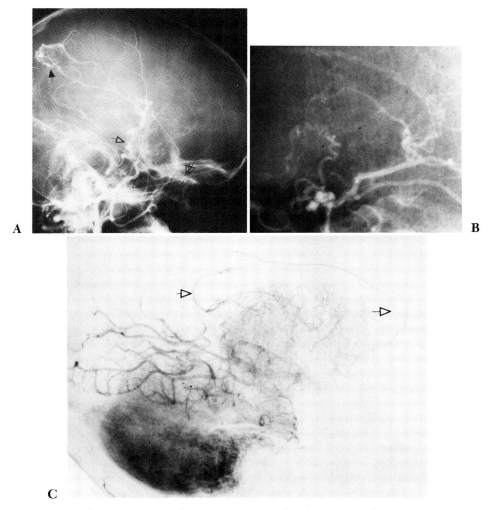

Fig. 14-61. Basal collateral circulation. **A,** Through the basal anterior perforating artery, arising from the proximal posterior communicating artery (open arrow). Note the transdural meningeal–posterior cerebral anastomoses (solid arrow) and the transdural ethmoidal–anterior cerebral anastomoses (double arrows). **B,** Large tortuous posterior perforating arteries of the basilar tip and the posterior choroidal arteries. **C,** Diffuse posterior thalamic and basal ganglionic perforating arteries produce a dense blush of the basal ganglia and supply both the anterior and the posterior callosal arteries (arrows). A diffuse collateral blush can be seen arising from the basilar and cerebellar arteries, providing a dense pial collateral network around the cerebellum and the posterior cerebral artery pathway.

lostriates off the anterior cerebral and middle cerebral (Fig. 14-53, *C*)

5. Posterior perforating arteries off the tip of the basilar (Fig. 14-61, *B*), posterior cerebral, and posterior choroidal arteries—including the posterior callosal (Fig. 14-61, *C*)

6. Basilar artery branches to the brain stem and cerebellum (Fig. 14-61, *C*)

Pial network

The following constitute vessels of the pial network:

1. Interarteriolar anastomoses (Fig. 14-62, *A*) between the anterior cerebral, middle cerebral, and posterior cerebral arteries (may create a diffuse cortical blush outlining the gyral pattern) (Fig. 14-62, *B*)

2. Pial vessel enlargement from brain stem and cerebellum passing upward from the brain stem to the cerebral pia (Fig. 14-61, *C*) (Weidner et al., 1965)

Transdural external carotid–internal carotid collaterals

The rete mirabile exists only in certain animals, not in man (de Gutiérrez-Mahoney and Schechter, 1972).

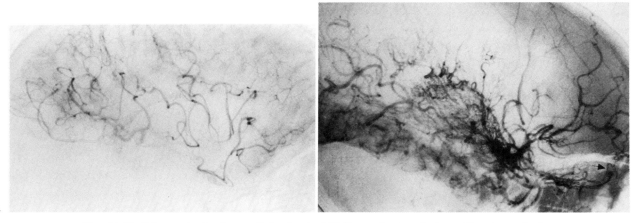

Fig. 14-62. Intracerebral artery collaterals. A, Middle cerebral occlusion with retrograde flow into the middle cerebral territory from the anterior cerebral and posterior cerebral arteries. **B,** In another child, partial middle cerebral and posterior cerebral occlusions with basal collaterals and an intense pial arteriolar blush of the occipital and temporal lobes. Note also the ethmoidal collaterals via the anterior meningeal artery (arrow).

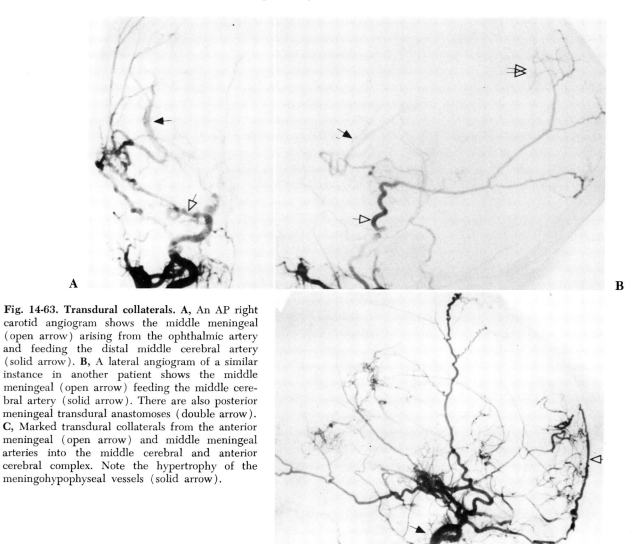

Fig. 14-63. Transdural collaterals. A, An AP right carotid angiogram shows the middle meningeal (open arrow) arising from the ophthalmic artery and feeding the distal middle cerebral artery (solid arrow). **B,** A lateral angiogram of a similar instance in another patient shows the middle meningeal (open arrow) feeding the middle cerebral artery (solid arrow). There are also posterior meningeal transdural anastomoses (double arrow). **C,** Marked transdural collaterals from the anterior meningeal (open arrow) and middle meningeal arteries into the middle cerebral and anterior cerebral complex. Note the hypertrophy of the meningohypophyseal vessels (solid arrow).

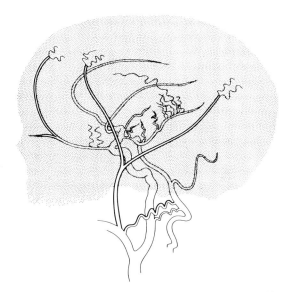

Fig. 14-64. Schematic representation of the major collateral pathways.

It is a profuse collection of small arteries related to the divisions of the fifth nerve passing within venous lakes from the internal maxillary arteries to the base of the brain (Daniel et al., 1953). We have identified small vessels linking the internal maxillary and infracavernous portions of the internal carotid artery within the carotid canal. The internal maxillary vessels tend to connect with a diffuse network around the internal carotid artery and the meningohypophyseal vessel, particularly the artery to the cavernous sinus.

Transdural collaterals form along the following channels and, in general, provide diffuse extracranial arterial feeders into equally diffuse pial arterioles—resulting in slow filling of the branches of the cerebral vessels distal to their occlusions (Fig. 14-63):

1. Ophthalmic to ethmoidal to anterior meningeal and anterior falcine to adjacent pial vessels of the anterior cerebral
2. Facial and sphenopalatine to ethmoidal to anterior cerebral collaterals
3. Middle meningeal to anterior and middle cerebrals
4. Posterior meningeal to occipital
5. Anterior and posterior temporals to meningeal collaterals

Fig. 14-64 is a schematic outline of the collateral pathways available in all types of vascular stenoses or occlusions. The reader is reminded that acute iatrogenic or traumatic occlusions do not readily form collaterals. We believe that occlusions and stenoses in childhood which lead to acute hemiplegia of unknown origin are slow and insidious and allow for

collateral circulation to develop. The acute episode leading to hemiplegia is the final and intolerable insult on an already compromised blood flow. Fields and co-workers (1965) provide a detailed account of the embryological and anatomical basis for the collaterals of the brain; these collaterals are legion.

Early filling of the deep venous system, the internal cerebral vein, and the galenic vein occurs by virtue of the profuse basal arteriolar vascularity with basal ganglionic venous drainage. Subependymal venous drainage from the cortex then occurs, and the thalamostriate and atrial veins not seen in the early phase are filled. Rupture of some of the transdural collaterals may result in a subdural hematoma, but this occurrence is uncommon. The chronic vascular changes beneath a subdural membrane (Chapter 12) may add to the abnormal angiographic picture.

To assess the collateral pathway systems, we habitually perform both selective internal and selective external carotid angiography together with bilateral vertebral angiography.

Unilateral internal carotid or branch occlusions developed pial collaterals with retrograde flow to the distal side of the occlusion. Unless the circle of Willis was congenitally incompetent, development of basal collaterals was uncommon.

Especially in the young, *bilateral* stenoses or occlusions of the supraclinoid internal carotid artery were associated with profuse basal collateral arterioles. In older children, however, the transdural collaterals were more likely to form and were more profuse whereas the basal collaterals were less so.

• • •

In summary, the collaterals that develop assist in obtaining an angiographic understanding of the basic arterial stenosis or occlusion.

Miscellaneous cerebral vascular abnormalities

FOCAL CEREBRAL INFARCTION

The neuroradiology of cerebral infarction is predominantly confined to the adult age group. Cerebral infarction in children is related to birth anoxia, to cerebral infection or trauma, or to emboli arising from congenital heart disease. We have pointed out that neuroradiological evidence of focal infarction is usually absent in idiopathic arterial occlusions. Focal infarction is often seen at autopsy in children with cortical venous thromboses, meningitis, or encephalitis (Ford, 1973). Focal infarction may be de-

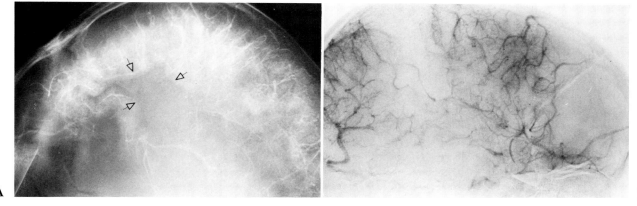

Fig. 14-65. Cerebral infarctions. A, A square area of infarction with complete loss of gyral cerebrogram (arrows). There also is early filling of deep veins. **B,** Two large areas of cerebral infarction with loss of cerebrogram in the frontal and posterior parietal regions of another child.

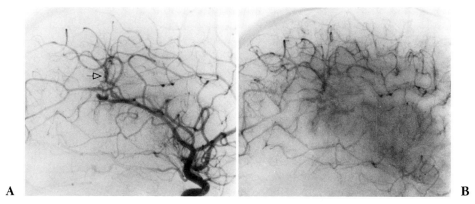

Fig. 14-66. Cerebral cicatrix. A posterior parietal postinfarct cicatrix (arrow) is associated with a profuse cerebrogram stain (**B**).

tected neuroradiologically in any *acute* form of intracranial arterial embolic or thrombotic lesions described previously or as a result of the uncommon identifiable primary intracranial arteritides that occur in children. The neuroradiological appearance depends on the interval between the onset of symptoms and the performance of the cerebral angiography.

The angiographic characteristics of infarcts are divided into two groups: those of the acute and those of the chronic stages.

In an *acute* infarct occlusion of the main or small branches of the cerebral arteries, usually the middle cerebral will be seen (Ring and Waddington, 1967; Davis et al., 1969). Taveras (1969) divided the findings of acute infarcts into an initial dilatation of the large arteries, an ensuing arteriolar block, and a subsequent vasodilatation:

1. The initial dilatation is due to the high carbon dioxide partial pressure and lowering of pH in the cerebral tissue and CSF around the infarct. This is commonly found in any cerebral insult in children—be it traumatic edema, encephalitis, or infarction. Small arterioles are seen to dilate and arise directly (at right angles) from the main arteries in the area rather than from the usual branching by arborization (Chapters 12 and 13).

2. The ensuing arteriolar block is due to vascular stasis (Denny-Brown and Meyer, 1957) and creates a local prolonged arteriolar phase. This leads to a local capillary blush or cerebrogram (Harwood-Nash, 1972). Proximal occlusion of larger branches will lead to slow filling by collaterals.

3. The subsequent vasodilatation in and around the area of infarction often leads to early filling of the regional veins due to a relative increase in the local blood flow rate. This appears within 12 days after the event (Taveras et al., 1969).

The nonspecific mass effect of cerebral edema at the area of infarction—which in children may develop within 24 hours after the onset of symptoms—may be very focal, often suggesting a more local lesion such as a hemorrhage, or may be quite diffuse

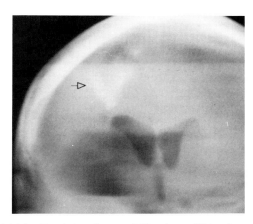

Fig. 14-67. **Postinfarction calcification.** This large right cerebral infarct with cerebral atrophy subsequently calcified (arrow).

and difficult to identify at angiography. Taveras and co-workers (1969) identified a mass in only fifteen of forty patients with an infarction.

In old infarcts, however, recanalization of the large vessel occlusion may have occurred. Furthermore, an area of cortical avascularity is now clearly seen (Fig. 14-65). The occlusion of the main artery may persist, and collateral circulation will often be present and involve the intercerebral pial vascular network. A cerebral cicatrix may be visualized creating an irregular starlike orientation of cerebral vessels in the area associated with a small network of enlarged irregular pial arterioles (Fig. 14-66).

Postembolic or postthrombotic stenosis of a cerebral vessel will result in decreased perfusion of a low-caliber distal vessel with lengthening of the circulation time in this vessel.

Computed tomography (Chapter 8) in the acute stage will show an area of edema with greater or lesser displacement of the ventricles, depending on the site and extent of the infarction. In the chronic stage, an irregular non–space-occupying area with an absorption coefficient similar to that of cerebrospinal fluid is seen. Dilatation of an adjacent part of the ventricle may also be present.

In the *chronic* phase of a sufficiently large infarct, pneumoencephalography will show dilatation of that portion of the ventricle in the area of the infarct and may reveal dilated sulci over the affected cortex. The more proximal the arterial occlusion or the more diffuse the peripheral occlusion, the greater will be the degree of atrophy.

Discrete popcornlike subcortical calcifications may occur associated with sulcal dilatation and often with dilatation of the underlying part of the ventricle. This is calcification (Fig. 14-67) within an infarct or possibly a calcified granuloma; or it may be an old hema-

toma. The latter, however, is less likely. We call these calcifications cerebroliths.

ANGIODYSPLASIAS

André and co-workers (1974) have grouped the angiodysplasias into (1) phacomatoses, (2) connective tissue dysplasias, and (3) inborn errors of metabolism. The reader is referred to this extensive report for an in-depth discussion. We shall mention only a few of this large group, and only those that occur with any frequency in children. Even these, however, are quite uncommon and the remainder are either very rare in children or present in adults. Hilal and co-workers (1971b) consider a group under the term neurocutaneous syndrome that produce cerebral arterial occlusive disease in children.

Sturge-Weber's encephalotrigeminal angiomatosis

Sturge-Weber syndrome is a regional angiomatous phacoma characterized by a hemifacial angioma present at birth and confined to the subcutaneous extent of the branches of the trigeminal nerve.

The common site is within the first branch above the palpebral fissure. The syndrome is rarely bilateral. There is a related angiomatosis of the ipsilateral cerebral leptomeninges that rarely may involve the choroid of the eye. In our experience, some children have had bilateral leptomeningeal angiomas in association with unilateral facial involvement.

Poser and Taveras (1957) suggested three types of the syndrome. The *first* type is the classical disturbance of the angiomatosis with two or more features including convulsions, hemiparesis, hemiatrophy, and mental retardation. Convulsions may start in infancy but the serious clinical sequelae develop in early childhood. The *second* type, which is rare, occurs in children with no skin angiomatosis; but a leptomeningeal angiomatosis is present. Leptomeningeal involvement is detected either by calcification on the skull radiograph or by angiography. The *third* type involves the leptomeningeal angiomatosis and atypical facial hemangiomas. The leptomeningeal angiomatosis is always of the occipital lobe and commonly extends to involve the parietal and temporal lobes and rarely the entire cerebral hemisphere. The cerebellum is rarely affected (Peterman et al., 1958).

Calcification of the leptomeningeal angiomatosis is a characteristic radiological feature of the syndrome and starts in the occipital pole (Chapter 2). The calcification is always circumscribed by the angiomatous area itself and rarely occurs bilaterally. The calcification progresses forward with age and characteristically follows the contours of the gyri, the so-called "tramline" calcification. The cortex is not in-

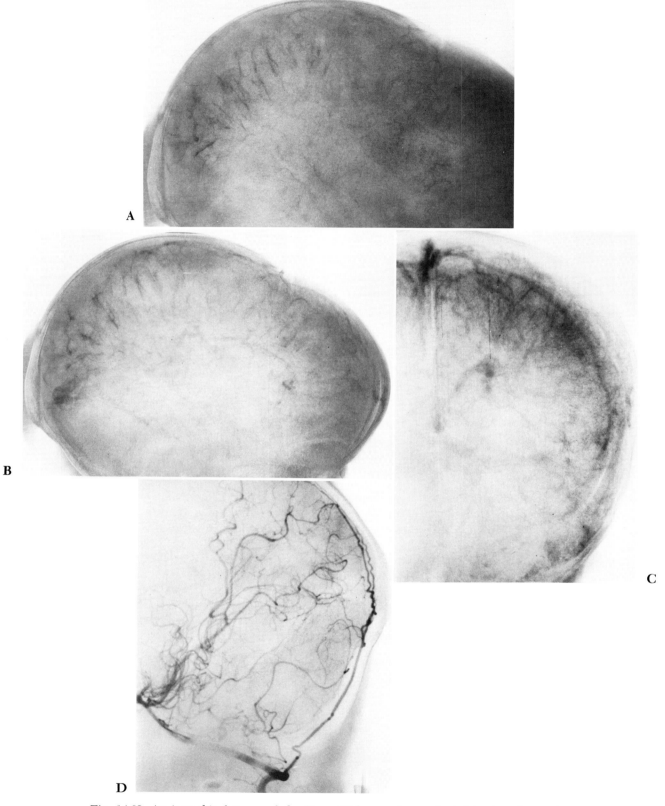

Fig. 14-68. Angiographic features of the Sturge-Weber syndrome. A, A lateral angiogram in an infant with intense staining of the leptomeninges of the left parieto-occipital cortex. B and C, In another infant, diffuse blush of the leptomeninges and rapid filling of large tortuous veins are evident. From the cortex, enlarged deep medullary veins drain into the deep venous system. D, Enlarged posterior meningeal artery feeding a malformation in the occipital lobes.

volved in the angiomatous process, but the calcification occurs as an anoxic watershed area at the second and third layers of the cerebral cortex (Cohen and Kay, 1941). Calcification of the vessels may also take place but is rarely specifically identified on skull radiographs. Calcification is commonly absent in infants and appears only after 1 to 2 years of age.

The radiological findings vary with the extent of the syndrome and the age of the child. They are more marked in older children and are commonly unilateral.

Skull radiography

Concomitant cerebral atrophy leads to decreased hemicranial size, particularly in the occipital region with a thickened diploic space (Chapter 2). Occipital tramline calcifications in the occipital region with variable forward extension are characteristic and rarely bilateral. Dilated ventricles may be more marked on the side of the angiomatosis, in particular around the occipital horn; and dilated sulci are present, indicating cerebral atrophy. Enlarged diploic venous channels due to the angiomatosis may be present in the occipital and parietal bones.

Angiography

Poser and Taveras (1957) and Bentson and co-workers (1971) describe in detail the characteristic angiographic signs of the Sturge-Weber syndrome (Fig. 14-68). There is a diffuse capillary blush over the occipital cortex extending forward to a variable degree. The cortical veins are irregular and follow bizarre courses; they are usually diminished in number and caliber. Large deep cerebral veins drain into large medullary veins. The meningeal arteries also may be enlarged (Fig. 14-68, D). Thromboses of the cortical veins and sagittal sinus may occur and even

thromboses of cortical arteries, but the latter are uncommon. Multiple altered tortuous and segmental ectasias and stenoses can occur (Hilal et al., 1971b), together with enlarged meningeal vessels. Associated subdural hematomas are rare and probably result from a rupture of these fragile abnormal leptomeningeal vessels.

It is necessary to perform angiography prior to an intended partial or complete hemispherectomy, a procedure that if performed in very young children will arrest severe chronic convulsions. Computed tomography with enhancement also may demonstrate the angiomatosis (Chapter 8).

Neurocutaneous melanosis

Neurocutaneous melanosis occurs with pigmented nevi in meningeal melanotic infiltration and is a rare disease (Hoffman, 1975). It produces a narrowing of the cerebral vessels with thrombotic occlusions. Areas of small vascular malformations may also be present.

Multiple neurofibromatosis

Hilal and co-workers (1971b) described three children in whom multiple neurofibromatosis was associated with basal cerebral arterial occlusions (Fig. 14-69). The internal carotid artery and distal branches were occluded, and there were occlusions of the basal collaterals similar to those in group 3 of the idiopathic arterial occlusions. Two children had been administered radiotherapy for an optic glioma, however, which may have had an occlusive arteritic effect.

Tuberous sclerosis

Hilal and co-workers (1971b) described a child with tuberous sclerosis in whom occlusions of the distal cerebral vessels and multiple segments of ec-

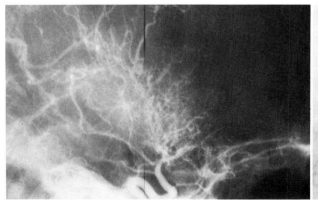 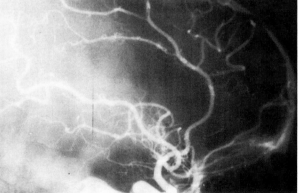

Fig. 14-69. Neurofibromatosis. This angiogram demonstrates bilateral cerebral arterial occlusions. The internal carotid artery is occluded on one side, with diffuse basal collaterals. Occlusions of the anterior branches of the middle cerebral artery and branches of the anterior cerebral artery are evident on the other side. Note the diffuse collateral vessels arising from the angular branch and the anterior cerebral artery. (Courtesy S. Hilal, M.D., New York.)

tasia and stenosis of the leptomeningeal arteries were seen. We have not identified these changes in any of the children with this disease on whom we have performed angiography.

Kinky-hair syndrome (Menkes)

Menkes and co-workers (1962) described a sex-linked recessive degenerative central nervous system disease with failure to thrive, severe psychomotor retardation, hypothermic crises, and seizures, together with white, coarse, crinkly hair. The syndrome was invariably fatal by 3 years of age. There were also low serum copper and ceruloplasmin levels and a defect in copper absorption.

Wesenberg and co-workers (1969) and later Adams and co-workers (1974) described symmetrical metaphyseal spurring and diaphyseal periosteal reaction of the long bones similar to those observed in the "abused child syndrome." Flaring of the ribs anteriorly and diffuse tortuous and irregular vessels occurred throughout the vascular system, particularly in the intracranial vessels. Marked cerebral atrophy and subdural effusions were also common. The striking tortuosity of the vessels represents the primary dysplasia, and the histology reveals fragmentation of the elastic lamina and marked intimal thickening.

The reader is reminded that a loop or whorl of the cervical internal carotid artery in infants is quite normal. In children who are giants due to eosinophilic adenoma of the pituitary, and who do not have arteriovenous malformations, large carotid arteries are also seen. Similar large carotid arteries occur in progeria.

Fibromuscular dysplasia

Fibromuscular dysplasia is not common in children. It may involve the renal, mesenteric, hepatic, and lumbar arteries as well as the carotid and vertebral arteries in the neck (Andersen, 1970). The angiographic appearance may vary from a single stenotic lesion to areas of arterial dilatation, long segmental stenoses both smooth and irregular, multiple short stenoses, and multiple aneurysms leading to a beaded appearance. This beaded appearance is similar to that seen in the middle cerebral arteries with childhood idiopathic cerebral arterial disease.

Extracranial carotid and vertebral involvement is far more common than intracranial involvement (Houser and Baker, 1968). Direct pathological confirmation is rare in the latter, however, and the diagnosis is usually by angiography alone (Andersen, 1970; Handa et al., 1970; Elias, 1971; Iosue et al., 1972). Renal artery fibromuscular dysplasia in adults may be associated with intracranial aneurysms (Palubinskas et al., 1966; Handa et al., 1970).

REFERENCES

Adams, P. C., Strand, R. D., Bresnan, M. J., and Lucky, A. W.: Kinky hair syndrome: serial study of radiological findings with emphasis on the similarity to the battered child syndrome, Radiology 112:401, 1974.

Aguilar, M. J., Gerbode, F., and Hill, J. D.: Neuropathologic complications of cardiac surgery, J. Thorac. Cardiovasc. Surg. 61:676, 1971.

Aicardia, J., Amsili, J., and Chevrie, J. J.: Acute hemiplegia in infancy and childhood, Dev. Med. Child Neurol. 11:162, 1969.

Allcock, J. M.: Aneurysms. In Newton, T. H., and Potts, D. G., editors: Radiology of the skull and brain. Vol. 2, book 4, Angiography, St. Louis, 1974, The C. V. Mosby Co.

Alpers, B. J.: Cerebral birth injuries. In Brock, S., editor: Injuries of the brain and spinal cord and their coverings, ed. 3, Baltimore, 1949, The Williams & Wilkins Co.

Amacher, A. L., and Shillito, J., Jr.: The syndromes and surgical treatment of aneurysms of the great vein of Galen, J. Neurosurg. 39:89, 1973.

Andersen, P. E.: Angiographic localization of small intracerebral hematomas, Acta Radiol. [Diagn.] 1:173, 1963.

Andersen, P. E.: Fibromuscular hyperplasia in children, Acta Radiol. [Diagn.] 10:205, 1970.

André, J. M., Picard, L., and Kissel, P.: Systematized angiodysplasias. Classification—nosology, J. Neuroradiol. 1:3, 1974.

Babson, S. G.: Spontaneous subarachnoid hemorrhage in infants and its relation to hydrocephalus, J. Pediatr. 25:68, 1944.

Bailey, O. T., and Hass, G. M.: Dural sinus thrombosis in early life. Recovery from acute thrombosis of the superior longitudinal sinus and its relation to certain acquired cerebral lesions in childhood, Brain 60:293, 1937a.

Bailey, O. T., and Hass, G. M.: Dural sinus thrombosis in early life. The clinical manifestations and extent of brain injury in acute sinus thrombosis, J. Pediatr. 11:755, 1937b.

Ballard, H. S., and Bondar, H.: Spontaneous subarachnoid hemorrhage in sickle cell anemia, Neurology 7:443, 1957.

Banker, B. Q.: Cerebral vascular disease in infancy and childhood. I. Occlusive vascular diseases, J. Neuropathol. Exp. Neurol. 20:127, 1961.

Barron, K. D., Siqueira, E., and Hirano, A.: Cerebral embolism caused by non-bacterial thrombotic endocarditis, Neurology 10:391, 1960.

Bax, M.: Acute hemiplegia in childhood; with a note on the management of the acute episode, Cerebral Palsy Bull. 3: 444, 1961.

Bax, M., and Mitchell, R.: Neuropathological finding in acute hemiplegia in childhood, Little Clubs Clinics in Developmental Medicine, No. 6, National Spastics Society, London, 1962, William Heinemann, Ltd.

Belber, C. J., and Hoffman, R. B.: The syndrome of intracranial aneurysm associated with fibromuscular hyperplasia of the renal arteries, J. Neurosurg. 28:556, 1968.

Benoit, B. G., and Wortzman, G.: Traumatic cerebral aneurysms; clinical features and natural history, J. Neurol. Neurosurg. Psychiatry 36:127, 1973.

Bentson, J. R., Wilson, G. H., and Newton, T. H.: Cerebral venous drainage pattern of the Sturge-Weber syndrome, Radiology 101:111, 1971.

Bergentz, S.: Studies on the genesis of post-traumatic fat embolism, Acta Chir. Scand. 123(supp. 282):1, 1961.

Berger, P. E., Harwood-Nash, D. C., and Fitz, C. R.: Computerized tomography: abnormal intracerebral collections of blood in children, Neuroradiology 11:29, 1976.

Bergouignan, M., and Arne, L.: A propos des anévrysmes des artères cérébrales associés à d'autres malformations, Acta Neurol. Psychiatrie [Belg.] 51:529, 1951.

Bickerstaff, E. R.: Aetiology of acute hemiplegia in childhood, Br. Med. J. 2:82, 1964.

Bigelow, N. H.: The association of polycystic kidneys with intracranial aneurysms and other related disorders, Am. J. Med. Sci. 225:485, 1953.

Boldrey, E., Maass, L., and Miller, E. R.: The role of atlantoid compression in the etiology of internal carotid thrombosis, J. Neurosurg. 13:127, 1956.

Braudo, M.: Thrombosis of the internal carotid artery in childhood after injuries in the region of the soft palate, Br. Med. J. 1:665, 1956.

Brisman, R., and Abbassioun, K.: Familial intracranial aneurysms, J. Neurosurg. 34:678, 1971.

Carmichael, R.: The pathogenesis of non-inflammatory cerebral aneurysms, J. Pathol. Bacteriol. 62:1, 1950.

Carter, S., and Gold, A. P.: Acute infantile hemiplegia, Pediatr. Clin. North Am. 14:851, 1967.

Chang, V., Rewcastle, N. B., Harwood-Nash, D. C., and Norman, M. G.: Bilateral dissecting aneurysms of the intracranial internal carotid arteries in an 8-year-old boy, Neurology 25:573, 1975.

Clarke, P. R. R., Dicksen, J., and Smith, B. J.: Traumatic thrombosis of the internal carotid artery following a nonpenetrating injury and leading to infarction of the brain, Br. J. Surg. 43:215, 1955.

Cocker, J., George, S. W., and Yates, P. O.: Perinatal occlusion of the middle cerebral artery, Dev. Med. Child Neurol. 7:235, 1965.

Cohen, H. J., and Kay, M. N.: Associated facial hemangioma and intracranial lesion (Weber-Dimitri disease), Am. J. Dis. Child. 62:606, 1941.

Crawford, T.: Some observations on the pathogenesis and natural history of intracranial aneurysms, J. Neurol. Neurosurg. Psychiatry 22:259, 1959.

Cronqvist, S., Granholm, L., and Lundström, N.-R.: Hydrocephalus and congestive heart failure caused by intracranial arteriovenous malformations in infants, J. Neurosurg. 36:249, 1972.

Cronqvist, S., and Troupp, H.: Intracranial arteriovenous malformation and arterial aneurysm in the same patient, Acta Neurol. Scand. 42:307, 1966.

Dalgaard, O. Z.: Bilateral polycystic disease of the kidneys: a follow-up of two hundred and eighty-four patients and their families, Copenhagen, 1957, Einar Munksgaard Forlag.

Daniel, P. M., Dawes, J. D. K., and Pritchard, M. M. L.: Studies on the carotid rete and its associated arteries, Philos. Trans. R. Soc. Lond. [Biol. Sci.] 237:173, 1953.

Davie, J. C., and Coxe, W.: Occlusive disease of the carotid artery in children, Arch. Neurol. 17:313, 1967.

Davis, D. O.: Personal communication, 1974.

Davis, D. O., Rumbaugh, C. L., and Gilson, J. M.: Angiographic diagnosis of small-vessel cerebral emboli, Acta Radiol. [Diagn.] 9:264, 1969.

de Gutiérrez-Mahoney, C. G., and Schechter, M. M.: The myth of the *rete mirabile* in man, Neuroradiology 4:141, 1972.

Denny-Brown, D., and Meyer, J. S.: Cerebral collateral circulation. II. Production of cerebral infarction by ischemic anoxia and its reversibility in early stages, Neurology 7:567, 1957.

de Saussure, R. L., Scheibert, C. D., and Hazouri, L. A.: Astrocytoma grade III associated with profuse subarachnoid bleeding as its first manifestation, J. Neurosurg. 8:236, 1951.

Dooley, J. M., Jr., and Smith, K. R., Jr.: Occlusion of the basilar artery in a 6-year-old boy, Neurology 18:1034, 1968.

Drummond, D. S., Salter, R. B., and Boone, J.: Fat embolism in children: its frequency and relationship to collagen disease, Can. Med. Assoc. J. 101:200, 1969.

du Boulay, G. H.: Some observations on the natural history of intracranial aneurysms, Br. J. Radiol. 38:721, 1965.

Duman, S., and Stephens, J. W.: Post-traumatic middle cerebral artery occlusion, Neurology 13:613, 1963.

Ekbom, K., and Greitz, T.: Syndrome of hydrocephalus caused by saccular aneurysm of the basilar artery, Acta Neurochir. 24:71, 1971.

Elias, W. S.: Intracranial fibromuscular hyperplasia, J.A.M.A. 218:254, 1971.

Ellington, E., and Margolis, G.: Block of arachnoid villus by subarachnoid hemorrhage, J. Neurosurg. 30:651, 1969.

Ferris, E. J., and Levine, H. L.: Cerebral arteritis: classification, Radiology, 109:327, 1973.

Fields, W. S., Bruetman, M. E., and Weibel, J.: Collateral circulation of the brain, Monogr. Surg. Sci. 2:183, 1965.

Foltz, E. L., and Ward, A. A.: Communicating hydrocephalus from subarachnoid bleeding, J. Neurosurg. 13:546, 1956.

Ford, F. R.: Diseases of the nervous system in infancy, childhood and adolescence, ed. 6, Springfield, Ill., 1973, Charles C Thomas, Publisher.

Ford, F. R., and Schaffer, A. J.: The etiology of infantile acquired hemiplegia, Arch. Neurol. Psychiatry 18:323, 1927.

Frantzen, E., Jacobsen, H. H., and Therkelsen, J.: Cerebral artery occlusions in children due to trauma to the head and neck, Neurology 11:695, 1961.

Freud, S. 1897. In Box, M., 1961.

Fuchsig, P., Brücke, P., Blümel, G., and Gottlob, R.: A new clinical and experimental concept on fat embolism, N. Engl. J. Med. 276:1192, 1967.

George, A. E., Kishore, P. R. S., and Chase, N. E.: Primary diseases of the cerebral blood vessels, Semin. Roentgenol. 6:34, 1971a.

George, A. E., Lin, J. P., and Morantz, R. A.: Intracranial aneurysm on a persistent primitive trigeminal artery; case report, J. Neurosurg. 35:601, 1971b.

Gold, A. P., Hammill, J. F., and Carter, S.: Cerebrovascular diseases. In Farmer, T. W., editor: Pediatric neurology, New York, 1964a, Harper & Row, Publishers.

Gold, A. P., Ransohoff, J., and Carter, S.: Vein of Galen malformation, Acta Neurol. Scand. 40(supp. 11):1, 1964b.

Gomes, M. M., and Bernatz, P. E.: Arteriovenous fistulas: a review and ten-year experience at the Mayo Clinic, Mayo Clin. Proc. 45:81, 1970.

Gomez, M. R., Whitten, C. F., Nolke, A., Bernstein, J., and Meyer, J. S.: Aneurysmal malformation of the great vein of Galen causing heart failure in early infancy; report of five cases, Pediatrics 31:400, 1963.

Goree, J. A., and Dukes, H. T.: The angiographic differential diagnosis between the vascularized malignant glioma and the intracranial arteriovenous malformation, Am. J. Roentgenol. Radium Ther. Nucl. Med. 90:512, 1963.

Handa, J., and Handa, H.: Progressive cerebral arterial occlusive disease: analysis of 27 cases, Neuroradiology 3:119, 1972.

Handa, J., Kamijyo, Y., and Handa, H.: Intracranial aneurysm associated with fibro-muscular hyperplasia of renal and internal carotid arteries, Br. J. Radiol. 43:483, 1970.

Harwood-Nash, D. C.: The cerebrogram and the spinal cordogram, Am. J. Roentgenol. Radium Ther. Nucl. Med. 114: 773, 1972.

Harwood-Nash, D. C., and Fitz, C. R.: The angiography of vascular anomalies in the newborn and infant. In Sano, K., and Ishii, S., editors: Recent progress in neurological surgery, New York, 1974a, American Elsevier Publishing Co., Inc.

Harwood-Nash, D. C., and Fitz, C. R.: Complications of pediatric arteriography. In Gyepes, M. T., editor: Angiography in infants and children, New York, 1974b, Grune & Stratton, Inc.

Harwood-Nash, D. C., McDonald, P., and Argent, W.: Cerebral arterial disease in children; an angiographic study of 40 cases, Am. J. Roentgenol. Radium Ther. Nucl. Med. 3: 672, 1971.

Heinz, E. R., Schwartz, J. F., and Sears, R. A.: Thrombosis in the vein of galen malformation, Br. J. Radiol. 41:424, 1968.

Henderson, W. R., and Gomez, R. D.: Natural history of cerebral angiomas, Br. Med. J. 4:571, 1967.

Hilal, S. K.: Personal communication, 1974.

Hilal, S. K., Mount, L., Correll, J., Trokel, S., and Wood, E. H.: Therapeutic embolization of vascular malformations of the external carotid circulation—clinical and experimental results, IX Symposium neuroradiologicum, Göteberg, Aug., 1970.

Hilal, S. K., Solomon, G. E., Gold, A. P., and Carter, S.: Primary cerebral arterial occlusive disease in children. I. Acute acquired hemiplegia, Radiology 99:71, 1971a.

Hilal, S. K., Solomon, G. E., Gold, A. P., and Carter, S.: Primary cerebral arterial occlusive disease in children. II. Neurocutaneous syndromes, Radiology 99:87, 1971b.

Hiller, F.: Cerebral hemorrhage in hyperergic angitis, J. Neuropathol. Exp. Neurol. 12:24, 1953.

Hoare, R. D.: Arteriovenous aneurysm of the posterior fossa, Acta Radiol. 40:96, 1953.

Hoffman, H. J.: Personal communication, 1975.

Holden, A. M., Fyler, D. C., Shillito, J., Jr., and Nadas, A. S.: Congestive heart failure from intracranial arteriovenous fistula in infancy; clinical and physiologic considerations in eight patients, Pediatrics 49:30, 1972.

Holland, H. W., and Thomson, J. L. G.: Aneurysm of the middle meningeal artery, Clin. Radiol. 16:334, 1965.

Housepian, E. M., and Pool, J. L.: A systematic analysis of intracranial aneurysms from the autopsy file of the Presbyterian Hospital 1914 to 1956, J. Neuropathol. Exp. Neurol. 17:409, 1958.

Houser, O. W., and Baker, H. L., Jr.: Fibromuscular dysplasia and other uncommon diseases of the cervical carotid artery: angiographic aspects, Am. J. Roentgenol. Radium Ther. Nucl. Med. 104:201, 1968.

Houser, O. W., Baker, H. L., Jr., Rhoton, A. L., Jr., and Okazaki, H.: Intracranial dural arteriovenous malformations, Radiology 105:55, 1972.

Houser, O. W., Baker, H. L., Jr., Svien, H. J., and Okazaki, H.: Arteriovenous malformations of the parenchyma of the brain; angiographic aspects, Radiology 109:83, 1973.

Hsia, D. Y.: Idiopathic hyperlipemia; inborn errors of metabolism, Chicago, 1959, Year Book Publishers, Inc.

Huckman, M. S., and Davis, D. O.: Intracerebral hemorrhage. In Newton, T. H., and Potts, D. G., editors: Radiology of the skull and brain. Vol. 2, book 4, Angiography, St. Louis, 1974, The C. V. Mosby Co.

Humphrey, J. G., and Newton, T. H.: Internal carotid occlusion in young adults, Brain 83:565, 1960.

Iosue, A., Kier, E. L., and Ostrow, D.: Fibromuscular dysplasia involving the intracranial vessels; case report, J. Neurosurg. 37:749, 1972.

Isler, W.: Acute hemiplegias and hemisyndromes in childhood, Clin. Dev. Med., no. 41, 42, 1971.

Iwanowski, L., and Olszewski, J.: The effects of subarachnoid injections of iron-containing substances on the central nervous system, J. Neuropathol. Exp. Neurol. 19:433, 1960.

Jacob, J. C., Maroun, F. B., Heneghan, W. D., and House, A. M.: Uncommon cerebrovascular lesions in children, Dev. Med. Child Neurol. 12:446, 1970.

Johnson, D. R., and Chalgren, W. S.: Polycythemia vera and the nervous system, Neurology 1:53, 1951.

Joynt, R. J., Zimmerman, G., and Khalifeh, R.: Cerebral emboli from cardiac tumors, Arch. Neurol. 12:84, 1965.

Kalbag, R. M., and Woolf, A. L.: Cerebral venous thrombosis, London, 1967, Oxford University Press.

Kaplan, H. A., Aronson, S. M., and Browder, E. J.: Vascular malformations of the brain; an anatomical study, J. Neurosurg. 18:630, 1961.

Kerr, C. B.: Intracranial haemorrhage in haemophilia, J. Neurol. Neurosurg. Psychiatry 27:166, 1964.

Krayenbühl, H., and Siebenmann, R.: Small vascular malformations as a cause of primary intracerebral hemorrhage, J. Neurosurg. 22:7, 1964.

Krayenbühl, H. A., and Yaşargil, M. G.: Cerebral angiography, London, 1968, Butterworth & Co. (Publishers), Ltd.

Kricheff, I. I., Madayag, M., and Braunstein, P.: Transfemoral catheter embolization of cerebral and posterior fossa arteriovenous malformations, Radiology 103:107, 1972.

Kudo, T.: Juvenile occlusion of the circle of Willis, Clin. Neurol. 5:607, 1965.

Laitinen, L.: Arteriella aneurysm med subarachnoidallblödning hos barn, Nord. Med. 71:329, 1964.

Leeds, N. E., and Rosenblatt, R.: Arterial wall irregularities in intracranial neoplasms. The shaggy vessel brought into focus, Radiology 103:121, 1972.

Lessell, S., Ferris, E. J., Feldman, R. G., and Hoyt, W. F.: Brain stem arteriovenous malformations, Arch. Ophthalmol. 86:225, 1971.

Lindblom, K.: Roentgenographic study of vascular channels of the skull, with special reference to intracranial tumors and arteriovenous aneurysms, Acta Radiol., supp. 30, p. 1, 1936.

Litvak, J., Yahr, M. D., and Ransohoff, J.: Aneurysms of the great vein of Galen and midline cerebral arteriovenous anomalies, J. Neurosurg. 17:945, 1960.

Locksley, H. B.: Report on the cooperative study of intracranial aneurysms and subarachnoid hemorrhage. Sect. V, I. Natural history of subarachnoid hemorrhage, intracranial aneurysms, and arteriovenous malformations, J. Neurosurg. 25:219, 1966.

Locksley, H. B., Sahs, A. L., and Sandler, R.: Report on the cooperative study of intracranial aneurysms and subarachnoid hemorrhage. Sect. III. Subarachnoid hemorrhage unrelated to intracranial aneurysm and A-V malformation, J. Neurosurg. 24:1034, 1966.

Luessenhop, A. J., Kachmann, R., Jr., Shevlin, W., and Ferrero, A. A.: Clinical evaluation of artificial embolization in the management of large cerebral arteriovenous malformations, J. Neurosurg. 23:400, 1965.

Madonick, M. J., and Savitsky, N.: Subarachnoid hemorrhage in melanoma of the brain, Arch. Neurol. Psychiatry 65:628, 1951.

Margolis, M. T., and Newton, T. H.: Collateral pathways between the cavernous portion of the internal carotid and external carotid arteries, Radiology 93:834, 1969.

Margolis, M. T., Newton, T. H., and Hoyt, W. F.: Cortical branches of the posterior cerebral artery, Anatomic-radiologic correlation, Neuroradiology 2:127, 1971.

Matson, D. D.: Intracranial arterial aneurysms in childhood, J. Neurosurg. 23:578, 1965.

Matson, D. D.: Neurosurgery of infancy and childhood, ed. 2, Springfield, Ill., 1969, Charles C Thomas, Publisher.

McCormick, W. F.: The pathology of vascular ("arteriovenous") malformations, J. Neurosurg. 24:807, 1966.

McCormick, W. F.: Vascular disorders of nervous tissue: anomalies, malformations, and aneurysms. In Bourne, G. H., editor: The structure and function of nervous tissue, vol. 3, New York, 1969, Academic Press, Inc.

McCormick, W. F., Hardman, J. M., and Boulter, T. R.: Vascular malformations ("angiomas") of the brain, with special reference to those occurring in the posterior fossa, J. Neurosurg. 28:241, 1968.

McCormick, W. F., and Nofzinger, J. D.: "Cryptic" vascular malformations of the central nervous system, J. Neurosurg. 24:865, 1966.

McDonald, C. A., and Korb, M.: Intracranial aneurysms, Arch. Neurol. Psychiatry 42:298, 1939.

McRae, D. L., and Valentino, V.: Pneumographic findings in angiomata of the brain, Acta Radiol. 50:18, 1958.

Menkes, J. H., Alter, M., Steigleder, G. K., Weakley, D. R., and Ho Sung, J.: A sex-linked recessive disorder with retardation of growth, peculiar hair, and focal cerebral and cerebellar degeneration, Pediatrics 29:764, 1962.

Mishkin, M. M., and Schreiber, M. N.: Collateral circulation. In Newton, T. H., and Potts, D. G., editors: Radiology of the skull and brain. Vol. 2, book 4, Angiography, St. Louis, 1974, The C. V. Mosby Co.

Moore, E. W., Thomas, L. B., Shaw, R. K., and Freireich, E. J.: The central nervous system in acute leukemia, Arch. Intern. Med. 105:451, 1960.

Morgan, W. L., and Bland, E. F.: Bacterial endocarditis in the antibiotic era with special reference to the later complications, Circulation 19:753, 1959.

Morley, T. P., and Barr, H. W. K.: Giant intracranial aneurysms: diagnosis, course, and management, Clin. Neurosurg. 16:73, 1969.

Murtagh, F., and Baird, R. M.: Circumscribed intraventricular hematoma in infants, J. Pediatr. 59:351, 1961.

Nassar, S. I., and Correll, J. W.: Subarachnoid hemorrhage due to spinal cord tumors, Neurology 18:87, 1968.

New, P. F. J.: True aneurysm of the middle meningeal artery, Clin. Radiol. 14:236, 1963.

New, P. F. J.: Myxomatous emboli in brain, N. Engl. J. Med. 282:396, 1970.

Newton, T. H., and Cronqvist, S.: Involvement of dural arteries in intracranial arteriovenous malformations, Radiology 93:1071, 1969.

Newton, T. H., and Troost, B. T.: Arteriovenous malformations and fistulae. In Newton, T. H., and Potts, D. G., editors: Radiology of the skull and brain. Vol. 2, book 4, Angiography, St. Louis, 1974, The C. V. Mosby Co.

Newton, T. H., Weidner, W., and Greitz, T.: Dural arteriovenous malformation in the posterior fossa, Radiology 90:27, 1968.

Nishimoto, A., and Sugiu, R.: Hemangiomatous malformation of bilateral internal carotid artery at the base of the brain;

preliminary report, Proc. Ann. Meet. Neuroradiol. Assoc. Jap. 5:2, 1964.

Nishimoto, A., Sugiu, R., and Mannami, T.: Hemangiomatous malformation of bilateral internal carotid artery at the base of the brain, Brain Nerve 17:750, 1965.

Nishimoto, A., and Takeuchi, S.: Abnormal cerebrovascular network related to the internal carotid arteries, J. Neurosurg. 29:255, 1968.

Nishimoto, A., and Takeuchi, S.: Moyamoya disease; abnormal cerebrovascular network in the cerebral basal region. In Vinken, P. J., and Bruyn, G. W., editors: Handbook of clinical neurology, vol. 12, New York, 1972, American Elsevier Publishing Co., Inc.

Norman, R. M., and Urich, H.: Dissecting aneurysm of the middle cerebral artery as a cause of infantile hemiplegia, J. Pathol. Bacteriol. 73:580, 1957.

O'Brien, M. S., and Schechter, M. M.: Arteriovenous malformations involving the galenic system, Am. J. Roentgenol. Radium Ther. Nucl. Med. 110:50, 1970.

Osler, W., 1889. In Box, M., 1961.

Ozonoff, M. B., and Burrows, E. H.: Intracranial calcification. In Newton, T. H., and Potts, D. G., editors: Radiology of the skull and brain. Vol. 1, book 2, The skull, St. Louis, 1971, The C. V. Mosby Co.

Padget, D. H.: The cranial venous system in man in reference to development, adult configuration, and relation to the arteries, Am. J. Anat. 98:307, 1956.

Palubinskas, A. J., Perloff, D., and Newton, T. H.: Fibromuscular hyperplasia; an arterial dysplasia of increasing clinical importance, Am. J. Roentgenol. Radium Ther. Nucl. Med. 98:907, 1966.

Patel, A. N., and Richardson, A. E.: Ruptured intracranial aneurysms in the first two decades of life; a study of 58 patients, J. Neurosurg. 35:571, 1971.

Paterson, J. H., and McKissock, W.: A clinical survey of intracranial angiomas with special reference to their mode of progression and surgical treatment; a report of 110 cases, Brain 79:233, 1956.

Perlstein, M. A., and Hood, P. N.: Etiology of postneonatally acquired cerebral palsy, J.A.M.A. 188:850, 1964.

Perret, G., and Nishioka, H.: Report on the cooperative study of intracranial aneurysms and subarachnoid hemorrhage. Sect. VI. Arteriovenous malformations, J. Neurosurg. 25:467, 1966.

Peterman, A. F., Hayles, A. B., Dockerty, M. B., and Love, J. G.: Encephalotrigeminal angiomatosis (Sturge-Weber disease), J.A.M.A. 167:2169, 1958.

Picard, L., Floquet, J., André, J. M., Montaut, J., and Salamon, G.: The Moyamoya syndrome; anatomico-pathological study, J. Neuroradiol. 1:113, 1974a.

Picard, L., Levesque, M., Crouzet, G., Simon, J., and André, J. M.: Neuroradiological aspects of some angiodysplasias. II. The "moyamoya" syndrome, J. Neuroradiol. 1:47, 1974b.

Pitner, S. E.: Carotid thrombosis due to intraoral trauma; an unusual complication of common childhood accident, N. Engl. J. Med. 274:764, 1966.

Poppen, J. L., and Avman, N.: Aneurysms of the great vein of Galen, J. Neurosurg. 17:238, 1960.

Poser, C. M., and Taveras, J. M.: Cerebral angiography in encephalo-trigeminal angiomatosis, Radiology 68:327, 1957.

Potter, E. L.: Pathology of the fetus and infant, ed. 2, Chicago, 1961, Year Book Medical Publishers, Inc.

Pouyanne, H., Arné, L., Loiseau, P., and Mouton, L.: Considérations sur deux cas de thrombose de la carotide interne chez l'enfant, Rev. Neurol. 97:525, 1957.

Presley, G. D., Stinson, I. N., and Sidbury, J. B.: Homocystinuria, Am. J. Ophthalmol. 66:884, 1968.

Pribram, H. F. W., Hudson, J. D., and Joynt, R. J.: Posterior fossa aneurysms presenting as mass lesions, Am. J. Roentgenol. Radium Ther. Nucl. Med. 105:334, 1969.

Raimondi, A. J.: Personal communication, 1975.

Ring, B. A., and Waddington, M. M.: The neglected cause of stroke: intracranial occlusion of the small arteries, Radiology 88:924, 1967.

Rodda, R. A., and Calvert, G. D.: Post-mortem arteriography of cerebral arteriovenous malformations, J. Neurol. Neurosurg. Psychiatry 32:432, 1969.

Rubinstein, M. K., and Cohen, N. H.: Ehlers-Danlos syndrome associated with multiple intracranial aneurysms, Neurology 14:125, 1964.

Rumbaugh, C. L., Bergeron, R. T., Fang, H. C. H., and McCormick, R.: Cerebral angiographic changes in the drug abuse patient, Radiology 101:335, 1971.

Rumbaugh, C. L., and Potts, D. G.: Skull changes associated with intracranial arterio-venous malformations, Am. J. Roentgenol. Radium Ther. Nucl. Med. 98:525, 1966.

Runnels, J. B., Gifford, D. B., Forsberg, P. L., and Hanbery, J. W.: Dense calcification in a large cavernous angioma; case report, J. Neurosurg. 30:293, 1969.

Russell, D. S.: The pathology of spontaneous intracranial haemorrhage, Proc. R. Soc. Med. 47:689, 1954.

Sahs, A. L.: Intracranial aneurysms and subarachnoid bleeding—a co-operative study, Philadelphia, 1969, J. B. Lippincott Co.

Sarkari, N. B., Holmes, J. M., and Bickerstaff, E. R.: Neurological manifestations associated with internal carotid loops and kinks in children, J. Neurol. Neurosurg. Psychiatry 33:194, 1970.

Schwartz, M. J., and Baronofsky, I. D.: Ruptured intracranial aneurysm associated with coarctation of the aorta, Am. J. Cardiol. 6:982, 1960.

Scott, B. B., Seeger, J. F., and Schneider, R. C.: Successful evacuation of a pontine hematoma secondary to rupture of a pathologically diagnosed "cryptic" vascular malformation; case report, J. Neurosurg. 39:104, 1973.

Sharpe, W., and Maclaire, A. S.: Intracranial hemorrhage in the newborn, Am. J. Obstet. Gynecol. 9:452, 1925a.

Sharpe, W., and Maclaire, A. S.: Further observations of intracranial haemorrhage in the newborn, Surg. Gynecol. Obstet. 41:583, 1925b.

Shillito, J., Jr.: Carotid arteritis: a cause of hemiplegia in childhood, J. Neurosurg. 21:540, 1964.

Shucart, W. A., and Wolpert, S. A.: An aneurysm in infancy presenting with diabetes insipidus; case report, J. Neurosurg. 37:368, 1973.

Simpson, D. A., and Robson, H. N.: Intracranial haemorrhage in disorders of blood coagulation, Aust. N.Z. J. Surg. 29:287, 1960.

Smith, R. R., Kees, C. J., and Hogg, I. D.: Agenesis of the internal carotid artery with an unusual primitive collateral, J. Neurosurg. 37:460, 1972.

Starrs, R. A.: Subacute bacterial endocarditis presenting as subarachnoid haemorrhage (report of a case with recovery), Ann. Intern. Med. 31:139, 1949.

Stehbens, W. E.: Pathology of the cerebral blood vessels, St. Louis, 1972, The C. V. Mosby Co.

Stockman, J. A., Nigro, M. A., Mishkin, M. M., and Oski, F. A.: Occlusion of large cerebral vessels in sickle-cell anemia, N. Engl. J. Med. 287:846, 1972.

Sullivan, H. G., Vines, F. S., and Becker, D. P.: Sequelae of indirect internal carotid injury, Radiology 109:91, 1973.

Suwanwela, C., Suwanwela, N., Charuchinda, S., and Hongsaprabhas, C.: Intracranial mycotic aneurysms of extravascular origin, J. Neurosurg. 36:552, 1972.

Suzuki, J., and Takaku, A.: Cerebrovascular "moyamoya" disease; disease showing abnormal net-like vessels in the base of the brain, Arch. Neurol. 20:288, 1969.

Szancer, S.: Acute cerebral venous occlusion manifested by spontaneous subarachnoid hemorrhage, Neurology 5:675, 1955.

Takeuchi, K.: Occlusive disease of the carotid artery, Recent Adv. Res. Nerv. Syst. (Tokyo) 5:511, 1961.

Taveras, J. M.: Multiple progressive intracranial arterial occlusions; a syndrome of children and young adults, Caldwell lecture, 1968, Am. J. Roentgenol. Radium Ther. Nucl. Med. 106:235, 1969.

Taveras, J. M., Gilson, J. M., Davis, D. O., Kilgore, B., and Rumbaugh, C. L.: Angiography in cerebral infarction, Radiology 93:549, 1969.

Teabeaut, J. R.: Subdural hematoma of non-traumatic origin, N. Engl. J. Med. 245:272, 1951.

Thompson, J. R., Harwood-Nash, D. C., and Fitz, C. R.: Cerebral aneurysms in children, Am. J. Roentgenol. Radium Ther. Nucl. Med. 118:163, 1973.

Thompson, R. A., and Pribram, H. F. W.: Infantile cerebral aneurysm associated with ophthalmoplegia and quadriparesis, Neurology 19:785, 1969.

Tyler, H. R., and Clark, D. B.: Cerebrovascular accidents in patients with congenital heart disease, Arch. Neurol. Psychiatry 77:483, 1957.

Vapalahti, P. M., Schugk, P., Tarkkanen, L., and af Björkesten, G.: Intracranial arterial aneurysm in a three-month-old infant; case report, J. Neurosurg. 30:169, 1969.

Walton, J. N.: Subarachnoid haemorrhage, Edinburgh, 1956, E. & S. Livingstone, Ltd.

Weidner, W., Crandall, P., Hanafee, W., and Tomiyasu, U.: Collateral circulation in the posterior fossa via leptomeningeal anastomoses, Am. J. Roentgenol. Radium Ther. Nucl. Med. 95:831, 1965.

Weir, B. K. A., Allen, P. B. R., Miller, J. D. R.: Excision of thrombosed vein of Galen aneurysm in an infant, J. Neurosurg. 29:619, 1968.

Wesenberg, R. L., Gwinn, J. L., and Barnes, G. R., Jr.: Radiological findings in the kinky-hair syndrome, Radiology 92:500, 1969.

Wilson, C. B.: Aneurysms of the superficial temporal artery, Am. J. Roentgenol. Radium Ther. Nucl. Med. 105:331, 1969.

Wilson, C. B., and Roy, M.: Calcification within congenital aneurysms of the vein of Galen, Am. J. Roentgenol. Radium Ther. Nucl. Med. 91:1319, 1964.

Wisoff, H. S., and Rothballer, A. B.: Cerebral arterial thrombosis in children, Arch. Neurol. 4:258, 1961.

Wolman, L.: Cerebral dissecting aneurysms, Brain 82:276, 1959.

Wolpert, S. M.: The trigeminal artery and associated aneurysms, Neurology 16:610, 1966.

Wyburn-Mason, R.: Arteriovenous aneurysm of the mid-brain and retina, facial naevi, and mental changes, Brain 66:163, 1943.

CHAPTER 15

Intracranial cysts

Benign or congenital cysts of the brain were considered by Robinson (1971) to be "obscured by two things: one of imprecise pathological description, and the other of terminological inexactitude." The task of the neuroradiologist is to establish that such cysts are not neoplastic, contain fluid of some sort, and reveal a mass effect. We shall thus attempt to provide an objective neuroradiological approach to the geography and character of these cysts in children.

> *CSF-containing cysts*
>   Encysted ventricle
>   Porencephalic cyst
>   Arachnoid cyst
> *Non–CSF-containing cysts*
>   Neoplastic cyst
>   Inflammatory cyst (purulent or parasitic)
>   Colloid, ependymal, and other cysts

We define an intracranial cyst as a well-circumscribed fluid-containing cavity that exhibits a mass effect and displaces normal structures. A cyst need not be a closed cavity per se but may communicate with and enlarge via pressure or pulsatile force from a hydrocephalic ventricle or the subarachnoid space respectively. The fact that a cyst exhibits a mass effect implies dynamic expansile growth. A large freely communicating CSF cistern is not a cyst and does not displace intracranial structures. A blood-containing cavity, a hematoma, is not considered to be a cyst. By common usage, postinflammatory or posttraumatic subdural nonhemorrhagic fluid collections are also not called cysts.

Cysts may contain CSF (e.g., an arachnoid or a porencephalic cyst) or a viscous high-protein fluid as exists in a craniopharyngioma or a cystic astrocytoma. A cyst can contain pus (e.g., a chronic abscess) or parasitic fluid and detritus (e.g., a hydatid cyst). Small fluid-containing cysts can be part of a larger neoplasm (e.g., teratoma or dermoid), or a large neoplastic cyst may contain a small solid neoplastic nidus (as occurs in many cystic astrocytomas).

Cysts may be formed within the CSF pathway by occlusion of the portals of a subarachnoid cistern or by isolation of part over the cerebral convexities. An encysted ventricle, or indeed the ventricular system as a whole, is a dynamic CSF-containing mass—dynamic because of CSF production by its choroid plexuses—and, due to a valvelike orifice which permits only ingress of CSF (in a pulsatile fashion), an encysted part of the subarachnoid space also assumes a dynamic mass effect.

Cysts form a significant portion of intracranial mass lesions in children. The largest intracranial mass lesions that occur are cysts. Decompression or removal may offer the neurosurgical promise of a complete cure. Only by computed tomography, however, can neuroradiologists establish with certainty whether indeed a mass is a fluid-containing cyst and, if so, what the probable character of its contained fluid is.

The neuroradiological investigation of an intracranial cyst, primarily the same as for any intracranial mass, is to establish the geography and character of the cyst. Some cysts, however, communicate freely with the CSF pathway in a uni- or bidirectional fashion; and such communications will be identified by radionuclide studies, pneumoencephalography, or ventriculography. The precise pathogenesis and often the true pathology of many CSF-containing cysts may not be conclusively determinable, and usually by inference alone will the neuroradiologist then provide the probable histological type of a cyst as well as establish its geography.

Notwithstanding these inadequacies, it behooves the neuroradiologist to be aware of the nuances of each type of intracranial cyst; for such an awareness will often greatly assist the further actions of the consulting neurosurgeon.

CEREBROSPINAL FLUID–CONTAINING CYSTS
Encysted ventricle

Encystment of a ventricle by occlusion of its CSF outlet, as occurs to the lateral ventricle and the fora-

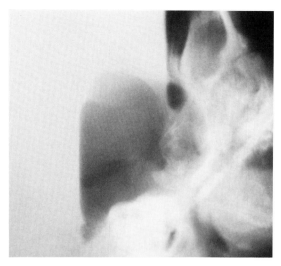

Fig. 15-1. Coarctation of a temporal horn. This was subsequent to a meningitis and ventriculitis. The other normal temporal horn can be faintly seen. There is air in the frontal subdural space.

men of Monro respectively, is not rare and is usually due to adhesions after intraventricular infection or hemorrhage or to the pressure effect of an extrinsic mass lesion; however, atresia or congenital occlusion of the foramen of Monro is quite rare (Blatt and Berkmen, 1969). An asymmetrical intracranial mass lesion due to the dilated ventricle will result. This enlargement of a ventricle constitutes intraventricular hydrocephalus, for the total volume of the ventricular system is increased.

Coarctation of the temporal horn by adhesions (Fig. 15-1), by extrinsic compression, or rarely by congenital transventricular cerebral tissue bands or *atresia* of the body of the lateral ventricle (Cloward, 1969) creates an intrinsic temporal mass due to dilatation of the cystic temporal horn—whose choroid plexus continues to produce CSF. Coarctation of the body of the ventricle is rare.

Encystment of the lateral ventricle as a whole is more common (Fig. 15-2, *A*) and results from occlusion of the foramen of Monro by intrinsic ventricular adhesions, a subependymal mass such as tuberous sclerosis, or an extrinsic mass such as craniopharyngioma. If the encystment is chronic, particularly in the

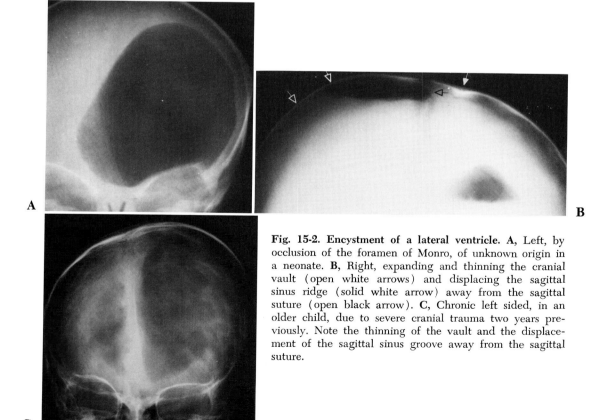

Fig. 15-2. Encystment of a lateral ventricle. A, Left, by occlusion of the foramen of Monro, of unknown origin in a neonate. **B,** Right, expanding and thinning the cranial vault (open white arrows) and displacing the sagittal sinus ridge (solid white arrow) away from the sagittal suture (open black arrow). **C,** Chronic left sided, in an older child, due to severe cranial trauma two years previously. Note the thinning of the vault and the displacement of the sagittal sinus groove away from the sagittal suture.

first few years of life, expansion of the ipsilateral skull vault will occur. The bone will thin, and the sagittal sinus will be displaced away from the midline (Fig. 15-2, *B* and *C*), particularly if the encystment occurs in utero or in early infancy (Nixon and Ravin, 1974).

Computed tomography will demonstrate a CSF-containing mass; carotid angiography will reveal an intrinsic temporal lobe mass with elevation of the proximal middle cerebral artery and sylvian branches and stretching of the temporal arteries over and around the mass. There will be straightening and some upward displacement of the supraclinoid internal carotid artery and medial displacement of the anterior choroidal and posterior communicating arteries and basal vein of Rosenthal. Contralateral displacement of the internal cerebral vein occurs to a lesser extent. In an enlargement of the temporal horn alone, the anterior cerebral artery is usually not displaced from midline. On an AP angiogram a dilated lateral ventricle will produce slight or massive displacement of the internal cerebral vein and the anterior cerebral artery away from the midline, the ventricle often herniating beneath the falcine edge and flattening the anterior cerebral artery. As in any hydrocephalic ventricle, the middle cerebral branches are displaced laterally and stretched. Depression of the anterior choroidal and posterior communicating arteries on the same side occurs.

Ventriculography by puncture of the encysted ventricle (Figs. 15-1 and 15-2) will graphically demonstrate ventricular enlargement and failure of air to pass out the foramen of Monro. Subsequent needling of the other ventricles may be difficult and is not usually indicated if massive infrafalcine herniation is present. Unilateral dilatation of the lateral ventricle without dynamic mass effect is due to cerebral atrophy and is not a cyst.

Inordinate enlargement of the third or fourth ventricle can occur with intraventricular obstructive hydrocephalus (Fig. 6-2) and will present a formidable cystic mass. At angiography, the uninformed neuroradiologist may misdiagnose such enlargement and accompanying herniations as the cause rather than the effect of hydrocephalus. Massive dilatation of the suprapineal recess (Fig. 6-2) (Lavender and du Boulay, 1965) and herniation of the third ventricle into the infratentorial compartment or retroclivally will also provide spectacular angiographic displacements—the result, not the cause, of the aqueductal stenosis. Computed tomography will identify these mass effects as CSF-containing cavities, and ventriculography will conclusively establish their true configuration and character. Similarly, occlusion of the orifice of the fourth ventricle by adhesions (particularly in infants) will result in an unusually en-

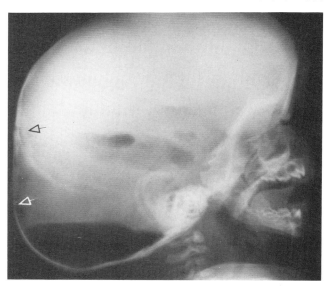

Fig. 15-3. **Dandy-Walker cyst.** A ventriculogram reveals marked dilatation of the fourth ventricle within a grossly expanded vault of the posterior fossa. Note the classical torcular displacement (black arrow) above the lambda (white arrow). This inversion is not seen in acquired cysts of the posterior fossa.

larged fourth ventricle, the enlargement being out of proportion to that of the third and lateral ventricles (Fig. 6-2). Angiography alone will demonstrate a large central mass, in reality the fourth ventricle, and the unwary diagnostician may infer it to be a cause rather than an effect of hydrocephalus.

Congenital occlusion of the fourth ventricular outlet (Chapter 16), the Dandy-Walker cyst, is a massive dilatation of the ventricle that expands the posterior fossa (Fig. 15-3). The acquired occlusions of the foramen of Magendie never produce such massive fourth ventricular dilatation. A variant of the Dandy-Walker syndrome is present in dysgenesis of the inferior vermis; a large midline inferior fourth ventricular diverticulum is formed as a developmental abnormality—herniation of an expanded inferior medullary velum (D'Agostino et al., 1963). Computed tomography will reveal the Dandy-Walker cyst as a CSF-containing pouch, and no normal fourth ventricle will be visualized. Ventriculography will depict a short aqueduct entering the CSF-containing cyst. Ventriculography best demonstrates the Dandy-Walker variants (Chapter 16). The angiographic appearance of the posterior inferior cerebellar artery, superior cerebellar artery, hemispheric branches, and draining veins betrays a large central posterior fossa mass.

In severe long-standing intraventricular obstructive hydrocephalus the ventricular ependymal wall can rupture and produce a false diverticulum of the

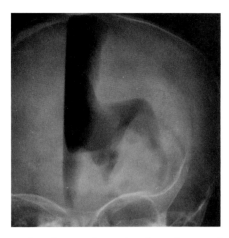

Fig. 15-4. False diverticulum of a lateral ventricle. Chronic hydrocephalus caused a false diverticulum of the medial wall into the interhemispheric sulcus.

ventricle extending through white matter and often rupturing into the subarachnoid space (Russell, 1949). This usually occurs at the medial wall of the trigone or occipital horn and creates a large cerebral "cyst" (Fig. 15-4). The ventricular diverticulum that occurs with hydrocephalus may not communicate with the subarachnoid space but may dissect the white matter in a tonguelike fashion adjacent to the ventricles (Northfield and Russell, 1939; Granholm and Rådberg, 1965). It is difficult to differentiate these diverticula, which in our experience are rare, from deeply placed porencephalic cysts; and the differentiation may be just a matter of semantics. In our opinion, air ventriculography is the only investigation to clearly define the abnormality.

In the absence of hydrocephalus, a large spheroid cyst of the cavum vergae or septum pellucidum is rare (Hughes et al., 1955; Zülch, 1965). When it occurs with hydrocephalus (Heiskanen, 1973), we believe the hydrocephalus enlarges the cyst; therefore

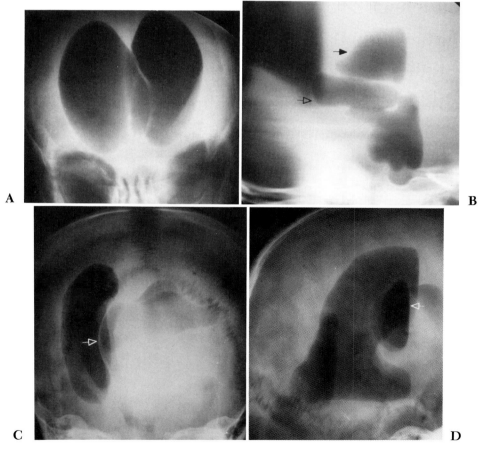

Fig. 15-5. Encysted cavum. A, Cystic dilatation of the cavum septi pellucidi caused by hydrocephalus in an infant. B, A sagittal tomogram of an infant with hydrocephalus due to aqueductal stenosis shows an enlarged suprapineal recess (open arrow) and a cystic cavum vergae (solid arrow). C and D, Hydrocephalus and a large cystic cavum vergae (arrows).

it may be considered to be just an extension of the hydrocephalic ventricles into another potential space (Fig. 15-5). Hydrocephalus with inordinate enlargement of the cyst due to a probable one-way valve effect may potentiate hydrocephalic enlargement of a lateral ventricle by compression of the foramen of Monro.

Porencephalic cyst

The discussion of porencephalic cysts will be confined to cysts that produce significant mass lesions within the brain. From the neuroradiological point of view, a porencephalic cyst is a CSF-containing nonneoplastic cavity or multiple cavities (polyporencephaly) of the brain large enough to create a mass effect and associated with hydrocephalus. It communicates or may have communicated with a ventricle but rarely will communicate with the subarachnoid space. It is not lined by true ependyma, and it contains no choroid plexus. It is not a dynamic space-occupying lesion in the absence of significant hydrocephalus; furthermore, even at operation, it is often difficult to differentiate from an arachnoid cyst as occurs within the sylvian fissure. Diffuse cystic disease of the white matter in infancy (Stevenson and McGowan, 1942; Wolf and Cowen, 1955; Armstrong and Norman, 1974) not communicating with the ventricles and not acting like a significant mass lesion is excluded from this neuroradiological consideration of porencephaly.

The pathological viewpoint contains many intricate and often conflicting impressions. Wolf and Cowen (1955), Naef (1958), and Norman (1963) provide extensive summaries of the theories of the formation of porencephalic cysts, large and small. Heschl (1859) originally stated that a porencephalic defect was the result of cerebral disease in fetal development; however, he later suggested that it was a cerebral process due to an occlusive vascular abnormality.

Yakovlev and Wadsworth (1946) subdivided porencephaly into two simple groups.

One group was termed *schizencephaly*. In these cysts, failure of development of the cerebral mantle in early fetal life leads to symmetrical cerebral clefts involving the whole depth of the cerebrum and usually situated in the zone of cleavage of the primary cerebral fissures. The commonest site is in the region of the sylvian fissure, extending into the parietal and frontal lobes. The cysts are lined by primitive gyri. If hydrocephalus supervenes, ventriculography will outline the large cystlike cavities. Because their chance of survival is poor, infants with these cysts are rarely referred for neuroradiological investigation.

The second group, far more commonly seen at neuroradiology, was termed *encephaloclastic poren-*

cephaly. These cysts are circumscribed defects resulting from destruction of cerebral tissue by cerebral vascular occlusions, primarily intracranial inflammatory processes or trauma leading to areas of direct cerebral damage. They may also be associated with generalized infantile circulatory disturbance and anoxia. Due to anoxia, cerebral vascular occlusion, or direct cerebral damage, apparently the birth process plays a dominant role in the cause of porencephaly. Benda (1945) described porencephaly in clinical and pathological studies as being often a direct sequela of cerebral birth injuries. The immature unmyelinated cerebrum probably allows much greater and more rapid dissolution after a necrotizing lesion of the brain due to any cause than is permitted in older children or adults (Norman et al., 1958; Courville, 1959; Allen, 1964). If this necrotic area then communicates with the ventricular system and if the ventricles are hydrocephalic, a dynamic cystic cavity and a mass effect may result. The cerebellum and brain stem are rarely involved by such processes.

Courville (1959) discussed cerebral damage to the fetus and infant occurring in one of three periods:

In the *antenatal* period, anoxia acts via the maternal circulation (toxemia, anemia, poisons), through the placenta (infections, premature separation), or by interfering with the circulation of the umbilical cord.

Anoxia in the *paranatal* period may be due to maternal hemorrhage, abruptio placentae, cord abnormalities, newborn respiratory difficulties, intracranial hemorrhage or edema, or vascular thromboses.

The early *postnatal* period features vascular occlusions and intracranial hemorrhage and edema, including respiratory anoxia. Cocker and co-workers (1965) described postnatal middle cerebral arterial occlusions due to emboli probably arising in the fetal veins of the placenta. Marburg and Casamajor (1944) described intracranial venous and sinus thromboses due to the birth process leading to porencephaly. Norman and co-workers (1958) provided pathological evidence of arterial occlusive disease leading to porencephaly and were later supported by Myers (1969), who investigated porencephaly after fetal cerebral vascular occlusion.

Our angiographic studies of infants and young children with porencephaly provide objective in vivo evidence of the vascular occlusive pathogenesis of porencephaly (Fig. 15-6). The cause of many such occlusions, whether in the antenatal, natal, or postnatal period, still remains conjectural.

In our experience, many infants had difficult deliveries with possible cerebral anoxia as a consequence. Some had neonatal meningitis, often associated with cortical venous or sinus thromboses, and

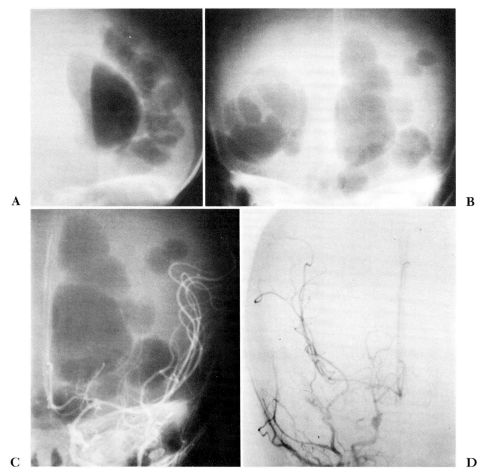

Fig. 15-6. Angiography and porencephaly. A and **B,** Hydrocephalus and multiple porencephalic cysts in the frontal lobes of an infant with severe postpartum anoxia. **C** and **D,** Bilateral carotid angiograms demonstrate no peripheral branches arising from the anterior cerebral arteries. The right middle cerebral artery is displaced inwardly by a porencephalic cyst that bulges through the sylvian triangle and presents as an extracerebral mass (**D**). All intracranial vessels are of small caliber.

others had significant postnatal head injuries. As a rule, the cysts are identified during the course of the investigation for hydrocephalus. Large areas of cortical brain atrophy can be detected in birth-damaged children without hydrocephalus. These are not dynamic cysts but superficial dilated subarachnoid spaces or dilated ventricles due to brain atrophy.

Posttraumatic intracerebral hemorrhage or cerebral infarction at any age may communicate with the ventricular system and together with hydrocephalus enlarge the ventricles (Cantu and LeMay, 1967). Porencephalic cysts are often associated with that part of the brain underlying a growing skull fracture through which protrudes a cyst of the leptomeninges (Chapter 12). The porencephalic cyst must not be confused with the cyst of the leptomeninges.

Transcerebral needle ventricular tapping will lead to dilatation of the needle tract to form a poren-

cephalic cyst, the so-called "puncture porencephaly," *only* if the ventricular cerebrospinal fluid pressure is high (Fig. 15-7). Lorber and Grainger (1963) and Lorber and Emery (1964) first described in detail the pathological and radiological characteristics of small cysts occurring after single punctures for ventriculography or multiple punctures for intraventricular antibiotic instillations. In our experience, only six infants have developed such cavities after more than 1,000 ventriculograms; and in each patient the hydrocephalus could not be shunted after the ventriculogram due to clinical contraindications. If the hydrocephalus is adequately shunted within 24 to 48 hours, these porencephalic cysts do not develop after ventricular puncture for ventriculography. Failure to shunt adequately will, unfortunately, inevitably result in a high incidence of puncture porencephaly.

Hydranencephaly is probably the ultimate form

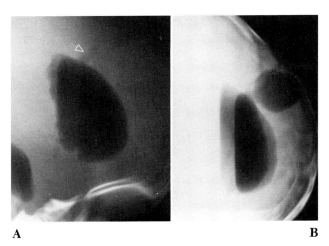

A   B

Fig. 15-7. Puncture porencephaly. A ventricular tap in the diagnosis of hydrocephalus shows air passing up into the needle track (**A,** arrow). Due to clinical circumstances, no shunt was performed and a large frontal porencephalic cyst (**B**) formed at the site of the initial ventricular tap.

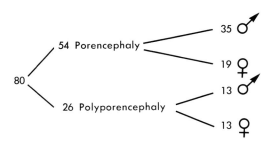

Fig. 15-8. Sex and porencephaly.

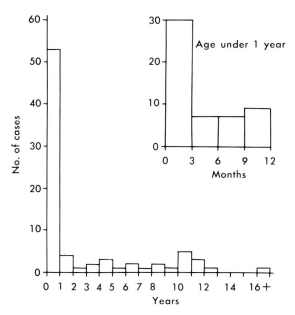

Fig. 15-9. Age and porencephaly.

of bilateral porencephaly. The cerebral hemispheres are converted into translucent thin-walled chambers lined by leptomeninges and a shell of gliosed tissue (Norman, 1963). There is no ependymal lining. The thalami may be preserved, the choroid plexus continues to function, and the cerebellum is usually normal. Prenatal bilateral internal carotid occlusions occur, probably due to intrauterine cerebral infection (Hamby et al., 1950; Halsey and Chamberlin, 1971). Intrauterine vascular thrombosis is suggested as a cause by Myers (1969), who occluded both internal carotid arteries in fetal monkeys and thereby produced hydranencephaly in the newborn monkeys. Lindenberg and Swanson (1967) suggested that postpartum cerebral edema from any cause, leading to anoxia, may compress the internal carotid arteries at their entrance into the subarachnoid space and result in infantile hydranencephaly due to massive nonlethal destruction of both cerebral hemispheres. We believe this should be referred to as massive cerebral atrophy, not hydranencephaly, for the middle cerebral and anterior cerebral arteries and branches are still visible at angiography.

Cytomegalic inclusion disease and toxoplasmosis may lead to massive cerebral destruction; but polyporencephaly (Mavin and Angerine, 1968), hydrocephalus, and/or cerebral atrophy rather than hydranencephaly result.

During a four-year period, we have identified one or more porencephalic cysts in eighty infants and children. Many other infants and children during the same period were found at autopsy to harbor porencephalic cysts; the latter children were not investigated neuroradiologically at the time the porencephalic cysts developed. We did not include in this series six infants in whom we found hydranencephaly, the extreme form of porencephaly. We shall describe them separately.

Characteristics

Age and sex. The male more than the female bears the brunt of this abnormality, forty-eight (60%) to thirty-two (40%) (Fig. 15-8). Approximately three quarters of the infants under 1 year of age were males. Porencephaly is common in infancy. Fifty-three patients (66%) were less than 1 year of age (Fig. 15-9), and two thirds of these were very young (between 1 day and 3 months).

Cause. The specific causes of the porencephalic cysts were often difficult to define. Infantile intracranial infection, difficult delivery, and postnatal craniocerebral trauma were the main causes implicated.

Large porencephalic cysts were identified by neuroradiological methods in twelve infants during the first week of life; and in half of these, the hemicranium was enlarged and the falx and sagittal sinus were displaced to some degree from the sagittal suture—changes similar to those described for encysted ventricles (Fig. 15-2). We inferred that the cyst was present in the antenatal period.

The majority of the few cysts that developed in older children were related to craniocerebral trauma or were found serendipitously as we investigated a child with chronic hydrocephalus. Only six children had puncture porencephaly. Angiography demonstrated that cerebral arterial occlusions were directly related to the porencephalic cysts, suggesting that the final focal insult common to many causes is cerebral infarction (Fig. 15-6). All the children with

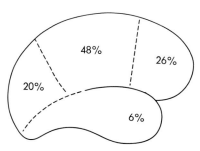

Fig. 15-10. Frequency of porencephalic involvement within the cerebral lobes.

porencephalic cysts either were currently or had previously been afflicted with a hydrocephalus of varying degree.

Site and character. The parietal lobe was commonly involved (48%) (Fig. 15-10), the frontal and occipital lobes less so (26% and 20%), and the temporal lobe rarely (6%). We have not identified a porencephalic cyst of the cerebellum or brain stem. The majority of cerebral porencephalic cysts were situated in the superficial gray matter and in the white matter, less commonly in the basal ganglia. Single cysts often involved part of more than one lobe and were usually smoothly cystic or lobulated, the lobules communicating with each other.

Polyporencephaly, a disease of infants in which multiple discrete cysts communicate with the ventricles, occurred in twenty-six (33%) of the children in the series. Twenty-two of these patients were under 1 year of age. Whereas single porencephalic cysts were commoner in boys, polyporencephaly occurred with equal frequency in both boys and girls. Of the fifty-three infants under 1 year of age, twenty-two had polyporencephaly. The polyporencephaly was unilateral in nineteen, bilateral in seven.

Agenesis of the corpus callosum and a large cerebral cyst or cysts communicating with the lateral ventricle occurred in nine children. The cyst was not a dilated third ventricle. Five children had large cysts

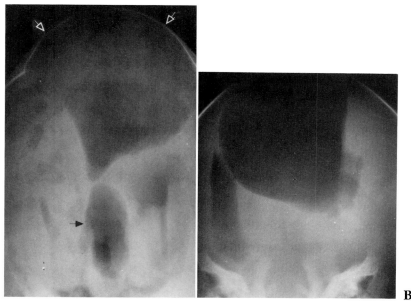

A   B

Fig. 15-11. Agenesis of the corpus callosum and porencephaly. A, A huge midline cyst caused ballooning of the vault (open arrows) and communicated with the left lateral ventricle in an infant with absent corpus callosum. Note the large interposed third ventricle (solid arrow). B, A huge posteriorly placed cyst communicates with the left lateral ventricle in a neonate. The corpus callosum is absent.

located in the medial aspect of the posterior parietal lobe (Fig. 15-11). These may have been ventricular diverticula, for they did not communicate with the subarachnoid space and there was no marked hydrocephalus. We have identified in the same area cysts that we think are arachnoid cysts that are also associated with an absent corpus callosum. This identification was made at surgery; the cysts impinged on the subarachnoid space, not the ventricular system, and were lined by arachnoid. Though at ventriculography or pneumoencephalography a porencephalic cyst might have seemed to be identical with an arachnoid cyst, in patients who underwent surgery

the former was found not to be lined by arachnoid. Zingesser and co-workers (1964) reported a case of what they called an interhemispheric arachnoid cyst and agenesis of the corpus callosum, and they reviewed the few previously reported cases; however, their case appears to have been more like a porencephalic cyst.

There were only four children in our series with an absent corpus callosum and a porencephalic cyst in the frontal and anterior parietal regions. One child had a single cyst and three had polyporencephaly; and all but one had cysts in the distribution of the anterior cerebral artery (Fig. 15-12). This anterior

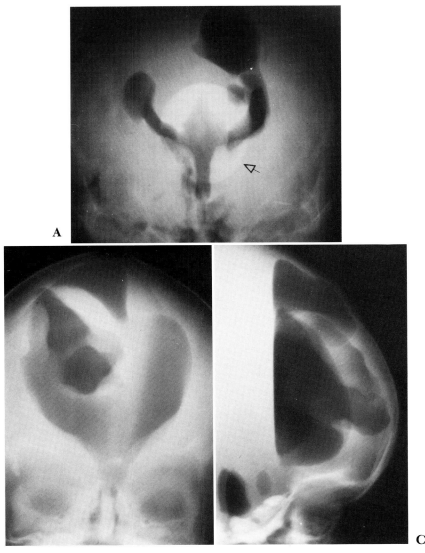

Fig. 15-12. Absent corpus callosum and porencephalic cysts. A, In the left lateral ventricle, with a posteriorly placed encephalocele (arrow). The cyst is in the territory fed by the anterior cerebral artery. **B** and **C,** With severe hydrocephalus. Again the cysts are within the distribution of the anterior cerebral artery. At autopsy the corpus callosum was seen to be destroyed. This complex probably has an acquired arterial ischemic basis.

cerebral artery pattern and our observed angiographic findings of anterior cerebral branch occlusions associated with the foregoing abnormalities lend credence to the theory that a fetal vascular abnormality of the anterior cerebral artery leads to destruction or atrophy of a partially or completely formed corpus callosum. Zingesser and co-workers (1964), however, point out that the anterior cerebral is not formed at the time of the development of the corpus callosum (at 12 weeks); and they therefore consider the theory of de Morsier (1954) that agenesis of the corpus callosum is due to developmental defective vascularity is not quite valid.

Neuroradiology

The neuroradiology of a porencephalic cyst is of an avascular mass in the cerebrum associated with some degree of hydrocephalus. The mass contains CSF, communicates freely with the ventricles, and displaces vessels. It is related to vascular occlusions.

Abnormalities of the skull are usually due to the underlying hydrocephalus, not to the cyst itself. If, however, the cyst is large (particularly in infants) or superficial and chronic (in older children), vault abnormalities do occur (Fig. 15-13). In infants a considerable area of the vault is markedly enlarged and thinned, commonly the parietal area, often creating a clinically obvious enlargement of the hemicranium. An encysted lateral ventricle may produce similar changes (Fig. 15-2, B and C). In older children a superficial chronic cyst will create local thinning and ballooning of the overlying vault. If the sagittal sinus groove is displaced from the sagittal suture, the cyst is presumed to have been present since infancy for such displacement is not possible after infancy. The falx, however, can be markedly angled away from

its base at the sagittal sinus. Large convexity arachnoid cysts and chronic unilateral subdural hygromas or hematomas or superficial low-grade cystic gliomas may create a similar appearance.

Computed tomography (Chapter 8) is now indispensable for the investigation of possible intracranial cysts. It provides specific localization of cysts situated apart from dilated ventricles and establishes their CSF content.

Air ventriculography is recommended to further define the site and possible obstruction within the ventricular system leading to the underlying hydrocephalus. It will also locate a possible porencephalic cyst (Fig. 15-14) or polyporencephaly (Fig. 15-15) and define whether some or all of the cysts connect with each other or with the ventricular system. A cyst may so enlarge as to further occlude the ventricular CSF pathways and increase the degree of hydrocephalus.

We have found that some polyporencephalic cysts do not freely fill with air at ventriculography, thereby appearing to be discrete solid mass lesions (Fig. 15-16). Large hydrocephalic ventricles containing many intraventricular septa and loculations due to previous ventriculitis (Chapter 13) or intraventricular hemorrhage can closely resemble multiple polyporencephalic cysts. Careful inspection will differentiate extraventricular cysts (outside the general outline of the ventricles) from intraventricular loculations.

Because surgery of porencephaly and polyporencephaly attempts to create an intercommunication of all cysts with each other and with the ventricular cavity, which is then shunted, the computed tomogram and the ventriculogram must be closely corre-

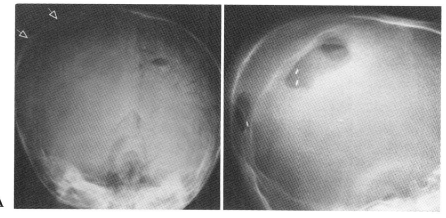

A **B**

Fig. 15-13. Skull deformities and a porencephalic cyst. A, Large right sided chronic, producing ballooning of the right cranial vault (arrows). This child had hydrocephalus and aqueductal stenosis. **B,** Lateral view after marsupialization of the cyst into the ventricle and shunting of the ventricle.

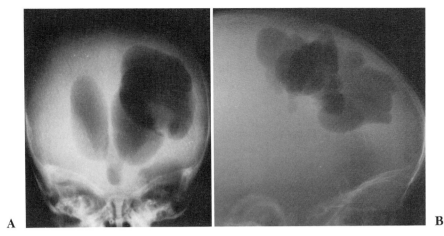

Fig. 15-14. Porencephalic cysts. A, Large left-sided single. **B,** Large frontoparietal, within the anterior cerebral artery distribution and containing many septa.

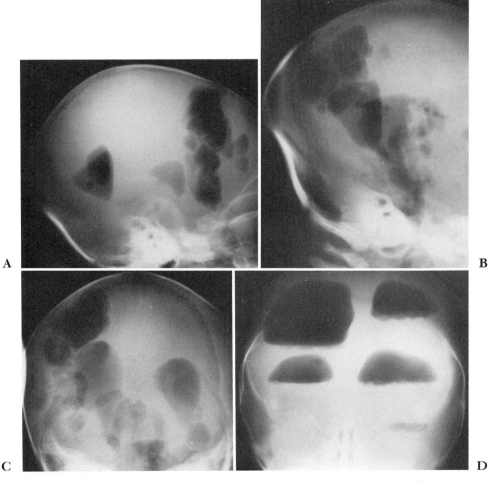

Fig. 15-15. Polyporencephalic cysts. A to **C,** Small and intercommunicating, filled with air. **D,** Huge bilateral supraventricular, concurrent with hydrocephalic dilated ventricles.

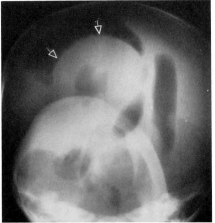

Fig. 15-16. **Ventriculography and noncommunicating porencephalic cysts. A,** In a child with a huge occipital encephalocele, polyporencephaly, and a large noncommunicating porencephalic cyst (arrows). **B,** An AP tomogram in another child shows a right-sided cyst, not filled with air, displacing the right ventricle (arrow) and indeed the entire ventricular system to the left. **C,** An angiogram in the same patient as in **B** reveals marked depression of the middle cerebral artery and an abnormal and stretched anterior cerebral artery (black arrow). Note the bulging of the vault (white arrows) due to the cyst.

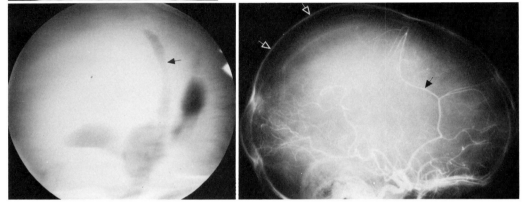

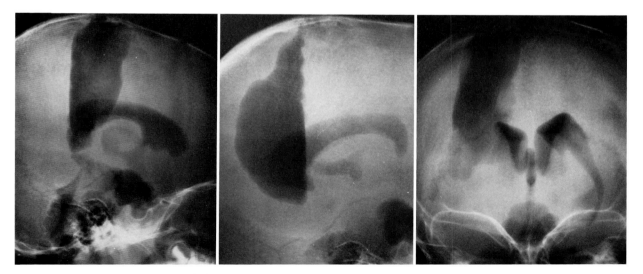

Fig. 15-17. **Porencephalic cyst and normal ventricles.** The cyst is mainly within the distal vascular supply of the right anterior cerebral artery and has filled via the ventricles (which are of normal size). A previous hydrocephalus of some degree is supposed, though its mass effect is now minimal.

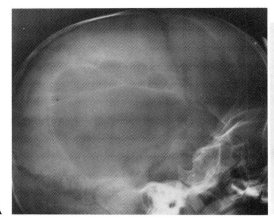 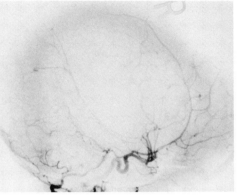

A   B

Fig. 15-18. Sylvian fissure porencephaly. A, This cyst filled with air during pneumoencephalography and contains a number of loculations. B, A carotid angiogram shows marked distortion of the middle cerebral artery with depression of the angular branch and stretching of the vessels over the cyst in the sylvian triangle. Such cysts closely resemble arachnoid cysts.

lated. An uncommon finding at ventriculography is a huge porencephalic cyst filled with air via relatively normal-sized ventricles (Fig. 15-17). We find it difficult to explain why this cavity should be so large yet have little mass effect. Unidirectional flow of CSF, creating a discrete expansile pulse effect, is supposed.

Pneumoencephalography of infants with suspect congenital cerebral malformations in the absence of hydrocephalus rarely will show large often bilateral air-filled cerebral defects in the sylvian fissure (Fig. 15-18). These may represent schizencephaly. If unilateral, an arachnoid cyst should be suspected.

Cerebral angiography will delineate the underlying hydrocephalus and the large space-occupying intracerebral cyst or cysts but will not demonstrate all the smaller cysts. The total angiographic picture may be quite bizarre in polyporencephaly.

The porencephalic cyst (or cysts) can displace superficial cerebral vessels around it, creating a relatively avascular area (Figs. 15-16, *C,* and 15-18, *B*). Though abnormal, some vessels will also be seen to course over the cyst and confirm its intracerebral location. On the lateral angiogram, care must be taken not to confuse the cortical vessels passing over a porencephalic cyst with the superficial vessels beneath an arachnoid cyst.

We have often identified some form of arterial occlusion or disordered venous drainage in the region of the cyst or cysts. These occlusions commonly involve the middle cerebral (Fig. 15-19) and anterior cerebral (Fig. 15-6) but rarely the posterior cerebral arteries. Cysts within the middle cerebral territory were identified in 55% of the children who had porencephalic cysts and were examined by angiog-

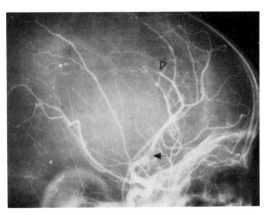

Fig. 15-19. Porencephalic cyst and cerebral arterial occlusions. The distal anterior cerebral artery (open arrow) and the frontoparietal and posterior parietal branches of the middle cerebral artery are occluded at their origins. The remaining branches are stretched over a large frontoparietal porencephalic cyst. Note the persisting thrombus in the proximal anterior cerebral artery (solid arrow).

raphy—the anterior cerebral being involved in 33%, the posterior cerebral in 12%. These occlusions develop either proximally in the main trunk or in branches. Intraluminal thrombi or the occlusions can occur distally in the fine arterial branches (Fig. 15-6). A single large branch may have polyporencephalic cysts directly related. The trunk will exhibit few or no smaller branches. Discrete thrombi may be identified (Fig. 15-19).

Thus it is often a moot point whether the arterial occlusion per se, together with hydrocephalus, produced the area of cerebral necrosis destined to become a porencephalic cyst or whether a cerebral in-

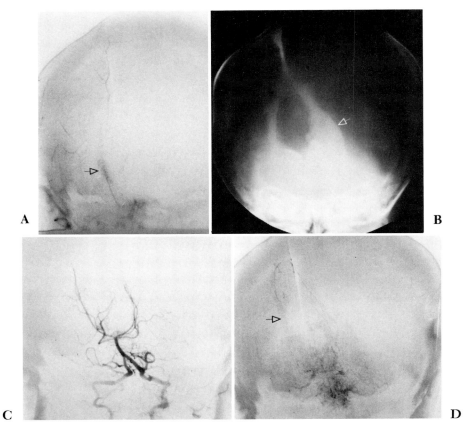

Fig. 15-20. **Hydranencephaly. A,** A right carotid angiogram shows no cortical vessels over the right hemisphere; however, some external carotid vessels are seen. Note the stretched anterior choroidal artery feeding the lateral choroid plexus (arrow). **B,** A ventriculogram demonstrates no cortical tissue other than some remnants of the inferior occipital lobe (arrow). **C** and **D,** A vertebral angiogram reveals the normal posterior fossa with abnormal posterior cerebral arteries feeding the remaining occipital lobes (**D,** arrow). Note the cerebellar blush in **D.**

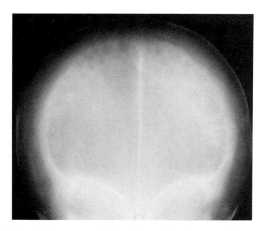

Fig. 15-21. **Hydranencephaly.** A ventriculogram demonstrates a single large air-filled space containing a midline "septum" due to the falx.

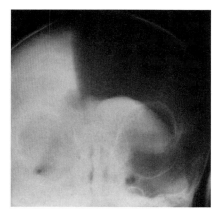

Fig. 15-22. **Subdural hygroma simulating hydranencephaly.** A huge left-sided air-filled hygroma compressed the left cerebral hemisphere. This must not be confused with hydranencephaly.

sult (e.g., infection, trauma) independently produced cerebral necrosis by direct cerebral destruction or by secondary action on cerebral vessels resulting in thrombosis. On the AP angiogram a superficial parietal ovoid porencephalic cyst may simulate a subdural hematoma and produce the characteristic lens-shaped surface deformity of a hematoma (Freeman and Gold, 1964; Ryvicker and Leeds, 1973).

Hydranencephaly is massive destruction of the cerebral hemispheres by prenatal bilateral internal carotid arterial occlusion. In our angiographic experience with six infants who had hydranencephaly, the supraclinoid internal carotid arteries were occluded distal to the anterior choroidal artery.

A small tangle of vessels may feed a nubbin of cerebrum in the inferior frontal region similar to that described by Poser and co-workers (1955); but more often a remnant of the occipital lobes will be fed via the posterior cerebral arteries from the basilar artery (Fig. 15-20). The choroid plexus is often preserved. The basilar artery is always normal. The falx may be intact, creating a spurious septum pellucidum or intraventricular septum as seen at ventriculography (Fig. 15-21). Massive dilatation of the ventricles is usually diagnosed initially and no cortical mantle is seen around the vault. No third ventricle, aqueduct, or fourth ventricle is identified; rather a rounded basal ganglionic impression into the air-filled spaces is seen. The head may or may not be enlarged and is rarely microcephalic.

Angiography is the only way to differentiate this huge CSF-filled structure from massive dilated hydrocephalic ventricles. Hydrocephalus will have a full complement of middle cerebral and anterior cerebral branches, albeit stretched, and these will be present no matter how thin the cortical mantle is. Hydranencephaly will not have such vessels. Huge subdural hygromas (Fig. 15-22) must not be confused with hydranencephaly. Angiography will depict a normal but compressed cerebral vascular supply (Chapter 13) in the former.

Intracranial arachnoid cyst

The intracranial arachnoid cyst exists between the brain substance and dura and contains clear CSF-like fluid. Its precise location between pia and arachnoid within layers of the arachnoid, or between arachnoid and dura, is often not easily discernable at operation or autopsy. The outer membrane does not adhere to dura, and the walls should not contain the capillary proliferations seen in subdural hematomas or effusions. Subdural effusions contain cloudy or yellow high-protein fluid and are not arachnoid cysts (Robinson, 1955). Leptomeningeal cysts, which are herniations of arachnoid through a dural tear

and fracture causing a growing fracture, also are not arachnoid cysts.

The lining of most arachnoid cysts appears to resemble arachnoid. Robinson (1971), who termed these sacs *arachnoid malformations*, provided an extensive description of the entities. Cysts lined by clearly defined ependyma are ependymal cysts, not arachnoid cysts. Many arachnoid cysts do not present clinically and are often found serendipitously.

We believe arachnoid cysts exist in two forms:

A *primary* or congenital cyst is enclosed by two layers of clearly defined arachnoid and does not freely communicate with the subarachnoid space. This type was first described by Starkman and co-workers (1958), who assumed it to be a derangement of the normal mechanism of leptomeningeal formation. Abnormal passage of CSF into the fetal perimedullary mesenchyme results in an encystment of fluid, which becomes truly intra-arachnoid. An intra-arachnoidal site has been confirmed by Holst (1965), Anderson and Landing (1966), and Wilson and Bertan (1966). We believe this type occurs in the sylvian fissure and the middle fossae.

A *secondary* or acquired cyst, which in our experience is the commonest type in children, is a result of the entrapping of subarachnoid or cisternal space by arachnoid adhesions and the unidirectional inward flow of CSF—creating a dynamic mass effect, in reality a subarachnoid cyst. This is the mechanism proposed by Trowbridge and French (1952) and by Dott (1962) and admittedly is a simplistic approach invoking the presence of the ubiquitous "flap-valve" orifice to limit the pulsatile ingress of CSF. Enclosing adhesions may result from the developmental disorganization of arachnoid in the fetus, as proposed by Starkman and co-workers (1958), or from the prenatal or postnatal subarachnoid inflammation or hemorrhage.

Pneumoencephalography or radionuclide studies will show that acquired cysts often communicate with the subarachnoid space, which (contrary to the report of Robinson, 1971) we have found to be a frequent occurrence. The cysts are most common within the cisterns, around the sella and posterior third ventricle, and in the posterior fossa. They may also occur in the middle fossa and less often over the hemispheres. We believe primary or congenital forms are more prevalent in the middle fossa. Secondary cysts are lined by a markedly thickened arachnoid. In our series, at surgery or autopsy some cysts were discovered by chance. Similar findings have been reported by Little and co-workers (1973).

Another theory of the pathogenesis of intracranial arachnoid cysts (Robinson, 1971) has proposed that these middle fossa malformations arise because of poor development of the anterior temporal lobe and that in place of the temporal lobe a collection of CSF forms. If this idea is correct, the cysts are secondary in type. The theory continues by postulating that the collection of fluid then acts like a space-occupying mass due to the pulsatile activity of the brain and hence of the CSF. The anterior temporal lobe is hypoplastic, and its cerebral substance is thinned. In some cases the ependymal lining of the temporal horn is contiguous with the inner membrane of the cyst, whereas in others the sylvian fissure and structures medial to the temporal lobe are exposed by the cyst. Equally plausible is our idea that the cyst forms first and then compresses the temporal lobe, all in a very chronic fashion at an early age.

Bleeding into the cyst due to trauma can occur (Robinson, 1971). Cerebral trauma only with no fracture can result in an arachnoid tear and a large subdural extra-arachnoid collection of CSF (Tiberin and Gruszkiewicz, 1961), a so-called "CSF-oma" or hygroma.

In a number of other cases in our experience, the cyst was lined by an arachnoid-like tissue containing some disordered glial ependyma-type cells but no true ependymal cells—similar to the cysts described by Lewis (1962) and Harrison (1971). Because these cysts had the neuroradiological appearance of secondary arachnoid cysts, however, they were included as such in our series. We have seen only two true ependymal cysts similar to those reported by Hamby and Gardner (1935), Zülch (1965), Jakubiak and co-workers (1968), and Tandon and co-workers (1972).

In 1900, Blake described a pouch that extended as an evagination of the roof of the fourth ventricle superiorly and posteriorly into the retrocerebellar space. As a consequence, other ependyma-lined cysts of the posterior fossa have been given the name *Blake's pouch*. Such evaginations can accompany inferior vermian hypoplasia with a pouchlike extension of the fourth ventricle containing CSF, more commonly called a Dandy-Walker variant (Fig. 15-23).

Large partially ependyma-lined cysts different from true neuroepithelial cysts may appear to be within the anterior third ventricle and closely simulate invaginated suprasellar cysts. Though they communicate with the third ventricle, contain CSF, and are dynamic mass lesions (Fig. 15-24), their origin remains an enigma. Ependyma-lined third ventricular cysts may also produce the bobble head syndrome, but we believe these to be encysted portions of the anterior aspect of the third ventricle that apparently develop prenatally or soon after birth. The neurological differentiation of such cysts from suprasellar arachnoid cysts is often extremely difficult. At pneumoencepha-

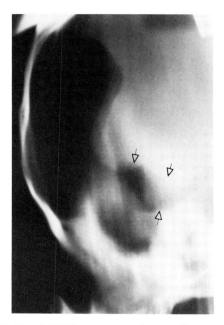

Fig. 15-23. Dandy-Walker variant. A partially formed fourth ventricle (arrows) herniates into the posterior fossa to form a large cyst. Note that the inferior vermis is absent. This is a Dandy-Walker variant pouch lined by ependyma.

lography the ependyma-lined cyst may fill with air from the third ventricle, suggesting a unidirectional flow of CSF and producing the expanded cystlike cavity (Fig. 15-24).

Harrison (1971) suggested that instances of embryonic rests of glial tissue may exist in the subarachnoid tissue, particularly around the base of the brain, and be the origin of ependyma-lined arachnoid cysts. Trowbridge and French (1952) also postulated that some arachnoid cysts form from embryonic rests in arachnoid, which may develop rudimentary secretory organs and even a highly developed choroid plexus. A cyst forms because the free flow of fluid has been impeded. Bouch and co-workers (1973) have described the postmortem findings in three adults each with a large ependyma-lined cyst in the frontal and parietal regions. The cysts did not communicate with the ventricles but did create a large mass effect. The authors suggested that an embryological defect had occurred and led to atopic ependymal cell isolation within cerebral tissue. Though at autopsy many of the arachnoid cysts in our patients showed ependyma-like linings at the junctions with the ventricles, none was an isolated cyst completely lined by true ependymal cells.

Be these as they may, the foregoing theories are not entirely conclusive or comprehensive. Disregarding the semantics of pathogenesis and pathology, we are of the opinion that a practical subdivision of arachnoid cysts does exist—and this is according to the specific

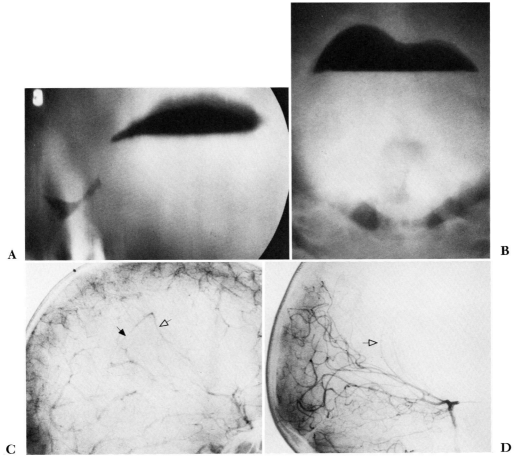

Fig. 15-24. Intra–third ventricular cyst, partially ependyma lined. A and **B,** A posteriorly displaced fourth ventricle and aqueduct. Air enters a large midline cyst which communicates freely with the lateral ventricles. The third ventricle is also inexplicably dilated. **C,** A carotid angiogram shows the internal cerebral vein, vein of Galen (open arrow), and straight sinus (solid arrow) to be markedly displaced superiorly. **D,** A vertebral angiogram reveals severe stretching and displacement of the posterior choroidal arteries (arrow) around the cyst. (See a similar case, Fig. 15-45.)

localization of the cyst within the subarachnoid space.

The neuroradiological characteristics of the cysts differ from site to site. Each cyst must have a dynamic *mass effect,* displacing normal structures (i.e., conforming to our definition of a cyst), which is due to both the increased size and the pulsatile effect on the surrounding brain by the CSF-contained mass. Thus a large subarachnoid space associated with atrophy of brain tissue will not displace normal structures but, in time, may lead to a thickened skull vault and a smaller hemicranium.

If present, *hydrocephalus* is due to the obstructive nature of the cysts. By its mass effect, an intracranial arachnoid cyst can cause an intraventricular obstructive hydrocephalus—with raised intracranial pressure.

Local bulging of the skull and/or displacement of intracranial structures occurs without a hydro-cephalus. Some cysts, particularly those that are supratentorial, may present serendipitously at skull radiography performed for other reasons; or they may present because the mother has noticed a local symptomless bulge or asymmetry in the head of her infant. Other cysts will lurk unnoticed for years and be discovered only at autopsy.

Intracranial arachnoid cysts are not common. Over a period of six years, forty-one infants and children with such a cyst were diagnosed by us and confirmed surgically. The incidence relative to that of paediatric brain neoplasms is approximately 1 to 10. Robinson (1971) estimated a 1% incidence among all space-occupying lesions. Anderson and Landing (1966) described eight infants and children with supratentorial arachnoid cysts, and Harrison (1971) reported fourteen such cases in infants and children (one of which was probably a Dandy-Walker cyst variant).

Characteristics

Age and sex. In our series, boys (twenty-nine, 70%) far outnumbered girls (twelve, 30%)—a ratio of 2.5 to 1. Robinson (1971), however, reported a collected ratio of 7 to 1. Two thirds of the girls were under 1 year of age; and three quarters had a posterior fossa cyst. In other words, nine of the seventeen posterior fossa cysts occurred in girls. Gilles and Rockett (1971) reported eleven children with retrocerebellar cysts, seven of whom were girls. Thus posterior fossa cysts are a common association with infant girls. A third of all the cysts (fourteen) were identified in infants under 1 year of age. Nine of these fourteen infants were under 3 months of age. No other age group was preponderant (Fig. 15-25).

A posterior fossa cyst is common among infants, occurring in ten of the fourteen infants under 1 year of age; and ten of the seventeen posterior fossa cysts occurring at all ages were in infants under 1 year of age. Furthermore, fourteen of the seventeen children with posterior fossa cysts were under 3 years of age whereas children with middle fossa cysts were older, varying in age from 5 to 10 years.

Little and co-workers (1973) reported a predomi-

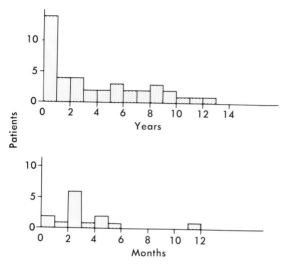

Fig. 15-25. Age and sex in arachnoid cysts. This study was comprised of forty-one children (twenty-nine boys and twelve girls).

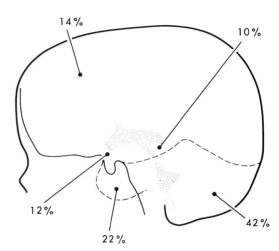

Fig. 15-26. Site of arachnoid cysts.

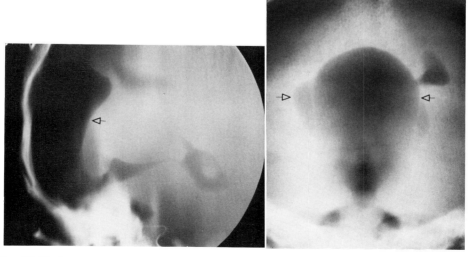

Fig. 15-27. Large cisterna magna. A pneumoencephalogram shows a normal fourth ventricle and aqueduct with a huge cisterna magna (arrows) that does not displace posterior fossa structures.

nantly adult series from the Mayo Clinic of twenty infratentorial arachnoid cysts in which five of the patients were under the age of 15, the youngest being 2 years of age. Four of the five were girls. Gilles and Rockett (1971) described eleven children with retrocerebellar cysts, eight of whom were less than 1 year of age.

Site. The middle fossa is said to be the most common site of an arachnoid cyst in children (Matson, 1969; Harrison, 1971), followed by the parasagittal area. This has not been our experience (Fig. 15-26), however. We found the posterior fossa to be the commonest location, being involved in seventeen patients (42%), the middle fossa in nine (22%), over the cerebral convexity in six (14%), the suprasellar region in five (12%), and posterior to the third ventricle in four (10%).

We believe that most arachnoid cysts in children are encysted arachnoid cisterns or spaces, together with a predominantly unidirectional CSF ingress. We are fully aware that a large cisterna magna is normal and common in children (Fig. 15-27) and can be particularly large with extraventricular obstructive hydrocephalus. This does *not* displace normal structures, however. It is not a dynamic system and must not be misdiagnosed as an arachnoid cyst, particularly if the only diagnostic study made is cerebral angiography.

A poorly performed ventriculography that identifies a posterior fossa air-containing cyst may not permit differentiation among a Dandy-Walker cyst, a posterior fossa arachnoid cyst, and a large cisterna magna. Great care must be taken to visualize the

fourth ventricle—which, if displaced anteriorly, will indicate that the cyst is arachnoid, not Dandy-Walker. Similarly, angiography will clearly establish the extracerebellar location of an arachnoid cyst. We believe that the literature abounds with many well-intentioned misdiagnoses of arachnoid cysts of the posterior fossa as Dandy-Walker cysts.

Posterior fossa. Under 1 year of age, cysts of the posterior fossa are usual. In our experience, the presence of bony skull changes due to a large cyst indicates that the cyst started prenatally.

Of the seventeen children who had posterior fossa cysts, the most common location was the posterior midline (eleven) with symmetrical or asymmetrical extensions laterally or superiorly over the cerebellar hemispheres. The majority of the cysts were quite large. Three occurred in the cerebellopontine angle, two occurred more superiorly over the cerebellar hemisphere (Fig. 15-28), and one (an extensive cyst in the cerebellopontine angle) extended between the clivus and the brain stem up through the tentorium to lie inferiorly and medially to the ipsilateral temporal horn (Fig. 15-29). From a statistical point of view, we considered this last cyst to be primarily a posterior fossa cyst.

Arachnoid cysts in the peripeduncular cistern (Blatt and Berkman, 1969) are uncommon and did not occur in our series. Cysts in the region of the quadrigeminal bodies are considered to be in the supratentorial compartment. One large suprasellar cyst extended anteroinferiorly from the brain stem, but we considered it to be a supratentorial cyst. Little and

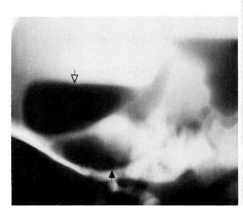
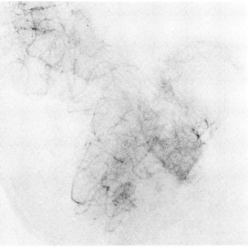

A   B

Fig. 15-28. A superior posterior fossa cyst. A, A ventriculogram demonstrates a large superiorly placed arachnoid cyst (open arrow) which communicated with the cisterna magna (solid arrow). **B,** The arteriolar phase of the vertebral arteriogram demonstrates the compressed blush of the cerebellum and a large avascular cystic space.

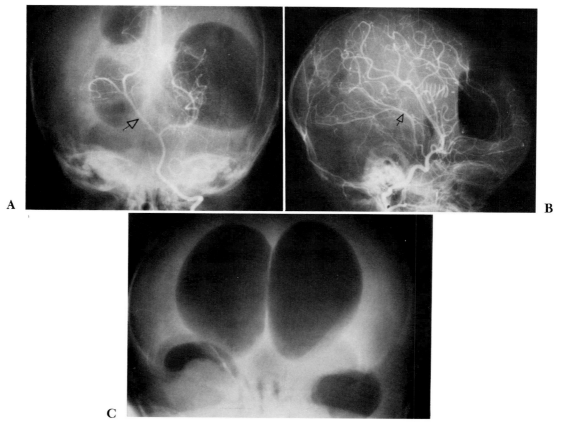

Fig. 15-29. **Cerebellopontine angle arachnoid cyst.** **A** and **B**, Displacing the basilar artery to the left and the superior cerebellar and right posterior cerebral arteries medially and superiorly (arrows). **C**, A ventriculogram shows extension into the right middle fossa and elevation of the right temporal horn. At operation, the tentorium was thinned and displaced superiorly and laterally by the cyst.

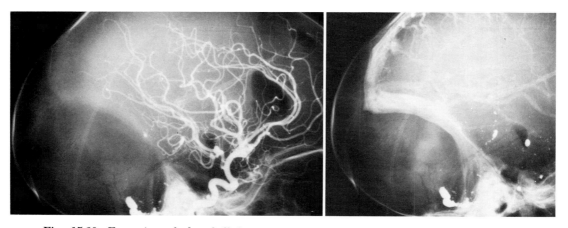

Fig. 15-30. **Expansion of the skull by a posterior fossa cyst.** The occipital and inferior parietal bones are expanded and thinned. The later venous phase of a carotid angiogram demonstrates the secondarily stretched posterior venous sinuses. Note that the torcular is still below the lambda. (These structures are inverted in a Dandy-Walker cyst.)

ticularly well seen in the basal and Towne projections

3. Elevation of the greater and lesser wings of the sphenoid, well seen in the Caldwell projection

An appearance similar to that of no. 3 may also be produced by a chronic subdural hematoma in the middle fossa, dysplasia of the greater wing of the sphenoid, or hamartomatous enlargement of the temporal lobe—as occurs with neurofibromatosis, a slow-growing or cystic temporal neoplasm, or an encysted temporal horn.

COMPUTED TOMOGRAPHY. CT (Chapter 8) demonstrates a cerebrospinal fluid–containing extracerebral mass within the middle fossa, together with possible ventricular displacement.

PNEUMOENCEPHALOGRAPHY AND VENTRICULOGRAPHY. Pneumoencephalography was performed on six of the nine children. Contrary to the experience of Anderson and Landing (1966)—in four children the air entered the cyst itself, which displaced the ventricular system (Figs. 15-34 and 15-37). It remained within the cyst regardless of posture changes, suggesting a one-way ingress of CSF and air.

Ventriculography was performed on two children in whom there was evidence of moderately raised intracranial pressure. A mild hydrocephalus due to distortion of the bases pedunculi and upper pons and aqueduct was demonstrated.

In seven children in whom bulging of the skull was present, the mass effect on the brain was either minimal or absent (Fig. 15-35). A converse relationship was shown in the two children in whom marked cerebral displacement occurred, for these children had almost no skull changes. The temporal horn was sometimes foreshortened, other times elevated and medially displaced. A sylvian cyst, however, displaces the temporal horn inferiorly and medially. Only the inferior portion of the third ventricle was

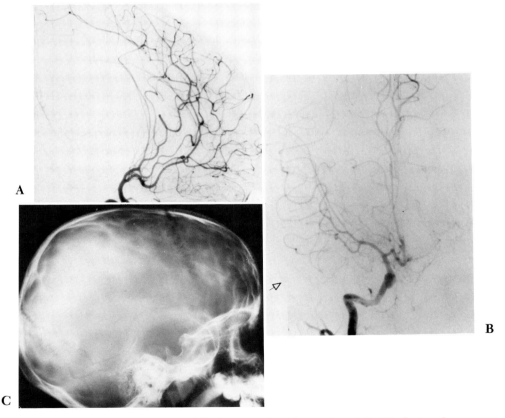

Fig. 15-38. Angiography and a middle fossa arachnoid cyst. A and B, Displacing the supraclinoid portion of the internal carotid artery anteriorly and medially, the horizontal portion of the middle cerebral artery superiorly and anteriorly, and the peripheral branches of the middle cerebral artery superiorly, anteriorly, and inwardly from the vault (arrow). Note that the anterior cerebral artery is not shifted. C, A skull radiograph of the same patient shows thin temporal and parietal bones with loss of the normal brain markings due to the peripheral cyst. The sutures are slightly split.

commonly displaced, and slight elevation and narrowing of the ipsilateral lateral ventricle were uncommonly seen.

ANGIOGRAPHY. The supraclinoid internal carotid artery may be displaced medially and anteriorly, the horizontal limb of the middle cerebral artery elevated, and the peripheral branches displaced and spread in a gentle superiorly convex curve (Fig. 15-38). Especially on an oblique angiogram, the peripheral vessels will be displaced from the inner table. A sylvian cyst may displace the temporal branches of the middle cerebral anteroinferiorly. A vascular rim of the cyst will not be present. The anterior cerebral will rarely be shifted (Fig. 15-38). The basal vein of Rosenthal and the anterior choroidal artery may also be displaced inwardly and superiorly (Fig. 15-39), and the sylvian veins similarly and forward (Fig. 15-39). Some cysts which create expansion of the bony confines of the middle fossa will have no mass effect on the cerebral tissue and the positions of the vessels will remain unchanged.

Arachnoid cysts in other locations

Convexity arachnoid cysts on the cerebrum occurred in six children—three in the frontoparietal region, one in the parieto-occipital region, and two

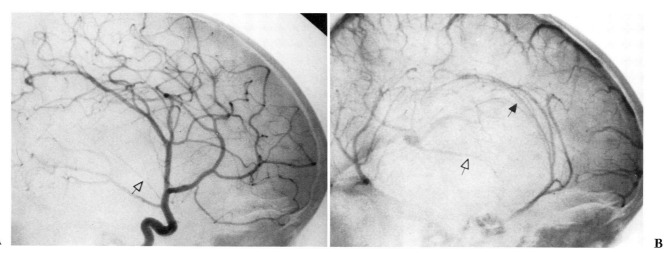

Fig. 15-39. Angiography and a middle fossa arachnoid cyst. A, Stretching and upward displacement of the anterior choroidal artery (open arrow) as well as the middle cerebral artery. B, In the venous phase the sylvian vessels (solid arrow) are similarly displaced superiorly and anteriorly and the basal vein of Rosenthal (open arrow) is displaced superiorly.

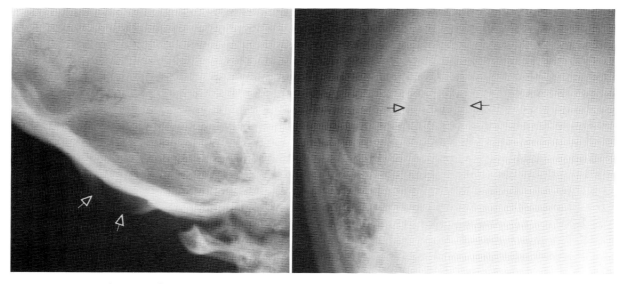

Fig. 15-40. Localized arachnoid cyst. Thinning of the occipital bone (arrows), with a clearly defined inner table margin, and marked thinning of the diploic space are evident.

in the interhemispheric sulcus. Each of the last two cysts was associated with an absent corpus callosum similar to a case reported by Zingesser and co-workers (1964). These last two differed from porencephalic cysts in the region associated with an absent corpus callosum by not communicating with the ventricles and at operation being lined by arachnoid; they could possibly have been formed by the rupturing of a ventricular diverticulum into the subarachnoid space, causing this space to become loculated, as occurred in a hydrocephalus described by Gruszkiewicz and Peyser (1965). Two primarily middle fossa cysts extended out to the parietal surface (Figs. 15-37 and 15-38); and one spread over the frontal lobe (Fig. 15-36).

A small convexity arachnoid cyst is well-defined and creates a focal erosion of the inner table (Figs. 15-40 and 15-41). The others cause mild to moderate expansion of the overlying vault with some thinning of the diploic space.

Suprasellar arachnoid cysts are relatively uncommon (Sansregret et al., 1969) and occurred in five children of our series. The arachnoid diverticula into the sella, creating an enlarged empty sella, as described by Kaufman (1968) and Zatz and co-workers (1969), have not occurred in our experience. The suprasellar cysts in our series were large to gigantic (Fig. 15-42) and either invaginated into or displaced posteriorly and superiorly the entire third ventricle (Fig. 15-43). They also encroached into the middle fossa or into the retroclival space (Fig. 15-43). All such cysts cause some hydrocephalus by obstruc-

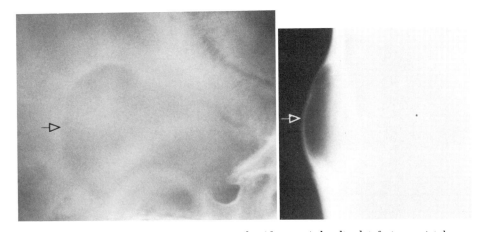

Fig. 15-41. Skull erosion and a convexity arachnoid cyst. A localized inferior parietal superficial arachnoid cyst creates a well-defined skull rim and marked thinning of the diploic space (arrows).

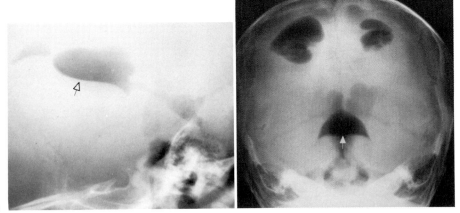

A   B

Fig. 15-42. Suprasellar arachnoid cyst. A pneumoencephalogram fails to demonstrate filling of an enormous cyst that displaced the third ventricle (arrows) superiorly and posteriorly. (This is not the fourth ventricle.)

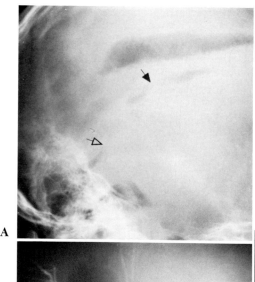

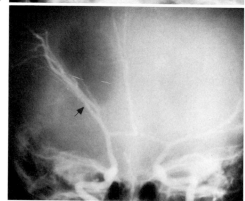

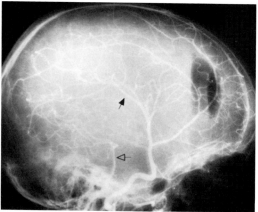

Fig. 15-43. Extension of a suprasellar arachnoid cyst. A, The encephalogram demonstrates gross backward displacement of the aqueduct (open arrow) and third ventricle (solid arrow) as well as markedly upward displacement. There is an associated hydrocephalus. B and C, The angiogram reveals retroclival extension with backward displacement of the basilar artery (open arrow) plus extension laterally into the right middle fossa, elevating the temporal lobe and middle cerebral artery superiorly and inwardly (solid arrows). At surgery, this cyst was thought to be primarily in the suprasellar area.

tion of the third ventricle, foramen of Monro, or aqueduct; they do not extend anteriorly under the frontal lobe as do craniopharyngiomas.

One child, illustrated in Fig. 15-43, exhibited inappropriate antidiuretic hormone secretion; and one manifested mild hypopituitary symptoms. Faris and co-workers (1971) described a 6-year-old boy with precocious puberty and a suprasellar arachnoid cyst; Segall and co-workers (1974) described five children with isosexual precocious puberty and a suprasellar cyst. A feature of these cysts is that they filled with air at ventriculography or pneumoencephalography—similar to only two cases in our experience, however (Fig. 15-44). These cysts must be differentiated from an encystment within the anterior aspect of the third ventricle, which is a large ependyma-lined sac that fills with air from the third ventricle (Fig. 15-45), or from the uncommon encysted cavum septi pellucidi occurring with hydrocephalus.

Strange rhythmic bobbing of the head is described with suprasellar cysts, particularly in infants (Benton et al., 1966; Patriquin, 1973). We have seen this bobbing only with large third ventricles due to aqueductal stenosis and hydrocephalus, however. Computed tomography will reveal the CSF content of these

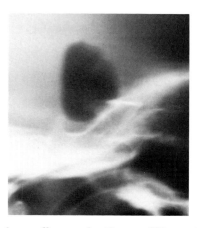

Fig. 15-44. Suprasellar arachnoid cyst filling with air. This example is relatively small.

cysts (Chapter 8); their mass effect is similar to that of a suprasellar cystic craniopharyngioma, a suprasellar teratoma, or indeed a large hypothalamic glioma. Dermoid cysts are extremely rare in this region.

Arachnoid cysts *posterior to the third ventricle* occurred in four children—two were infants under 1

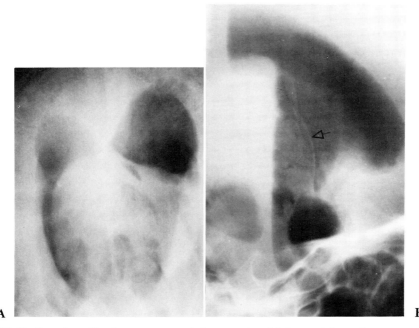

Fig. 15-45. Ependyma-lined encystment of the anterior third ventricle. A large cyst within the third ventricle initially did not fill with air (**A**) but subsequently showed an air-fluid level and thin wall (**B**, arrow) in the brow-up position. At operation, it was judged to be an encystment of part of the third ventricle, creating a large cyst that communicated with remnants of the third ventricle. (Similar to Fig. 15-24.)

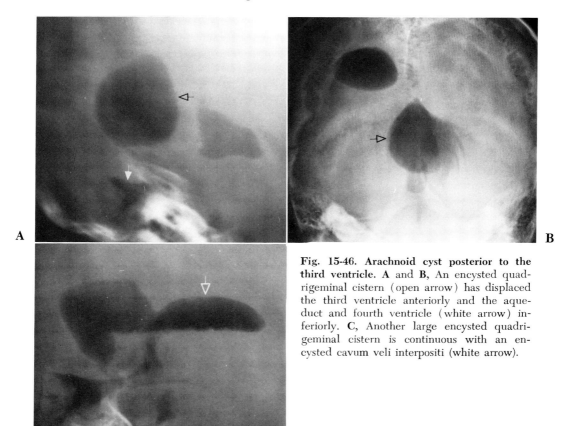

Fig. 15-46. Arachnoid cyst posterior to the third ventricle. A and **B,** An encysted quadrigeminal cistern (open arrow) has displaced the third ventricle anteriorly and the aqueduct and fourth ventricle (white arrow) inferiorly. **C,** Another large encysted quadrigeminal cistern is continuous with an encysted cavum veli interpositi (white arrow).

year of age, one was 3 years old, and the fourth was 5 years old. Similar cases have been reported by Lourie and Berne (1961) and Huckman and co-workers (1970). Great care must be taken not to misdiagnose as a posterior fossa arachnoid cyst an enlarged suprapineal recess—which is common in hydrocephalus due to aqueductal stenosis (Chapters 6 and 10), a dilated cistern of the vein of Galen and quadrigeminal cistern, or a cavum veli interpositi that freely communicates with the CSF in extraventricular obstructive hydrocephalus. We believe the so-called quadrigeminal arachnoid cysts are encysted quadrigeminal and galenic cisterns caused by arachnoid adhesions and creating a specific mass effect on the surrounding structures (Fig. 15-46).

Two of the four cysts filled with air during pneumoencephalography. Computed tomography revealed the CSF content of the cysts (Chapter 8), and ventriculography and angiography demonstrated an avascular posterior third ventricular mass. If large enough, such cysts will kink and obstruct the aqueduct and produce hydrocephalus (Fig. 15-46). Neoplasms in the pineal region or an arteriovenous malformation with a galenic varix may closely resemble the mass effect of these cysts; however, they can be differentiated by computed tomography and angiography. Some cysts in this region with more or less epithelial lining, the so-called epithelial cysts, do contain clear fluid; but true epithelial cysts have a high protein content.

CYSTS NOT CONTAINING CEREBROSPINAL FLUID
Neoplastic cyst

A cyst can occur in a neoplasm in many parts of the brain and have diverse appearances. It may be the major component of the neoplastic mass lesion (Chapter 11) (e.g., a cystic astrocytoma, a craniopharyngioma, a dermoid), or it may be small and multiple and scattered throughout the neoplasm (an ependymoma, some astrocytomas, a teratoma) (Ingraham and Bailey, 1946).

Astrocytoma and craniopharyngioma are the most common cystic neoplasms; 25% of astrocytomas and 80% of craniopharyngiomas contain significantly large cysts. Astrocytomas, however, outnumber craniopharyngiomas; therefore, on the basis of number alone, astrocytomas are the most common cystic neoplasm. Fifteen percent of ependymomas contain cysts, which are usually not large. In our experience, 10% of brain stem tumors were cystic.

Cystic craniopharyngiomas may invaginate into the third ventricle or into the middle fossa or even down and into the posterior fossa anterior to the brain stem (Chapter 11). Cystic astrocytomas may contain a well-defined vascular nodule identifiable by angiography and computed tomography. Only with computed tomography, however, can both a cystic component and a solid component of a neoplasm be conclusively demonstrated (Chapter 8). Inferential angiographic evidence of a cyst is (1) marked stretching of related cortical or cerebellar vessels with little tumor vascularity or (2) a well-defined nidus of vascularity in a relatively avascular mass effect. A cerebellar location with clinical evidence of recently increased intracranial pressure and hydrocephalus is further evidence that the cyst may be neoplastic (e.g., cystic astrocytoma). A cerebral neoplastic cyst may have a similar angiographic appearance with either meager vascularity or an avascular nodule. A cystic astrocytoma that impinges on and obstructs chiefly the fourth ventricle will have a smooth curved surface. A medulloblastoma or a solid astrocytoma will rarely have a similar surface appearance.

The neurosurgeon may decide to aspirate the cyst or cystic neoplasm in the cerebrum and instill some sterile micropaque barium (Chapter 11). This will coat the cyst wall and be phagocytized by the lining cells. If present, a mural nodule will thereby be demonstrated more graphically. Rarely will the cyst rupture spontaneously. We have seen only one neoplastic cyst that ruptured and subsequently filled with air at ventriculography or pneumoencephalography. Bleeding may occur into the neoplastic cyst; but, other than by computed tomography, which will detect the contained blood, it will not be identified as such by other neuroradiological methods.

Inflammatory cyst

A purulent abscess with a liquid necrotic center (Chapter 13) may be termed a cyst of sorts insofar as its mass effect is relieved by aspiration. Its clinical presentation and its angiographically intense compressive mass effect on the surrounding gyri will aid in the precise diagnosis.

A parasitic cyst—as exists in hydatid disease or cysticerosis (Chapter 13)—may lurk for years within the brain and often not present until it obstructs the CSF pathway, leading to hydrocephalus or seizures. If large and superficial, it may expand the vault. A hydatid cyst rarely calcifies. Angiography will reveal a large avascular mass but will not differentiate the mass from other benign cysts of the brain.

Small cysts from cysticercosis can occur in the ventricular cavity and are well demonstrated by ventriculography.

Colloid, ependymal, and other cysts

Colloid and ependymal cysts are best termed *neuroepithelial* cysts (Shuangshoti and Netsky, 1966).

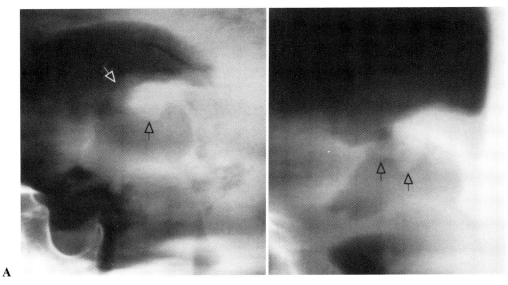

A   B

Fig. 15-47. Colloid cysts. The classical appearances of these small cysts just behind the foramina of Monro in the lateral and third ventricles (**A**, arrows) or in the third ventricle alone (**B**, arrows) can be seen. The cyst in **B** has produced a marked hydrocephalus by partially occluding the foramina.

From a neuroradiological point of view, they are rare in children, but they are common as chance findings at autopsy (Shuangshoti and Netsky, 1966). They originate from invaginations of the neuroepithelium into the ventricles or into the cerebrum or subarachnoid space during the development of the brain. The neck of these folded sacs may then be pinched off to form a cystic cavity.

Other neuroepithelial cysts are said to rise from neuroglial heterotopia in the cortex or subarachnoid space (Cooper and Kernohan, 1951). These cysts are lined by well-differentiated ependyma and contain a viscous high-protein fluid. Tufts of choroid plexus may also be present in the ependymal lining (Rand et al., 1964; Shuangshoti and Netsky, 1966). *We consider large cysts which have walls predominantly of arachnoid-like cells with islands of ependyma-like cells as described by Harrison (1971) to be arachnoid cysts, not ependymal cysts.*

The neuroradiological appearance of ependymal cysts in the sylvian fissure (Tandon et al., 1972) or in the cerebrum (Jakubiak et al., 1968; Bouch et al., 1973) is indistinguishable from that of porencephaly or an avascular neoplasm.

The most common site of the neuroepithelial cyst is beneath the fornices just posterior to the foramina of Monro, the so-called colloid cyst (Fig. 15-47). Few cases are diagnosed neuroradiologically in infancy or early childhood (Yenermen et al., 1958; Gemperlein, 1960; Buchsbaum and Colton, 1967; Little and Mac-Carty, 1974). The cyst is said to make up approximately 0.5% of all brain mass lesions at any age (Ferry and Kempe, 1968). It presents with hydrocephalus of both ventricles by totally or partially occluding the foramina of Monro and is best visualized by ventriculography (Bull and Sutton, 1949) or pneumoencephalography *after* shunting of the hydrocephalic ventricles. It forms a smooth and rounded or gently lobulated mass (Fig. 15-47). At angiography the internal cerebral vein may exhibit an anterior humplike deformity (Batnitzky et al., 1974).

Ependymomas that involve the posterior aspect of the third ventricle and papillomas of the choroid plexus are cauliflower-like fungating masses that may be highly vascular. Small teratomas are rare at this site (Ferry et al., 1972). Cysticercosis of the third ventricle is extremely rare (Allen and Lovell, 1932). Nodules of tuberous sclerosis arising in the lateral ventricular walls may extend into and occlude the foramen of Monro (Fitz et al., 1974).

The appearance of epithelium-lined cysts in the cerebellopontine angles (Gardner et al., 1960; Zülch, 1965) is similar to that of other cysts at this site (e.g., arachnoid cysts) or neoplasms. Ependyma-lined cysts may also occur over the quadrigeminal bodies (Hamby and Gardner, 1935) or be related to the pineal body (Gladstone and Wakely, 1940); they may be observed within the cerebellar vermis (Handa and Bucy, 1956) or above the cerebellum (Lewis, 1962).

Intrasellar epithelial cysts arising from Rathke's cleft (Fairburn and Larkin, 1964; Fager and Carter, 1966) are very rare. We have not seen any in children. They are distinct from craniopharyngiomas and are contained within the pituitary fossa. Weber and co-workers (1970) described three patients with intrasellar cysts not lined by epithelium, and these probably arose from hemorrhagic infarctions of the pituitary gland.

REFERENCES

Allen, N.: Developmental and degenerative diseases of the brain. In Farmer, T. W., editor: Pediatric neurology, New York, 1964, Paul B. Hoeber, Inc.

Allen, S. S., and Lovell, H. W.: Tumors of the third ventricle, Arch. Neurol. Psychiatry 28:990, 1932.

Anderson, F. M., and Landing, B. H.: Cerebral arachnoid cysts in infants, J. Pediatr. 69:88, 1966.

Armstrong, D., and Norman, M. G.: Periventricular leucomalacia in neonates; Complications and sequelae, Arch. Dis. Child. 49:367, 1974.

Batnitzky, S., Sarwar, M., Leeds, N. E., Schecter, M. M., and Azar-Kia, B.: Colloid cysts of the third ventricle, Radiology 112:327, 1974.

Benda, C. E.: The late effects of cerebral birth injuries, Medicine 24:71, 1945.

Benton, J. W. Nellhaus, G., Huttenlocher, P. R., Ojemann, R. G., and Dodge, P. R.: The bobble-head syndrome; report of a unique truncal tremor associated with third ventricular cyst and hydrocephalus in children, Neurology 16:725, 1966.

Blake, J. A.: The roof and lateral recesses of the fourth ventricle, considered morphologically and embryonically, J. Comp. Neurol. 10:79, 1900.

Blatt, E. S., and Berkmen, Y. M.: Congenital occlusion of the foramen of Monro, Radiology 92:1061, 1969.

Bouch, D. C., Mitchell, I., and Maloney, A. F. J.: Ependymal lined paraventricular cerebral cysts; a report of three cases, J. Neurol. Neurosurg. Psychiatry 36:611, 1973.

Buchsbaum, H. W., and Colton, R. P.: Anterior third ventricular cysts in infancy; case report, J. Neurosurg. 26:264, 1967.

Bull, J. W. D., and Sutton, D.: The diagnosis of paraphysial cysts, Brain 72:487, 1949.

Cantu, R. C., and LeMay, M.: Porencephaly caused by intracerebral hemorrhage, Radiology 88:526, 1967.

Cloward, R. B.: Atresia of the lateral ventricle, J. Neurol. Neurosurg. Psychiatry 32:624, 1969.

Cocker, J., George, S. W., and Yates, P. O.: Perinatal occlusion of the middle cerebral artery, Dev. Med. Child Neurol. 7:235, 1965.

Cooper, I. S., and Kernohan, J. W.: Heterotopic glial nests in the subarachnoid space: histopathologic characteristics, mode of origin and relation to meningeal gliomas, J. Neuropathol. Exp. Neurol. 10:16, 1951.

Courville, C. B.: Antenatal and paranatal circulatory disorders as a cause of cerebral damage in early life, J. Neuropathol. Exp. Neurol. 18:115, 1959.

D'Agostino, A. N., Kernohan, J. W., and Brown, J. R.: The Dandy-Walker syndrome, J. Neuropathol. Exp. Neurol. 22:450, 1963.

de Morsier, G.: Studies in cranial-encephalic dysraphia. I. Agenesia of the olfactory lobe (lateral, telencephaloschisis) and of the callous and anterior commissures (median, telencephaloschisis); olfacto-genital dysplasia, Schweiz. Arch. Neurol. Psychiatry 74:309, 1954.

Dott, N. M.: An introductory review; presidential address, Dev. Med. Child Neurol. 4:259, 1962.

Fager, C. A., and Carter, H.: Intrasellar epithelial cysts, J. Neurosurg. 24:77, 1966.

Fairburn, B., and Larkin, I. M.: A cyst of Rathke's cleft, J. Neurosurg. 21:223, 1964.

Faris, A. A., Bale, G. F., and Cannon, B.: Arachnoidal cyst of the third ventricle with precocious puberty, South. Med. J. 64:1139, 1971.

Farris, M. D. M.: Bitemporal bulging and thinning of the skull, Va. Med. Mon. 93:80, 1966.

Ferry, D. J., and Kempe, L. G.: Colloid cyst of the third ventricle, Milit. Med. 733:734, 1968.

Ferry, D J., Mylander, K., and Hardman, J.: Radiographic identification and surgical removal of a teratoid tumor of the roof of the third ventricle; case report, J. Neurosurg. 36:231, 1972.

Fitz, C. R., Harwood-Nash, D. C. F., and Thompson, J. R.: Neuroradiology of tuberous sclerosis in children, Radiology 110:635, 1974.

Freeman, J. M., and Gold, A. P.: Porencephaly simulating subdural hematoma in childhood, Am. J. Dis. Child. 107:327, 1964.

Gardner, W. J., McCormack, L. J., and Dohn, D. F.: Embryonal atresia of the fourth ventricle: the cause of "arachnoid cyst" of the cerebellopontine angle, J. Neurosurg. 17:226, 1960.

Gemperlein, J.: Paraphyseal cyst of the third ventricle, J. Neuropathol. Exp. Neurol. 19:133, 1960.

Gilles, F. H., and Rockett, F. X.: Infantile hydrocephalus: retrocerebellar "arachnoidal" cyst, J. Pediatr. 79:436, 1971.

Gladstone, R. J., and Wakeley, C. P. G.: The pineal organ, London, 1940, Bailliere, Tindall & Cox.

Granholm, L., and Rådberg, C.: Ventricular diverticulum in infantile hydrocephalus, Acta Radiol. 3:156, 1956.

Gruszkiewicz, J., and Peyser, E.: Supratentorial arachnoidal cyst associated with hydrocephalus, J. Neurol. Neurosurg. Psychiatry 28:438, 1965.

Halsey, J. H., and Chamberlin, H. R.: The morphogenesis of hydranencephaly, J. Neurol. Sci. 12:187, 1971.

Hamby, W. B., and Gardner, W. J.: An ependymal cyst in the quadrigeminal region; report of a case, Arch. Neurol. Psychiatry 33:391, 1935.

Hamby, W. B., Krauss, R. F., and Beswick, W. F.: Hydranencephaly: clinical diagnosis; presentation of seven cases, Pediatrics 6:371, 1950.

Handa, H., and Bucy, P. C.: Benign cysts of the brain simulating brain tumor, J. Neurosurg. 13:489, 1956.

Harrison, M. J. G.: Cerebral arachnoid cysts in children, J. Neurol. Neurosurg. Psychiatry 34:316, 1971.

Heiskanen, O.: Cyst of the septum pellucidum causing increased intracranial pressure and hydrocephalus; case report, J. Neurosurg. 38:771, 1973.

Heschl, R., 1859. In Yakovlev and Wadsworth, 1946.

Holst, S.: Congenital intracranial arachnoidal cysts; case reports and discussion of the pathogenesis, J. Oslo City Hosp. 15:114, 1965.

Huckman, M. S., Davis, D. O., and Coxe, W. S.: Arachnoid cyst of the quadrigeminal plate; case report, J. Neurosurg. 32:367, 1970.

Hughes, R. A., Kernohan, J. W., and Craig, W. M.: Caves and cysts of the septum pellucidum, Arch. Neurol. Psychiatry 74:259, 1955.

Ingraham, F. D., and Bailey, O. T.: Cystic teratomas and teratoid tumours of the central nervous system in infancy and childhood, J. Neurosurg. 3:511, 1946.

Jakubiak, P., Dunsmore, R. H., and Beckett, R. S.: Supratentorial brain cysts, J. Neurosurg. 28:129, 1968.

Kaufman, B.: The "empty" sella turcica—a manifestation of the intrasellar subarachnoid space, Radiology 90:931, 1968.

Lavender, J. P., and du Boulay, G. H.: Aqueduct stenosis and cystic expansion of the suprapineal recess, Clin. Radiol. 16:330, 1965.

Lewis, A. J.: Infantile hydrocephalus caused by arachnoid cyst; case report, J. Neurosurg. 19:431, 1962.

Lindenberg, R., and Swanson, P. D.: "Infantile hydranencephaly"—a report of five cases of infarction of both cerebral hemispheres in infancy, Brain 90:839, 1967.

Little, J. R., Gomez, M. R., and MacCarty, C. S.: Infratentorial arachnoid cysts, J. Neurosurg. 39:380, 1973.

Little, J. R., and MacCarty, C. S.: Colloid cysts of the third ventricle, J. Neurosurg. 39:230, 1974.

Lorber, J., and Emery, J. L.: Intracerebral cysts complicating ventricular needline in hydrocephalic infants: a clinicopathological study, Dev. Med. Child Neurol. 6:125, 1964.

Lorber, J., and Grainger, R. G.: Cerebral cavities following ventricular punctures in infants, Clin. Radiol. 14:98, 1963.

Lourie, H., and Berne, A. S.: Radiological and clinical features of an arachnoid cyst of the quadrigeminal cistern, J. Neurol. Neurosurg. Psychiatry 24:374, 1961.

Marburg, O., and Casemajor, L.: Phlebostasis and phlebothrombosis of the brain in the newborn and in early childhood, Arch. Neurol. Psychiatry 52:170, 1944.

Matson, D. D.: Neurosurgery of infancy and childhood, ed. 2, Springfield, Ill., 1969, Charles C Thomas, Publisher.

Mavin, J. J., and Angerine, J. M.: Congenital cytomegalic inclusion disease with porencephaly, Neurology 18:47, 1968.

Myers, R. E.: Brain pathology following fetal vascular occlusion: an experimental study, Invest. Ophthalmol. 8:41, 1969.

Naef, R. W.: Clinical features of porencephaly; a review of thirty-two cases, Arch. Neurol. Psychiatry 80:133, 1958.

Nixon, G. W., and Ravin, C. E.: Malposition of the attached portion of the falx cerebri and the superior sagittal sinus: an indicator of severe cerebral maldevelopment, Am. J. Roentgenol. Radium Ther. Nucl. Med. 122:44, 1974.

Norman, R. M.: Malformations of the nervous system, birth injury and diseases of early life. In Blackwood, W., McMenemey, W. H., Meyer, A., Norman, R. M., and Russell, D. S., editors: Greenfield's neuropathology, ed. 2, London, 1963, Edward Arnold (Publishers), Ltd.

Norman, R. M., Urich, H., and Woods, G. E.: The relationship between prenatal porencephaly and the encephalomalacias of early life, J. Ment. Sci. 104:758, 1958.

Northfield, D. W. C., and Russell, D. S.: False diverticulum of a lateral ventricle causing hemiplegia in chronic internal hydrocephalus, Brain 62:311, 1939.

Patriquin, H. B.: The bobble-head syndrome; a curable entity, Radiology 107:171, 1973.

Poser, C. M., Walsh, F. C., and Scheinberg, L. C.: Hydranencephaly, Neurology 5:284, 1955.

Rand, B. O., Foltz, E. L., and Alvord, E. C.: Intracranial telencephalic meningoencephalocele containing choroid plexus, J. Neuropathol. Exp. Neurol. 22:293, 1964.

Robinson, R. G.: Congenital cysts of the brain: arachnoid malformations, Prog. Neurol. Surg. 4:133, 1971.

Robinson, R. G.: Intracranial collections of fluid with local bulging of the skull, J. Neurosurg. 12:345, 1955.

Russell, D. S.: Observations on the pathology of hydrocephalus, Spec. Rep. Ser. Med. Res. Counc. no. 265, 1949,

Ryvicker, M., and Leeds, N. E.: Development cerebral intra-arachnoidal cysts, Radiology 109:105, 1973.

Sansregret, A., Ledoux, R., Duplantis, F., Lamoureux, C., Chapdelaine, A., and Leblanc, P.: Suprasellar subarachnoid cysts; radioclinical features, Am. J. Roentgenol. Radium Ther. Nucl. Med. 105:291, 1969.

Segall, H. D., Hassan, G., Ling, S. M., and Carton, C.: Suprasellar cysts associated with isosexual precocious puberty, Radiology 111:607, 1974.

Shuangshoti, S., and Netsky, M. G.: Neuroepithelial (colloid) cysts of the nervous system; further observations on pathogenesis, location, incidence, and histochemistry, Neurology 16:887, 1966.

Starkman, S. P., Brown, T. C., and Linell, E. A.: Cerebral arachnoid cysts, J. Neuropathol. 17:484, 1958.

Stevenson, L. E., and McGowan, L. E.: Encephalomalacia with cavity formation in infants, Arch. Pathol. 34:286, 1942.

Tandon, P. N., Roy, S., and Elvidge, A.: Subarachnoid ependymal cyst, J. Neurosurg. 37:741, 1972.

Tiberin, P., and Gruszkiewicz, J.: Chronic arachnoidal cysts of the middle cranial fossa and their relation to trauma, J. Neurol. Neurosurg. Psychiatry 24:86, 1961.

Trowbridge, W. V., and French, J. D.: Benign arachnoid cysts of the posterior fossa, J. Neurosurg. 9:398, 1952.

Weber, E. L., Vogel, F. S., and Odom, G. L.: Cysts of the sella turcica, J. Neurosurg. 33:48, 1970.

Wilner, H. I., and Kashef, R.: Unilateral arachnoidal cysts and adhesions involving the eighth nerve, Am. J. Roentgenol. Radium Ther. Nucl. Med. 115:126, 1972.

Wilson, C. B., and Bertan, V.: Cerebral leptomeningeal cysts of developmental origin, Am. J. Roentgenol. Radium Ther. Nucl. Med. 98:570, 1966.

Wolf, A., and Cowen, D.: Cerebral atrophies and encephalomalacias, Assoc. Res. Nerv. Ment. Dis. Proc. 34:199, 1955.

Wolpert, S. M., Haller, J. S., and Rabe, E. F.: The value of angiography in the Dandy-Walker syndrome and posterior fossa extra-axial cysts, Am. J. Roentgenol. Radium Ther. Nucl. Med. 109:261, 1970.

Yakovlev, P. I., and Wadsworth, R. C.: Schizencephalies; study of the congenital clefts in the cerebral mantle. I. Clefts with fused lips. II. Clefts with hydrocephalus and lips separated, J. Neuropathol. Exp. Neurol. 5:116, 169, 1946.

Yenermen, M. H., Bowerman, C. I., and Haymaker, W.: Colloid cyst of the third ventricle; a clinical study of 54 cases in the light of previous publications, Acta Neurovegetativa 17:211, 1958.

Zatz, L. M., Janon, E. A., and Newton, T. H.: The enlarged sella and the intrasellar cistern, Radiology 93:1085, 1969.

Zingesser, L., Schechter, M., Gonatas, N., Levy, A., and Wisoff, H.: Agenesis of the corpus callosum associated with an inter-hemispheric arachnoid cyst, Br. J. Radiol. 37:905, 1964.

Zülch, K. J.: Brain tumors, their biology and pathology, ed. 2, New York, 1965, Springer-Verlag New York, Inc.

Congenital malformations of the brain

The in vivo study of congenital malformations of the brain is not possible without neuroradiological techniques. These malformations are complex and show great variation between and within morphological groups. The rationale for in vivo studies is not merely to gain therapeutic benefit but also to identify and understand the dysgenesis, thereby enabling an insight into possible pathogenesis to be achieved. The practical rationale is for prognostic and genetic parental counseling.

Congenital malformations of the brain are deviations in form and structure; but they are induced during the brain's intrauterine development. Of interest to the neuroradiologist quite simply are those malformations that survive the birth process and continue to survive. We believe these constitute at least 50% of all congenital defects. Ebaugh and Holt (1963) stated that chromosomal deviations account for 10%; inheritance, either recessive or dominant, 20%; and intrauterine environmental influences such as infection, 10%. The majority of malformations, 60%, have no clear pathogenetic factor.

It is the *interaction* of the genetic and environmental factors that produces the ultimate malformation. The circumstance of environment may include factors affecting clusters of births with lesions of the central nervous system. For example, Fedrick and Wilson (1971) summarized reports of anencephaly, spina bifida, and hydrocephalus varying in incidence with year, month of conception, and area of residence of the mother. Blackwood and co-workers (1963) warned that the immature nervous system reacts differently from the adult nervous system and that abnormal segments of the immature system may be completely absorbed in utero, thus affecting the accuracy of deduced pathogenetic factors extrapolated from neuroradiologically observed morphological abnormalities.

The formation and folding of the neural plate of the embryo are complete by the end of the third week. The initiation of most congenital brain malformations occurs before the sixth week. Inflammatory reactions within the fetal brain are not usually seen before the sixth month. Thus dysgenesis may occur in the *formative* period of neural tube development (third week or before) or during the *maturation* and development of the tube; after this period the malformation may be due to nonlethal destruction, cessation of growth, or altered development of some part of the brain.

Classification

A classification of malformations of the brain applicable to the geographic demonstration of altered macroscopic morphology by neuroradiological methods must exclude disorders of cytogenesis. These disorders are at the molecular level of anatomy, arrangement, and function (e.g., abnormalities of the gene, inborn errors of metabolism, leukodystrophies, chromosomal abnormalities like trisomy 13-15, 18, XO, or XXY configurations). Our interest therefore lies in those malformations which are simplified or altered expressions of the usual form and structure of the brain.

There are two stages of formative alteration (Yakovlev, 1959):

The first is an *organogenetic* malformation, wherein an alteration of development occurs without an abnormality of histogenesis but with persistence of some embryonal form of brain structure. This group, usually occurring sporadically and with no evidence of heredity, includes Chiari malformation, schizencephaly, and anencephaly. Thus abnormalities of organogenesis consist of failures of migration of neuroblasts (e.g., heterotopias) and failures of prosencephalic cleavage (holoprosencephaly).

The other stage is a *histogenetic* malformation, wherein normal development of the brain occurs but with specific deviant cell differentiation. Such mal-

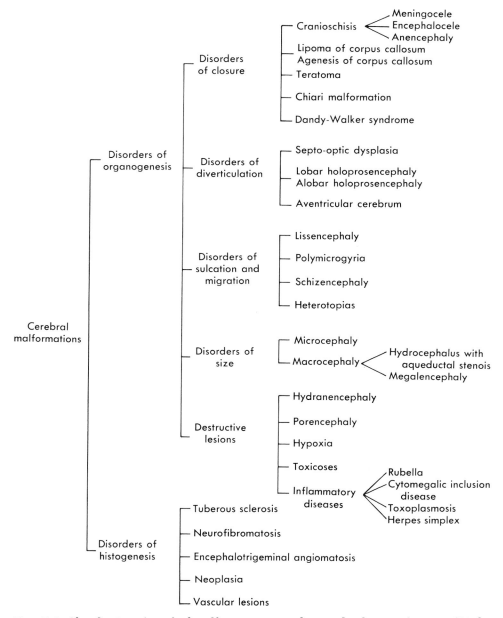

Fig. 16-1. Classification of cerebral malformations according to developmental stages. (Modified from DeMyer, W.: Birth Defects **7**:78, 1971.)

formations are usually hereditary and familial and include mixed cell deviations, hamartomas (e.g., neurofibromatosis), and tuberous sclerosis.

Acknowledging that in some malformations an overlap may occur within the simple classification, we have adopted the dendrogram form of classification (Fig. 16-1) developed by DeMyer (1971). Organogenesis, histogenesis, and cytogenesis overlap and are often interrelated. DeMyer based his classification on the two basic stages of morphogenesis described by Yakovlev (1959). His is a classification based on a formative rather than a causative patho-

genesis. We have described many of the malformations elsewhere. Unfortunately, the enigmatic eponym is inescapable in certain syndromes; and we shall use it only when an alternate short morphological title defies imagination or intellect.

ORGANOGENETIC MALFORMATIONS

Organogenesis may be altered by disorders of closure of the neural tube, disorders of diverticulation within the primary brain vesicles, disorders of sulcation of the hemispheres or neuroblast migration, disorders of brain size that may or may not be associated with somatic or biochemical syndromes, and finally intrauterine destructive lesions. Though many of these lesions are extremely rare and complex, others are relatively common within a large paediatric hospital practice and merit specific neuroradiological attention. Some have been detailed in other chapters.

Disorders of closure
Chiari malformation

The Chiari malformation is a complex congenital abnormality of the brain whose basis is a malformation of the lower brain stem and cerebellum. It is usually associated with a myelomeningocele. History has done injustice to Cleland (1883) and provided Arnold with an unsought eponymic prominence. Chiari (1891, 1896) described three variations of hindbrain malformations. We prefer the term *Chiari malformation.*

Wilkins and Brody (1971) provided an English translation of Chiari's original paper describing three types of brain stem and cerebellar abnormalities. The so-called Arnold-Chiari malformation applies in neuroradiological practice to the type II Chiari malformation:

1. *Type I* is a variable downward displacement of the tonsils and inferior cerebellum only into the vertebral canal without displacement of the medulla and fourth ventricle.
2. *Type II* is a similar variable downward displacement of the inferior cerebellum and tonsils but includes caudal displacement of the lower pons and medulla and a fourth ventricle elongated into the vertebral canal. A myelomeningocele accompanies this malformation. Type II is the most common type and is usually referred to as the Arnold-Chiari malformation.
3. *Type III* is a displacement of the medulla and fourth ventricle and virtually all of the cerebellum into an occipital and high cervical encephalomeningocele.

A type IV, consisting of hypoplasia of the cerebellum with no inferior displacement of structures, is sometimes included in descriptions of this malformation. We do not recognize the type IV as a Chiari malformation.

Morphogenesis. It is apparent to us that the malformations of the brain, cord, and spine as occur in the Chiari malformation have a common origin in early prenatal life, with no area of malformation being the direct result of another.

In short, the theories of morphogenesis of the Chiari malformation are presented with considerable lack of unanimity. Boulter (1967) gave an excellent review of the prevailing morphogenetic theories. Peach (1965a) divided the theories into three groups: (1) The first

proposed that the malformation is due to mechanical factors during embryonic life such as downward traction of the upper neural axis caused by the spinal cord's being fixed to the vertebral column at a myelomeningocele (Lichtenstein, 1942, 1958). This theory is now considered to be untenable (Russell, 1949; Barry et al., 1957; Peach, 1965a). (2) The second theory proposed not that the syndrome is a malformation but that embryonic hydrocephalus causes the downward displacement of posterior fossa structures. This theory was first advanced by Chiari in 1895. Gardner (1959) suggested as the only reason for a persistent hydrocephalus the fact that the normal embryonic cephalohydromyelia fails to decrease in volume because of continuing impermeability of the rhombic roof of the developing fourth ventricle. The lateral ventricles then dilate, compressing the tentorium inferiorly, decreasing the size of the posterior fossa, and thus also depressing the developing brain stem and cerebellum. Most Chiari malformations at birth, however, do not have hydrocephalus and the foramen of Magendie is often patent. (3) The third and most complex theory proposed that the malformation is a primary dysgenesis of the hindbrain.

These extensive point-and-counterpoint discussions leave no unified concept.

Russell (1949) considered the Chiari malformation to be a developmental dysplasia occurring at the third week of fetal life. Daniel and Strich (1958) suggested a failure of the pontine flexure to develop, together with an abnormal growth of the cerebellum and brain stem in early embryonic life, or failure of the inductive process to occur at about 28 days.

Barry and co-workers (1957) proposed a primary overgrowth of the entire central nervous system, starting at the fourth week, with active herniation of the brain stem and cerebellum through the foramen magnum into the cervical canal. It seems that such an overgrowth might cause the embryonic hydrocephalus to persist and lead to relatively large ventricles that would inferiorly displace the final attachment of the tentorium to the skull by the third month; but could not the occipital bone be hypoplastic per se and both these phenomena provide a small posterior fossa—especially since the occipital bone and hindbrain form at about the tenth week? The combined effect of brain stem and midbrain overgrowth within a too small posterior fossa might thus lead to neuroradiological and pathological features of the Chiari malformation. An enlargement of the massa intermedia and accessory anterior commissure could be part of this generalized overgrowth. The spinal cord involved in a myelomeningocele exhibits a similar overgrowth (Emery and Naik, 1968).

Williams (1971) suggested that brain herniation is

initiated by low intraspinal pressure due to leakage from a sump effect within a spinal dysraphia. The presence of raised levels of alpha fetal proteins in the amniotic fluid of fetuses with severe neural tube defects as early as 14 weeks (Milunsky et al., 1974) supports the theory that the Chiari malformation occurs early.

Gardner and co-workers (1972), Padget (1972), and Padget and Lindenberg (1972) favored an interrelationship and a common origin between the Chiari malformation and the Dandy-Walker syndrome—the former developing in an embryonic small posterior fossa, and the latter creating a large posterior fossa. Padget (1972) also suggested that encephaloschisis and myeloschisis result from the reopening of a closed embryonic neural tube, rather than from a failure of closure, and are associated with considerable secondary neural tissue disorganization and scarring.

The reader is referred to Norman (1963) and Peach (1965a) for further concise summaries of such theories.

Regardless of the foregoing hypotheses, it appears to us that whatever injurious agent acts on and impedes closure of the neural groove, the effect in causing the Chiari malformation alters the primary development of the hindbrain and distal neural axis simultaneously (myelomeningocele); and there is *no* direct cause-and-effect relationship between the two. Some change in growth of the brain stem, bases pedunculi, midbrain, and often the cerebrum (polymicrogyria) also results—but not necessarily of the cerebellar hemispheres—which leads to transtentorial upward and transforaminal downward herniation of the Chiari malformation.

Peach (1965a) postulated that the failure of the pontine flexure to develop, with an embryonic portion of the intraventricular cerebellum being depressed into the cervical canal, is a key feature of this altered morphogenesis.

Neuroradiology of the Chiari malformation

Type I. Our practice is to recognize the Chiari malformation as the type II form. We believe type I is

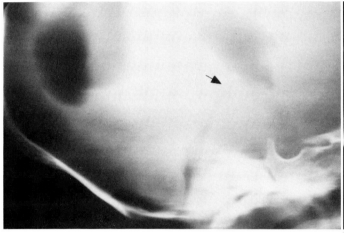

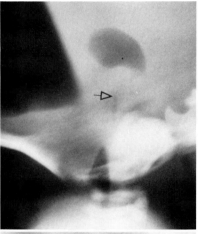

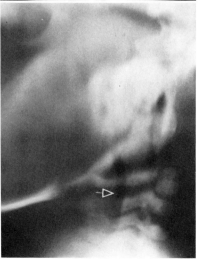

Fig. 16-2. Chiari malformation. A, Type I. Moderate hydrocephalus with an elongated, narrowed, and slightly kinked (arrow) aqueduct. The fourth ventricle is thin but normally positioned, the cisterna magna is small, and the tonsils are prolapsed. These findings must not be confused with those of a mass lesion in the posterior fossa. This patient had no spinal dysraphia. **B,** Type II. Significant hydrocephalus in a neonate with an elongated and thinned aqueduct (arrow) and the fourth ventricle positioned at the foramen magnum. **C,** Type II. The fourth ventricle (arrow) is markedly elongated and inferiorly positioned, extending down to the C5 level.

really an abnormally low orientation of the tonsils to the foramen magnum with a thinned but normally situated fourth ventricle (Fig. 16-2, *A*) and is not a mild form of type II. The aqueduct is elongated and narrowed, and a resultant hydrocephalus may be present. It is more properly considered under the general term *foramen magnum syndrome* and is probably due to bony cervical occipital dysplasia rather than to a hindbrain abnormality (Spillane et al., 1957). It might also be, primarily, an increased pressure within the posterior fossa (Brocklehurst, 1971).

Approximately 20% to 50% of the so-called type I Chiari malformations in adults have basilar impression (De Barros et al., 1968). This type presents in adulthood and is very rare in children under 10 years of age. It is not associated with spinal dysraphia (Greenfield, 1963) but rather with segmentation abnormalities of the upper cervical spine. At ventriculography, the fourth ventricle may appear to be a little thinner and elongated but not depressed (Fig. 16-2, *A*). At operation, there are peglike tonsils in the upper cervical cord associated with adhesions; and often a firm tethering fibrous band within the dura that passes across the tonsillar base at the foramen magnum. The association of hydrocephalus other than to a mild or moderate degree is not a feature.

Type II. This is the classical Chiari malformation; and, unless otherwise qualified, it is what we shall refer to as the Chiari malformation. It presents soon after birth or in early infancy. The pathology of the Chiari malformation is complex (Norman, 1963; Peach, 1965a,b; McCoy et al., 1967). The significant anatomical alterations that occur are as follows (Fig. 16-2, *B* and *C*), some of which are not neuroradiologically identifiable:

1. The pons is elongated, with partial or total displacement of the medulla into the cervical canal. The aqueduct (Fig. 16-2, *B*) and fourth ventricle also are elongated and narrowed, the majority of the ventricle being within the cervical canal (Fig. 16-2, *C*).

2. The cerebellum may wrap the pons laterally and anteriorly, enclosing the basilar artery, and may herniate superiorly through the tentorial hiatus. The tectum is prolonged upward and forms a beak at the colliculi (Daniel and Strich, 1958), often kinking the aqueduct and causing a slight aqueductal dilatation at the kink.

3. Fingerlike processes of the inferior cerebellar vermis are prolonged to varying degrees, often asymmetrically, together with the tonsils around the medulla and cervical cord. These processes are bound down by arachnoid and dural thickening (Alvord, 1961).

4. Often enlarged, the medulla ends abruptly; or it may fold the contiguous cervical cord, producing a characteristic Z shape. This kinking is due to the restraint by the cervical cord dentate ligaments, which prevent similar caudal displacement of the cord (Emery and MacKenzie, 1973). The upper cervical roots may have a horizontal or an upward course. An aqueductal stenosis or occlusion due to forking (rarely) (Russell, 1949), compression (commonly), or inflammatory gliosis (Cameron, 1957) occurs in every case. The stenosis may be converted into a complete occlusion by intracerebral hemorrhage or infection.

5. The brain often has an increased weight. The cerebrum may exhibit polymicrogyria.

Infants with the Chiari malformation commonly present neuroradiologically with at least a mild degree of hydrocephalus, but not necessarily a large head. We believe strongly that air ventriculography best demonstrates the abnormal morphology of the Chiari malformation complex. Skull radiographs prior to such ventriculography are essential. Angiography is rarely employed as the prime investigative procedure; and unless an aqueductal occlusion is thought clinically to be due to a posterior fossa mass lesion, we do not commonly use it as a subsequent investigation—except infrequently in older children whose hydrocephalus due to the Chiari malformation was investigated and treated elsewhere.

The spine. The Chiari malformation is *always* associated with some form of spinal dysraphia and rarely with merely a spina bifida of the lumbar or sacral region without abnormal cord coverings (Laurence, 1964). Although Peach (1964) and Teng and Papatheodorou (1964) each described one child with a Chiari malformation (type II) who they claimed had a normal spine, we have not seen such an example. The Chiari malformation will have an associated meningocele or, more commonly, a myelomeningocele, but the latter will always have an associated Chiari malformation (Norman, 1963); however, a simple meningocele may not.

In our experience, children presenting after infancy with a spina bifida alone and a low-fixed cord with or without a thick filum terminale as seen by myelography usually do not have a Chiari malformation and/or hydrocephalus. Spinal dysraphia occurs in the lumbar and sacral regions in approximately three quarters of these cases, and in the thoracic and lumbar regions in less than a quarter. Most dysraphic defects involve more than one spinal region. A purely thoracic meningocele or myelomeningocele is uncommon; but when it occurs, it is associated with a Chiari malformation.

Diastematomyelia is related to the Chiari malformation only because of its association with spinal

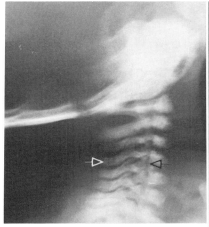

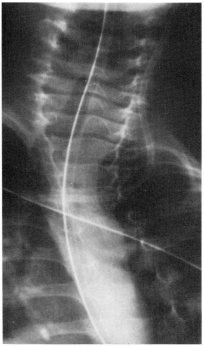

Fig. 16-3. Chiari malformation and a widened cervical canal. A, Widened sagittal diameter (arrows) due to extensively prolapsed tonsils. B, Widening of the cervical interpediculate distances down to Tl due to a Chiari malformation and hydromyelia. Note the slight widening of the thoracic interpediculate distances due to the hydromyelia.

dysraphia per se, and the same can be said for an associated hemivertebra. There is no direct cause-and-effect relationship.

Hydromyelia that is commonly associated with the Chiari malformation in infants is merely a thin patent central canal and is rarely identified by myelography (Harwood-Nash and Fitz, 1974). In older children who have a poorly treated hydrocephalus due to the Chiari malformation, however, it may develop into a formidable cyst in both diameter and extent and may expand the cervical and thoracic spinal canal (Harwood-Nash and Fitz, 1974). Moderate widening of the cervical spinal diameters (Fig. 16-3, A) at C1 to C6 is often present in the Chiari malformation; the mass effect of the herniated cerebellum and medulla is what causes this widening in infants, together with a possible large hydromyelia in older children.

Simple occipitalization of C1 is rarely associated with the type II Chiari malformation, but a nonossified posterior arch of C1 is often normally present and should not be mistaken for a spina bifida. Because of the herniated posterior fossa structures, the nonossified posterior arch later ossifies into a thinner than normal rim of bone. The Klippel-Feil syndrome (Fig. 16-4), together with a small occipital encephalocele, a cleft palate, and often congenital middle ear anomalies (particularly in females), is commonly associated with the Chiari malformation, usually type II; but if the encephalocele is large, the syndrome may also be associated with a type III

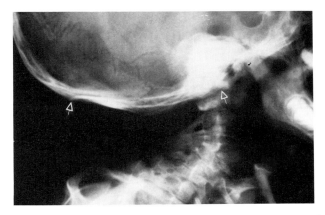

Fig. 16-4. Klippel-Feil syndrome and a Chiari type II malformation. A small encephalocele and an enlarged foramen magnum (arrows) are associated with a Chiari type II in an infant who has a Klippel-Feil syndrome of the cervical spine.

malformation (Hendrick et al., 1974). The Klippel-Feil complex in infants has some features similar to those in adults as described by Spillane and coworkers (1957).

MYELOGRAPHY. In children with spinal dysraphia, myelography will often reveal the cervical roots passing in an initially *upward* direction (Fig. 16-5), seen only in the Chiari malformation. When obtaining the films, therefore, the radiologist must be careful not to extend the head—for this will create a spurious upward course of the roots. The herniated tonsils

(Fig. 16-6) will be seen occupying the cervical canal to a lesser or greater extent in the Chiari malformation. Such prolapse of the tonsils may be clearly seen at oblique prone myelography or, if necessary, supine myelography. Contrast will not pass easily through the foramen magnum.

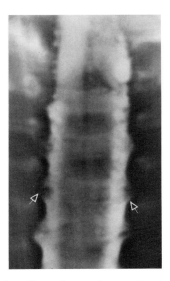

Fig. 16-5. Chiari malformation and upward extension of cervical roots. A Pantopaque myelogram reveals the low cervical roots (arrows) passing superiorly in a patient with a Chiari malformation.

The skull. A normal skull in an infant with the Chiari malformation must be very uncommon and has not occurred in our experience. Skull changes due to the addition of hydrocephalus from aqueductal stenosis and subarachnoid CSF obstruction broaden the spectrum of abnormalities present initially in, as well as during the subsequent natural history of, the Chiari malformation. We believe that the myelomeningocele, the Chiari malformation, and the *craniolacunia* form an inseparable triad; also that the craniolacunia (Fig. 16-7) is an intrinsic bony dysplasia of the membranous skull, with a common cause but a different form from dysplasia in other parts of the neural axis covering (i.e., the dysraphic spine, Chapter 18). It is thus an accompaniment and not a result of the Chiari malformation. We are furthermore of the opinion that all Chiari malformations have or have had an associated craniolacunia, which is rarely not obvious on skull radiographs at birth; its appearance varies from florid extensive lacunae to a subtle trabecular pattern in some part of the skull, particularly the occipital bone. It may be identified on maternal abdominal radiographs, only to have evanesced at birth. It disappears with increasing head size (Fig. 16-8) and age and is rarely present after 6 months of age.

Even though the ventricles may be moderately enlarged, the *head size* is usually normal at birth (Fig. 16-7, *A*). This paradox is explained by Padget (1972) as follows: some Chiari malformations have

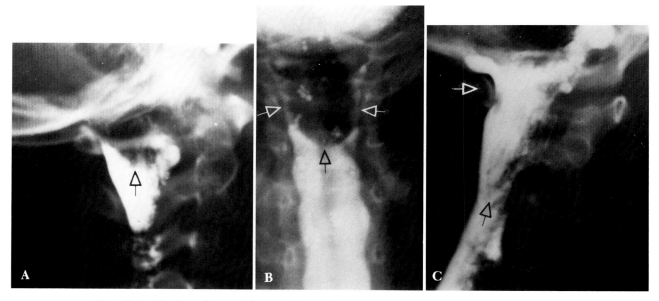

Fig. 16-6. Myelography and herniated tonsils. A, Lateral and, **B,** PA myelograms clearly demonstrate the outline of the inferiorly placed tonsils (arrows) in the Chiari malformation. **C,** A supine myelogram shows contrast passing around the herniated tonsils down to the level of C4 (black arrow). Note the impression on these tonsils by the posterior arch of the atlas (white arrow).

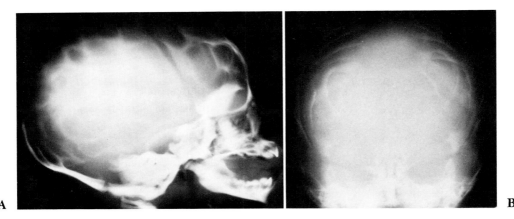

Fig. 16-7. Chiari malformation and craniolacunia. A neonatal skull with the Chiari malformation is often of normal size (**A**). Craniolacunia may be associated with a poorly ossified midline vault (**B**).

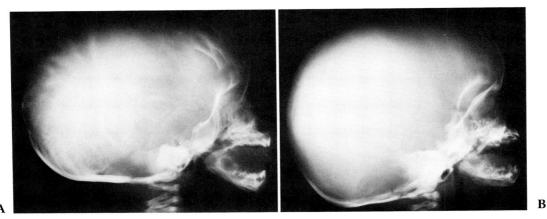

Fig. 16-8. Craniolacunia and hydrocephalus. Due to hydrocephalus (**B**), infantile craniolacunia will disappear with increasing age and with increasing head size. Note the flat occipital squamae often seen in the Chiari malformation.

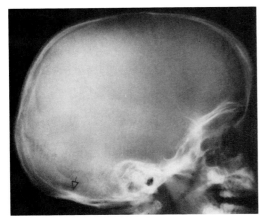

Fig. 16-9. Chiari malformation and a small posterior fossa. Note the large square head due to stenosis of the aqueduct; but the undersized clivus and the extremely low-placed torcular (arrow) indicate a small posterior fossa due to a Chiari malformation. The reduced size of the fossa is more pronounced in the Chiari than in a simple aqueductal stenosis.

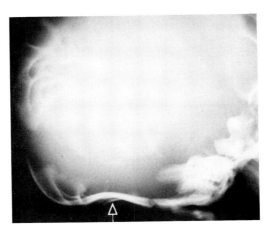

Fig. 16-10. Chiari malformation and convex occipital squamae. The Chiari malformation may also exhibit a slightly superiorly convex curve of the occipital squamae (arrow).

an embryologically small brain, or the ventricles never become small by the usual maturation and involution processes after early fetal life; however, in other Chiari malformations the cerebrum itself may be larger and heavier than normal.

The abnormal *configuration* of the skull consists of a low-placed inion, indicating at least a low posterior attachment of the tentorium at the torcular (Daniel and Strich, 1958) and thus implying a small posterior fossa (Fig. 16-9). No matter how extreme, hydro-

cephalus due to acquired aqueductal stenosis does not produce quite such a low position. In at least 50% of Chiari malformations, the occipital bone between the inion and the posterior foramen magnum will be quite flat (Fig. 16-8); in the rest it will retain varying degrees of its normal superiorly convex configuration (Fig. 16-10).

The greater the hydrocephalus and Chiari malformation, the straighter will be the portion of the occipital bone between the inion and the foramen magnum (Fig. 16-8, *B*). Platybasia or basilar invagination is not present in type II Chiari malformations. Increasing age and the success or failure of shunt procedures will alter skull abnormalities, regardless of cause. Scalloping of a posteriorly concave clivus, together with relative shortness of the clivus, is very common (Fig. 16-11). In older children, especially after successful shunting of the hydrocephalus, some remolding may occur.

An *enlarged foramen magnum*, usually pear shaped in a sagittal direction, is frequently observed; but a rounded posteriorly scalloped or asymmetrically shaped large foramen magnum may also occur (Fig. 16-12). Though uncommon, a normal foramen magnum may be present in infants (not in older children, however).

Scalloping of the posterior aspect of the petrous bone (Fig. 16-13) as seen on the basal skull radiograph (Kruyff and Jeffs, 1966) is not common in infants but is increasingly obvious as the child becomes older and is due to cerebellar compression. The rare parietal or high occipital encephalocele may be associated with the type II Chiari malformation. If a low occipital encephalocele occurs together with

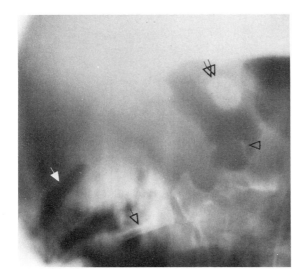

Fig. 16-11. Chiari malformation and the scalloped clivus. Note the short scalloped clivus (open arrow) with a low fourth ventricle (solid arrow), a large massa intermedia (double arrow), and the accessory commissure (arrowhead)—all characteristic of the Chiari malformation.

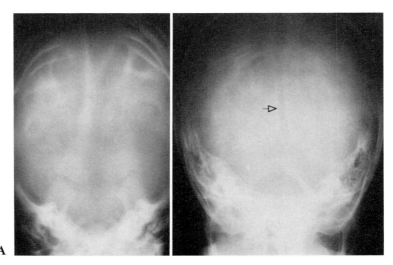

A   B

Fig. 16-12. Chiari malformation and a large foramen magnum. A, In a newborn child. B, In a 5-year-old child. Note the persistent occipital sinus groove (arrow) often seen with the Chiari malformation.

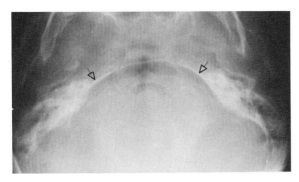

Fig. 16-13. Chiari malformation and petrous scalloping. Arrows denote petrous scalloping in a 6-year-old child with the Chiari malformation.

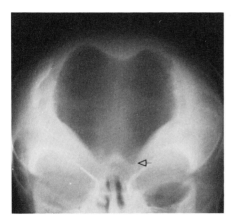

Fig. 16-14. Chiari malformation and the frontal horns. Note the enlarged frontal horns with an absent septum pellucidum but with a pointed floor (arrow).

Table 16-1. Skull abnormalities in Chiari malformation (type II)

	Infants	Children
Craniolacunia	Very common	Very rare
Low inion	Very common	Very common
Scalloped clivus	Very common	Common
Large head	Common	Very common
Large foramen magnum	Common	Very common
Petrous scalloping	Less common	Common
Normal skull	Very uncommon	Uncommon

cervical vertebral anomalies, a type III Chiari malformation will be present (Table 16-1).

COMPUTED TOMOGRAPHY. CT (Chapter 8) will identify the large ventricles but not the displaced fourth ventricle. A large massa intermedia may be seen projecting through the third ventricle. We have noted that the absorption coefficient for the midline cerebellum is especially increased in the Chiari malformation—to between 20 and 24 EMI units (i.e., greater than that for the normal cerebellar vermis).

VENTRICULOGRAPHY. The neuroradiological investigation of the Chiari malformation is by air ventriculography with tomography. It is our belief and recommendation that angiography has no place in the *initial* study of the Chiari malformation.

The ventricles are moderately enlarged at birth, even though the head may be of normal size (often with a bulging fontanelle); therefore no technical problem presents at ventriculography. Sufficient air and cerebrospinal fluid must be exchanged to provide an air-fluid level at least at the foramina of Monro in the brow-up position. If the ventricles are extremely large, approximately 40 cc of exchanged air will suffice. The "bubble" study is to be condemned.

Many of the pathological features of the Chiari malformation that we described previously are clearly demonstrated in vivo by ventriculography (Gooding et al., 1967; McCoy et al., 1967).

Lateral ventricles. The size of the lateral ventricles varies according to the age of the infant. If ventriculography is performed within days of birth, moderate dilatation is present and is particularly prominent in the frontal horns. At a later age or after the myelomeningocele or meningocele has been repaired (if possible) or if meningitis has supervened, the ventricles and the head become very large. This enlargement is due to increasing severity of occlusion of the aqueduct.

The shape of the *frontal horns* is characteristic insofar as the inferior angle is abnormally pointed (Gooding et al., 1967) and the frontal horns themselves are more bulbous (Fig. 16-14). These changes are due to a prominent head of the caudate nucleus and probably also to the deficient formation of the forceps minor, both of which help to form the normal shape of the frontal horns. Gooding and co-workers (1967) suggested that some medially directed force juxtaposes the hemispheres, thereby creating a deformity and the large massa intermedia; and they question whether similar abnormalities could occur in sagittal synostosis. Our experience with pneumoencephalography and sagittal synostosis, however, suggests that the answer is no. We believe the midbrain to be involved in the general hyperplasia of the brain stem and in the encephalocranial disproportion of the posterior fossa.

The *midbrain* may partially protrude into the posterior fossa through a wide tentorial hiatus, particularly if there is an associated marked hydrocephalus.

The *corpus callosum* is seldom absent. The roof of each lateral ventricle is a flatter than normal V—suggesting hypoplasia of the falx and a poorer falcine impression between the ventricles (Fig. 16-14). Heterotopic gray matter is rarely large enough to be visualized. Though the septum pellucidum may

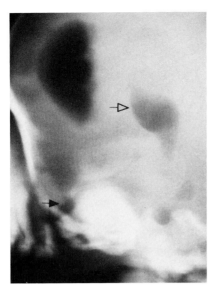

Fig. 16-15. Chiari malformation and upward displacement of the brain stem. The high position of the suprapineal recess of the third ventricle (open arrow), even in the face of moderate hydrocephalus, is probably due to upward transtentorial herniation of the cerebellum and brain stem as part of the Chiari malformation. Note the characteristically elongated inferiorly positioned fourth ventricle (solid arrow).

be absent (Fig. 16-14), a cystic septum is relatively common and its thin walls are often not obvious on standard ventriculograms without tomography. This is not specific to Chiari malformation.

The *third ventricle* is usually slightly enlarged initially and becomes even larger with advancing age and increasing aqueductal stenosis. Its size does not increase so much with enlargement of the lateral ventricles as occurs with acquired postinflammatory aqueductal stenosis in otherwise normal children. Its low position is due to the small posterior fossa. The suprapineal recess may enlarge enormously with increasing hydrocephalus. Upward displacement of the recess and floor of the third ventricle and the origin of the aqueduct (Fig. 16-15) may be seen in neonatal infants without marked hydrocephalus and is probably due to upward transtentorial herniation of the cerebellum and brain stem, which is reversed with increasing hydrocephalus.

Particularly if ventriculography is performed at an early age—the enlargement of the *accessory commissure* described by Gooding and co-workers (1967), occurring in the third ventricle adjacent to the lamina terminalis, is frequently seen (80%+). It may occur within the lamina terminalis and create a bulbous anterior outpouching, or it may be communicated to the lamina by a thin isthmus; in the latter instance, it is quite discrete within the third ventricular cavity, lying under the foramen of Monro (Fig. 16-16).

Though common in the Chiari malformation, this enlargement still is not absolutely specific, however. It also occurs in infants with simple hydrocephalus.

A large *massa intermedia* is common in infants with or without a Chiari malformation; but a Chiari malformation will often have a very large massa intermedia, which then appears to be more anteriorly placed (Fig. 16-17, A). The greater the hydrocephalus, the smaller becomes the massa. A small massa intermedia may be present de novo in a Chiari malformation (Fig. 16-17, B).

The changes in the *aqueduct* are quite specific. It is elongated and narrowed (Fig. 16-18, A) and may not readily permit the passage of air or oil. Generally a posterior kink and mild dilatation in the upper aqueduct at the approximate level of the colliculi reflect a tectal beaking (Fig. 16-18, B). The elongated aqueduct is quite vertical. This increase in aqueductal length may be partially due to squeezing of the upper fourth ventricle by the superior vermis, which segment is then taken up as part of the aqueduct. The superior medullary velum may be quite short and acutely curved or completely straightened (Fig. 16-18). The aqueduct is usually patent in neonates, but an abruptly tapered occlusion to air may be seen in its upper third.

With the infant in the brow-down position, a gentle tapping of the head and a 5-minute wait will often permit air to be visualized throughout the entire length of the aqueduct and into the fourth ventricle. If total occlusion is present (Fig. 16-16, C), the occlusion to air is usually abrupt and also appears near the third ventricle or within the upper segment of the aqueduct. We have failed to identify by air or positive contrast ventriculography any instance of a forked aqueduct with occlusion. Uncommonly will Pantopaque or Conray pass through the aqueduct in the Chiari malformation when air will not (Fig. 16-19).

The *fourth ventricle* is displaced inferiorly (Fig. 16-18). Sagittal tomography is essential for its accurate visualization. Its inferior limit is usually at C1 to C3, but we have observed the limit to be as low as C6. Demarcation of the junction between an inferiorly placed fourth ventricle and an accompanying hydromyelia may be quite difficult. If air fills the hydromyelia via the obex, the diameter of the hydromyelia and of the inferior fourth ventricle may be the same. Rarely are both the hydromyelia and the fourth ventricle quite large (Fig. 16-20, A). Though to identify an accompanying hydromyelia at ventriculography is unusual, positive contrast ventriculography (Fig. 16-20, B) will often permit such visualization on cervical spine radiographs taken 24 to 48 hours later (Harwood-Nash and Fitz, 1974).

situated below the foramen magnum (Fig. 16-28), and the origin of the PICA may also be displaced more inferiorly (Spillane et al., 1957; Greitz and Sjögren, 1963; Occleshaw, 1970). At postmortem examination, however, the loop is easily related not to the tonsils but to the herniated inferior cerebellar hemispheres. The tonsillar branch of the PICA is rarely visible in the Chiari malformation; but the hemispheric branches angle superiorly into the posterior fossa proper and are tightly applied to the inner table, a more reliable sign (Fig. 16-28). The actual herniation of the tonsils, which are thin peglike struc-

tures, was not usually identified angiographically but was inferred.

A more characteristic sign of the Chiari malformation, and probably the only truly reliable one, especially in small infants, is the horizontal (Fig. 16-25) or even downward (Fig. 16-29) orientation of the intraspinal portion of the vertebral artery just below the foramen magnum as seen in the AP projection. The artery will usually have an inferiorly convex loop. The distal vertebral arteries are then squeezed together and pass vertically for a short distance to form the origin of the basilar artery, often well below

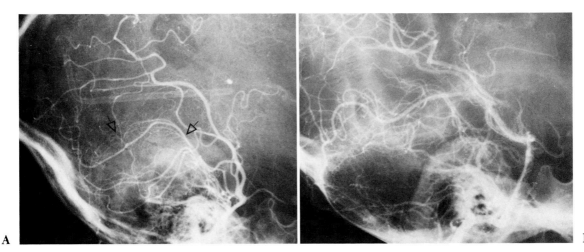

A   B

Fig. 16-27. Chiari malformation and the basilar artery. A, The tip of the artery is below the posterior clinoids, particularly with marked hydrocephalus. Note the small size of the cerebellum as indicated by the superior cerebellar artery (arrows). B, A type II Chiari malformation with a normally situated basilar artery.

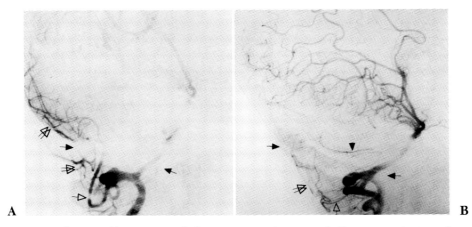

A   B

Fig. 16-28. Chiari malformation and the posterior inferior cerebellar artery. A, An inferior caudal loop of the PICA (open arrow) herniated below the foramen magnum (solid arrows). Some hemispheric branches (double arrows) are prolapsed and tightly applied to the foramen magnum and occiput, a reliable sign of inferior hemispheric herniation and the Chiari malformation. B, Marked downward displacement of the PICA (open arrow) and most of its branches (double arrow) below the level of the foramen magnum (solid arrows). The AICA is equally depressed (arrowhead).

the foramen magnum, particularly well seen on the straight AP vertebral angiogram and confirming angiographically the pathological observations made initially by Emery and Levick (1966) that this deformity is the result of displacement of the medulla inferiorly.

The *venous phase* of carotid and vertebral angiography reveals the straight sinus to be more vertical and often shorter than normal due to the wider tentorial hiatus and the smaller posterior fossa (Fig. 16-30). The torcular is extremely low, frequently only

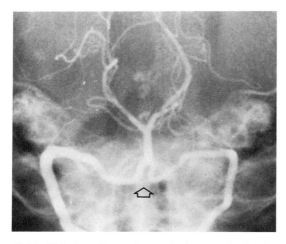

Fig. 16-29. Chiari malformation and the vertebrobasilar system. A characteristic sign of the Chiari malformation is approximation and often downward displacement of the distal vertebral arteries (arrow). Note the ∨ formation of the origin of the PCAs and their tight application to the brain stem.

a few centimeters behind the posterior tip of the foramen magnum; and the transverse sinuses pass anteriorly to the sigmoid sinus, which is situated a short distance above the rim of the foramen (Howieson and Norrell, 1969). The sagittal and transverse sinuses form a small open λ shape on the angled AP angiogram (Fig. 16-31). A midline occipital sinus may be seen passing down from the torcular around the foramen magnum to one or both sigmoid sinuses. Cerebellar and vermian veins will conform to the small size of the posterior fossa part of the cerebellum (Fig. 16-30), but rarely will the inferior cerebellar veins fill adequately on vertebral angiography; and if they do, they lose their usual recognizable pattern. The anterior pontomesencephalic vein will be displaced inferiorly with the basilar artery, particularly in light of hydrocephalus.

Dandy-Walker cyst

The Dandy-Walker syndrome is a congenital cystic dilatation of the fourth ventricle due to atresia at least of the foramen of Magendie, and possibly also the foramina of Luschka, associated with some form of vermian dysgenesis. Its exact in vivo identification demands precise neuroradiology to differentiate it from more common CSF-containing cysts or cisterns of the posterior fossa. The term *pseudo–Dandy-Walker syndrome* is not tenable and indicates only a poor understanding of the morphology of the Dandy-Walker syndrome and even poorer neuroradiology.

The possible morphogenesis of the Dandy-Walker cyst is said to be closely allied to that of the Chiari malformation and therefore probably to a disorder of closure of the neural tube (Gardner et al., 1972; Padget, 1972), but its precise morphogenesis has yet to be conclusively established. Boulter (1967) and Wolpert (1974) have provided an extensive

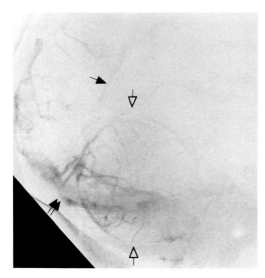

Fig. 16-30. Posterior dural sinuses and the Chiari malformation. The straight sinus is quite vertical (solid arrow) and often poorly filled. The torcular is extremely low (double arrow), and the vermian veins outline an extremely small cerebellum (open arrows).

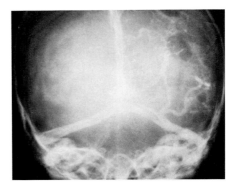

Fig. 16-31. Transverse sinuses and the Chiari malformation. The sinuses are inferiorly placed in the occiput and form an open λ. This configuration merely reflects the small posterior fossa.

discussion of the various theories, and we shall attempt to distill these.

The choroid plexus of the fourth ventricle forms at about the fourth week of embryonic development. Next, thinning of the rhombic roof of the fourth ventricle occurs; and the foramen of Magendie appears within the roof at the sixth week, just prior to the formation of the subarachnoid space (Blake, 1900; Weed, 1935). The superior vermis and then the inferior vermis, together with the cerebellum, start to develop at the sixth week. Primary foraminal atresia within the rhombic roof was proposed as the initiating factor by Dandy and Blackfan (1914), Taggart and Walker (1942), and later Gibson (1955).

The increasing size of the cystic fourth ventricle was supposed to inhibit cerebellar development. Gardner and co-workers (1972) considered the primary impermeability of the rhombic roof and persistent fetal hydrocephalus involving mainly the fourth ventricle to interfere with this development. Brodal and Hauglie-Hanssen (1959), however, believed that the hypoplasia of the vermis is primary along with the imperforate roof. These authors noted that the cerebellar anlagen fuse before the foramen of Magendie evolves. Benda (1954), who coined the eponym now used, considered the Dandy-Walker syndrome to be an embryonal maldevelopment and a failure of neural tube closure with diverticulation of the postmedullary velum (Padget, 1972). More recently, Padget (1972) considered it to be the result of a persistent separation of the cerebellar primordia by splitting (neuroschisis) of part of these primordia and scarring of the rhombic roof.

Certain points, however, are objectively defined and aid in the neuroradiological diagnosis of the Dandy-Walker cyst:

1. A variably large degree of *dilatation and deformity* of the fourth ventricle results from a cystic cavity of the entire fourth ventricle itself due to a large diverticulum of the inferior medullary velum (Gibson, 1955). The diverticulum has an intact upper fourth ventricular cavity. The cyst wall is lined on the inside by ependymal cells and pia arachnoid exteriorly. The choroid plexus is inferiorly placed.

2. The cerebellum is *small* and the inferior vermis is commonly *absent* or rudimentary; but the superior vermis, which forms first, is usually intact or is displaced superiorly.

3. The posterior fossa is very *large*.

4. Associated *cerebral malformations* are present— e.g., encephaloceles (McLaurin, 1964), extracranial anomalies (Juhl and Wesenberg, 1966), agenesis of the corpus callosum (Raimondi, 1971), holoprosencephaly, cerebral gyral and cerebellar folial abnormalities, heterotopias (Hart et al., 1972). Dandy-Walker cysts have occurred in siblings (Benda, 1954; D'Agostino et al., 1963).

5. A Dandy-Walker cyst is said *rarely* to have filled during lumbar pneumoencephalography (Strandgaard, 1970). Filling was probably via

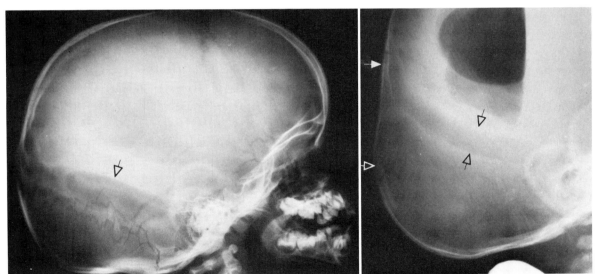

Fig. 16-32. Skull and the Dandy-Walker cyst. A, Severe thinning of the occipital and inferior parietal bones up to the level of the attachment of the dura of the transverse sinus (arrow). A well-formed sinus groove is not present as yet in this infant. The clivus is small and scalloped. **B,** Well-marked transverse sinus groove (open black arrows) with the torcular (solid arrow) high above the lambda (open white arrow).

patent foramina of Luschka. The lateral ventricles are surprisingly not so dilated as would be expected, indicating some egress of CSF from the cystic fourth ventricle.

Neuroradiology of Dandy-Walker syndrome

SKULL RADIOGRAPHY. The vault will be enlarged posteroinferiorly. In infants the inferior occipital bone has a superiorly concave instead of the normal inferiorly concave appearance and, together with the occipital squama, is thinned and ballooned (Bucy and Siqueira, 1937). The transverse sinus grooves are not easily visualized, but the torcular is displaced *above the lambda*.

A ridge on the inner table may be seen early in infancy delineating the upper lateral margin of the cyst and the tentorium where the tentorium meets the inner table at the transverse sinuses (Fig. 16-32, *A*). In older children the transverse sinuses are usually well seen (Fig. 16-32, *B*). The gross dilatation of the fourth ventricle that develops early in fetal life prevents the normal downward migration of the transverse sinuses and torcular to their ultimate orientation (which is attained at the third month of gestation); therefore the sinuses and torcular persist above the developing lambda in the vault. The sinuses are originally above the lambdoid sutures in the fetus. An acquired posterior fossa cyst can expand the occipital bone and create a high position of the sinuses and lambda, but there is never a torcular-lambdoid inversion because the cyst develops after the normal orientation of the sinuses at the inner table is established. Sinuses can never be displaced across sutures once both structures have formed.

This torcular-lambdoid inversion is pathognomonic of a Dandy-Walker cyst and is best seen in children older than 2 years, at which time the sinus grooves are well formed. Without treatment, the cystic expansion of the occipital bone will enlarge considerably in older children. The square-shaped head with bulging occiput (Fig. 16-32, *A*) is typical of a chronic mass lesion of the posterior fossa such as a Dandy-Walker cyst (Benda, 1954). The smaller diverticular variant of the Dandy-Walker syndrome may not be large enough to cause this inversion.

Due to hydrocephalus of the lateral ventricles, *skull size* in infancy may be increased; but the vault, other than the occipital area, may be of normal size. A similar discrepancy occurs in older children, which may be explained by patency of the foramina of Luschka and/or transependymal absorption of CSF in the lateral ventricles or in the wall of the cyst itself (Juhl and Wesenberg, 1966). Sutures are usually chronically split, the lambdoids more than the coronal, with elongated digitations—a finding usually

seen only in chronic large posterior fossa mass lesions or in occipital trauma.

The *clivus* is small and may be gently scalloped concave posteriorly (Fig. 16-32, *A*); the foramen magnum is rounded or oval from front to back but is not usually enlarged (refer to discussion of Chiari malformation). Scalloping of the petrous ridges is not seen.

COMPUTED TOMOGRAPHY. CT will reveal precisely a huge posterior fossa cyst, together with a small cerebellar remnant, and no fourth ventricle; the cyst contains cerebrospinal fluid. The ependymal diverticular form will have a detectable partial fourth ventricle, and there will be a wide communication between the cyst and the ventricle (Chapter 8).

VENTRICULOGRAPHY. Air ventriculography and/or computed tomography are performed before angiography. Air ventriculography will often reveal surprisingly moderate-sized lateral ventricles and a third ventricle as noted before. The ventricles may be huge, however, and the occipital horns of the lateral ventricles superiorly displaced by the high tentorium. An absent corpus callosum is commonly associated with a Dandy-Walker cyst or variant and will be clearly shown by ventriculography (Fig. 16-33). The aqueduct is taken up by the cystic expansion of the fourth ventricle, and air passes from the third ventricle directly into the dilated fourth ventricle (Fig. 16-34).

We have not found the aqueduct to be obstructed in the Dandy-Walker syndrome. This occurred in one of the cases reported by Raimondi and co-workers (1969). Careful rotation of the infant will enable the air to outline the entire cyst. The cyst often interposes itself between the tentorium and the superior cerebellar hemispheres and may even reach the colliculi (Fig. 16-35). A tongue of the cyst that herniates down through the foramen magnum behind the cord (Fig. 16-34) is *not* pathognomonic of a Dandy-Walker cyst but occurs in arachnoid cysts of the posterior fossa. Small superiorly and laterally placed impressions into the cysts will be seen on ventriculography and are due to the cerebellar remnants.

The diverticular variant of the Dandy-Walker syndrome has a large partially formed fourth ventricle, a wide foramen of Magendie and valleculae, absence of the inferior vermis, often small cerebellar hemispheres, and varying sizes and shapes of the cystic cavity (Fig. 16-36); however, the variant is never quite as large as the true Dandy-Walker cyst. Such diverticulations are rather difficult to differentiate by CT or air ventriculography alone from arachnoid cysts, especially cysts that communicate with the fourth ventricle.

On only one occasion have we observed ventricu-

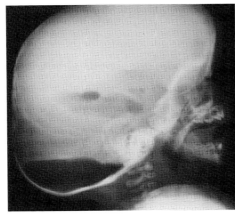

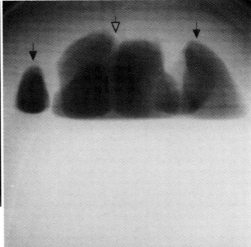

Fig. 16-33. Dandy-Walker cyst and an absent corpus callosum. A, The cyst is filled with air at ventriculography. B, The corpus callosum is absent in the same patient, and there is an enormous third ventricle (open arrow) herniating superiorly between the lateral ventricles (solid arrows). C, A large cyst (arrows) in an older child with absent corpus callosum. Note the herniation of the third ventricle superiorly between the lateral ventricles. Air has escaped from the fourth ventricle and is filling the sulci.

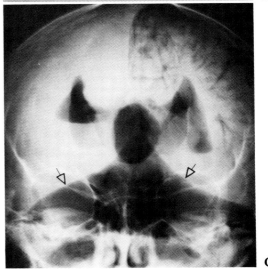

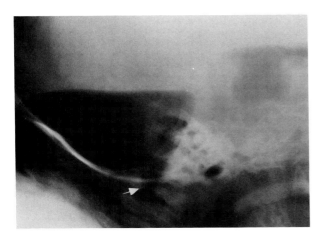

Fig. 16-34. Dandy-Walker cyst. Air passed immediately from the third ventricle anteriorly into the large cystic fourth ventricle. A little prolapsed tongue of the fourth ventricle (arrow) through the foramen magnum is not typical of a Dandy-Walker cyst but can also occur in arachnoid cysts of the posterior fossa.

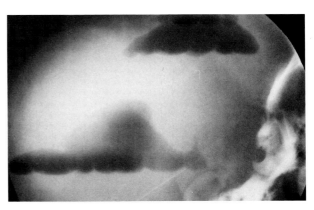

Fig. 16-35. Dandy-Walker cyst. The superior aspect of a large cyst may interpose itself anteriorly between the cerebellar remnant and the tentorium.

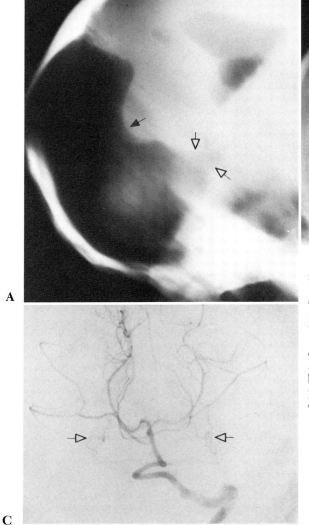

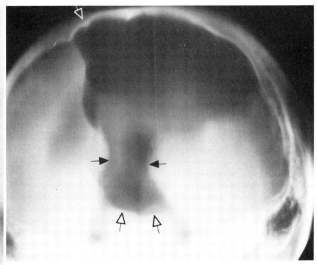

A

B

C

Fig. 16-36. Dandy-Walker variant. A, Large posterior fossa cyst with only the upper portion of the fourth ventricle (open arrows), no vermis, and a small impression of the remnants of the cerebellum superiorly (solid arrow). B, An AP tomogram shows the floor of the fourth ventricle (open black arrows), the widened valleculae (solid arrows), and a large cyst which has scalloped the occipital bone (open white arrow). C, An AP vertebral angiogram demonstrates marked kinking of the vertebrobasilar junction, no filling of the PICAs, but wide displacement of the AICAs (arrows). There also is no corpus callosum in this child.

lographic air to exit from a large Dandy-Walker cyst (Fig. 16-33, B), but from which orifice we were unable to say. We have not performed pneumoencephalography on any infants and children with the Dandy-Walker cyst and do not advise this recourse in children in whom such a cyst is suspected. Though postinflammatory or posthemorrhagic adhesions may occlude the outlets of the fourth ventricle and produce large lateral ventricles with an enlarged fourth ventricle, they never do so to the extent of a Dandy-Walker cyst. The fourth ventricle does not expand the bony confines of the posterior fossa.

On pneumoencephalography or ventriculography an infant may exhibit an inordinately large cisterna magna, particularly if a milder degree of extraventricular obstructive hydrocephalus is present (Chapter 15). This is quite normal.

ANGIOGRAPHY. Angiography will serve to determine whether a mass is intra–fourth ventricular or extra-cerebellar and whether vascular or not. In these instances it is helpful (Wolpert et al., 1970; Raimondi, 1971; Swischuk et al., 1972; LaTorre et al., 1973; Wolpert, 1974); but in our experience its correct interpretation has often been difficult. The size of the lateral ventricles may also be determined by angiography.

The angiographic evidence of a Dandy-Walker cyst is based primarily on the PICAs and may be quite variable, depending on the degree and form of the cyst.

1. In the diverticular form there is relatively little displacement of the SCAs and AICAs other than mild stretching and displacement. The retromedullary segment of the PICA is displaced anteriorly and often

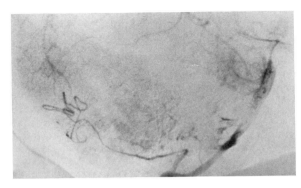

Fig. 16-37. Dandy-Walker cyst and the posterior inferior cerebellar artery. A long disorganized PICA passes laterally to form a tangle of vessels. No vermian artery is seen.

superiorly, and the vermian branch and often most of the hemispheric branches are absent. The inferior vermis itself is absent. The choroidal tuft, however, may be seen inferiorly and will be anteriorly placed.

2. When the cyst is grossly enlarged, the SCAs appear to be above the posterior cerebral arteries on the lateral angiogram and the hemispheric branches appear to feed the superior vermis and upper cerebellar hemispheres. The AICAs are small and with the basilar artery are displaced superiorly; the basilar is often quite elongated.

3. The PICAs may not be present or may be very small and pass laterally from their basilar or vertebral origin, losing their cranial and caudal or perimedullary curves (Fig. 16-37). They also tend to branch into fine vessels that disappear after a few centimeters. A vermian branch is not present. A small high cerebellar capillary blush is often seen and represents the superior vermis and remaining cerebellar hemispheres.

The *venous phase* shows a flattened vein of Galen which is elevated and often bowed inferiorly concave, together with the straight sinus, and a high torcular above the lambda. The transverse sinuses angle steeply down to the sigmoid sinus and cross the lambdoid suture; each may often have an inferiorly concave bend forming a large λ (the Chiari malformation forms a low small λ). An arachnoid cyst may cause transverse sinus enlargement, but the changes are confined to below the lambdoid sutures. The superior cerebellar and anterior pontomesencephalic veins are displaced superiorly and anteriorly, and the inferior vermian vein is absent.

The *differential diagnosis* of Dandy-Walker cysts includes posterior fossa arachnoid cysts and a normally large cisterna magna (Chapter 15). Precise neuroradiology is required to differentiate these conditions.

At ventriculography, a posterior fossa arachnoid cyst may communicate with or obstruct the fourth ventricle; but angiography will reveal a normal complement of cerebellar vessels displaced anteriorly and superiorly, often to a considerable degree, creating a small cerebellum. This displacement, however, is from an extracerebellar mass lesion.

The cisterna magna may normally be quite enlarged in infants and small children and may even herniate through a defect in the tentorium. It does not balloon the occipital bone, however, though its margins may groove the inner table (as does a Dandy-Walker variant cyst, Fig. 16-36). Large vermian or intra–fourth ventricular neoplasms will displace intact vessels and often be vascular. A cystic astrocytoma will expand the occipital bone on one side, but usually only to a minor degree.

Absence of the corpus callosum

The corpus callosum may be absent due to a primary embryonic agenesis or a dysgenesis secondary to acquired intrauterine encephalomalacia. Absence may be partial or complete and be associated with additional intracranial malformations. Agenesis is considered to be a disorder of closure.

The corpus callosum and its abnormalities were presented by Bull (1967)—who detailed its history, development, anatomy, malformations, and neoplasms. Brun and Probst (1973) and Probst (1973) outlined a similar and most detailed description and the reader is strongly urged to consult these studies.

The callosal commissural fibers, the great connecting system between the cerebral hemispheres, have their origin at the upper end of the developing lamina terminalis of the telencephalon—which appears at the third month of embryonic development. These commissural fibers with the developing hemispheres converge fanlike medially to concentrate at the midline and form a dense aggregation of brain tissue. As the primitive cerebral hemispheres grow out and then posteriorly, the callosal aggregate of commissural connections persists in a backward extension as a discrete midline band. The anterior genu, then the body, and finally the posterior splenium develop by the fifth month.

Two deviations from this developmental pattern may occur, however (Fig. 16-38):

1. The initial connections between the commissural fibers across the midline may fail to take place—possibly because of some unknown chemical or mechanical factors affecting the fetus (Rakic and Yakovlev, 1968)—leading to *complete agenesis* of the corpus callosum. A large callosal bundle of fibers passing anteroposteriorly on the medial aspect of the ventricles but disconnected from each other persists (Norman, 1963).

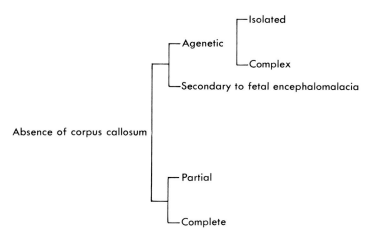

Fig. 16-38. Absence of the corpus callosum.

This abnormality may be further divisible into *isolated* agenesis and *complex* agenesis. The latter is associated with additional congenital malformations such as the following: polymicrogyria or white matter heterotopias within the anterior cerebral artery territory (Norman, 1963), midline intracerebral lipomas (Sutton, 1949; Sabourard et al., 1967), encephaloceles (Van Nouhuys and Bruyn, 1964; Pollack et al., 1968; Harwood-Nash, 1972), interhemispheric arachnoid cysts (Zingesser et al., 1964), microcephaly (Brun and Probst, 1973), Dandy-Walker cyst (Van Epps, 1953), the Chiari malformation, the cyclopia-holoprosencephaly complex (Yakovlev, 1959; Loeser and Alvord, 1968a,b; Warkany, 1971), septo-optic dysplasia (de Morsier, 1962).

What causes this aberration of embryogenesis is not certain. Heredity (Zellweger, 1952) seems to play a part, as we have observed in two brothers. Naiman and Fraser (1955) observed corpus callosal agenesis in identical twin sisters, and Ziegler (1958) observed it in three brothers. Elliott and Wollin (1961) reported absence of the corpus in a patient with tuberous sclerosis. True arrhinencephaly with absence of the corpus occurs in trisomy 13-15.

2. A formed corpus callosum may be subjected to some acquired fetal insult—leading to encephalomalacia and callosal destruction or hypoplasia *(partial agenesis)*. Such insults may be vascular with infarction in the anterior cerebral pathway (Loeser and Alvord, 1968a,b; Brun and Probst, 1973) or inflammatory (Friedman and Cohen, 1947; Marburg, 1949).

Marburg (1949) suggested that vascular infarction occurs after the corpus callosum has developed because the anterior cerebral artery is not fully differentiated when the corpus starts to form. The long callosal paramedian bundle characteristic of isolated agenesis is not present, however. Such acquired absence may be total or partial and may be associated with microcephaly (Brun and Probst, 1973) or with hydrocephalus and/or porencephaly (including macrocrania due to aqueductal occlusion or the Chiari malformation). Macrocrania may also be due to an interhemispheric arachnoid cyst. We have angiographic evidence to show the concomitance of vascular infarction and medial porencephalic cysts. To differentiate the primary and secondary forms of absence of the corpus callosum by neuroradiological means alone, however, may be quite difficult.

We have identified partial agenesis of the corpus callosum in both the posterior segment (splenium), as described by Bull in 1967, and the anterior segment, as described by Banergee and Sayers in 1972; and Probst in 1974; and we are in possession of two examples of each type.

Neuroradiology of corpus callosal absence. It is our policy to perform pneumoencephalography (or ventriculography if hydrocephalus is suspected) and angiography in the study of this often puzzling malformation. Our experience numbers twenty cases of complete absence and four cases of partial absence of the corpus callosum. Patients who present with hydrocephalus are usually infants, and the absence is often discovered serendipitously (Koch and Doyle, 1957). Some patients are mentally aberrated nonhydrocephalic children; others are microcephalic children, on whom pneumoencephalography is first performed.

SKULL RADIOGRAPHY. This procedure may reveal microcrania, a normal-sized skull, or macrocrania; or it may demonstrate the association of a median cleft syndrome with evidence of a cleft palate, hypotelorism, and trigonocephaly. In some infants, however, particularly if the absent corpus callosum is concomitant with a transsphenoidal or transnasal en-

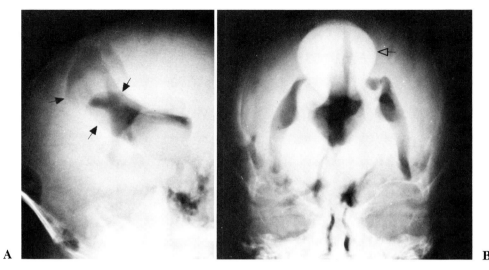

Fig. 16-39. Parietal encephalocele with an absent corpus callosum. The suprapineal recess (**A,** arrows) enters the encephalocele. Note the absence of the corpus callosum and the encephalocele (**B,** arrow).

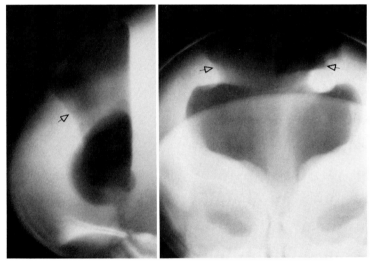

Fig. 16-40. Huge third ventricle and an absent corpus callosum. Lateral and AP views show a huge superiorly herniated ventricle (arrows) in the interhemispheric compartment.

cephalocele (Pollock et al., 1968; Suwanwela and Suwanwela, 1972), hypertelorism will be present. Craniolacunia with a myelomeningocele indicates a Chiari malformation and may occur (rarely) when the corpus is absent. A Dandy-Walker syndrome with a large posterior fossa also may accompany the condition (Fig. 16-33). An associated parietal or transethmoidal encephalocele may be present, or an elevated third ventricle and suprapineal recess may provide ventricular extension into a parietal encephalocele (Fig. 16-39).

Macrocrania is due to hydrocephalus with the Chiari or Dandy-Walker malformations or more commonly to aqueductal stenosis or a large midline arachnoid cyst. Hydrocephalus may be complicated by large porencephalic cysts (Chapter 15) or a superior extension of the third ventricle (Fig. 16-40) (Brocklehurst, 1973).

COMPUTED TOMOGRAPHY. CT (Chapter 8) will reveal a disordered collection of cerebrospinal fluid–filled spaces and alone may not provide good evidence of an absent corpus callosum. A large midline cerebrospinal fluid–containing "cyst," however (i.e., the third ventricle), may suggest it as a probable diagnosis.

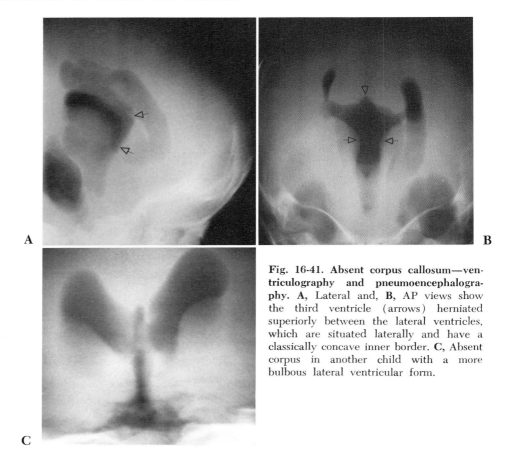

Fig. 16-41. Absent corpus callosum—ventriculography and pneumoencephalography. A, Lateral and, B, AP views show the third ventricle (arrows) herniated superiorly between the lateral ventricles, which are situated laterally and have a classically concave inner border. C, Absent corpus in another child with a more bulbous lateral ventricular form.

PNEUMOENCEPHALOGRAPHY OR VENTRICULOGRAPHY. Either of these is the diagnostic procedure of choice and will detail the entire ventricular geography of the malformation (Fig. 16-41). The classical neuroradiological criteria as described by Davidoff and Dyke (1934) are applied to the isolated complete agenesis:

1. Marked separation of the lateral ventricles
2. Narrow frontal horns (unless hydrocephalus is present)
3. Sharply angled lateral peaks of the frontal horns and bodies of the lateral ventricles
4. Relative dilatation of the occipital horns with a concavity to the medial border of the ventricles
5. Elongation of the foramina of Monro
6. General dilatation of the third ventricle with a varying degree of interposition between the lateral ventricles

The sharp outward angulation of the lateral ventricles is due to the lack of a support normally provided the ventricles by the forceps major and minor and the corona radiata as occurs with an intact corpus callosum. The ventricles may, however, be quite bulbous (Fig. 16-41, C). Furthermore, there is no septum pellucidum. The medial concavity results from the longitudinal callosal bundle. Deformities of the ventricular outline caused by gray matter heterotopias are relatively common.

The dilatation and upward extension of the third ventricle are greatly variable. We have observed third ventricles occupying virtually the entire inter–cerebral hemispheric region, even extending posterosuperiorly into a parietal meningocele (Fig. 16-39). It may not be possible to differentiate the ventricular lumen from an air-filled medially placed arachnoid (Fig. 16-42, A) or porencephalic (Fig. 16-42, B) cyst. In some instances, however, the size and upward extension of the ventricle may be quite modest (Fig. 16-41, C).

Anterior partial absence of the corpus callosum is probably due to a focal encephalomalacic process, and only the anterior third ventricle herniates upward between the frontal horns and anterior body of the lateral ventricles (Fig. 16-43, A and B) (Probst, 1974). Posterior partial absence is probably due to an incomplete formation of the corpus, and the posterior third ventricle herniates posterosuperiorly (Fig. 16-43, C and D). Absence of the corpus anteriorly or posteriorly may closely simulate a callosal neoplasm or mass lesion (Probst, 1974).

In some cases of corpus callosal absence—due to

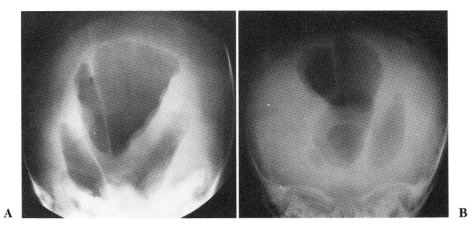

Fig. 16-42. Associated cysts and an absent corpus callosum. A, Large arachnoid cyst. B, Large multiloculated porencephalic cyst above the third ventricle. Unless pneumoencephalography fills the cyst (as in A) or ventriculography fills it (as in B), the two types usually cannot be differentiated by neuroradiological means alone.

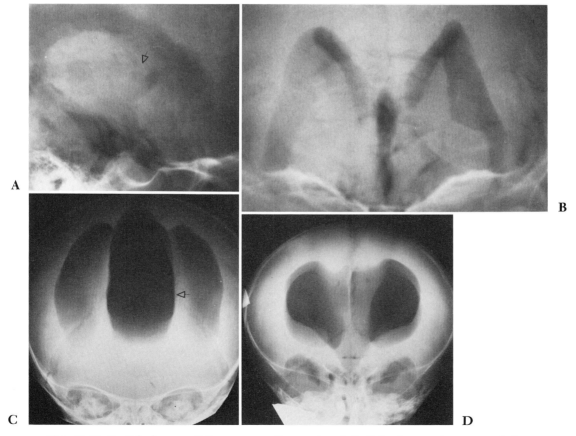

Fig. 16-43. Partial absence of the corpus callosum. A and B, Only the anterior aspect of the third ventricle herniates superiorly (arrow). In this patient the posterior corpus was seen to be intact. C and D, Posterosuperior prolapse of the third ventricle (arrow) due to absence, except for an intact anterior portion, of the corpus (D). Note the septum pellucidum, indicating formation of the anterior corpus.

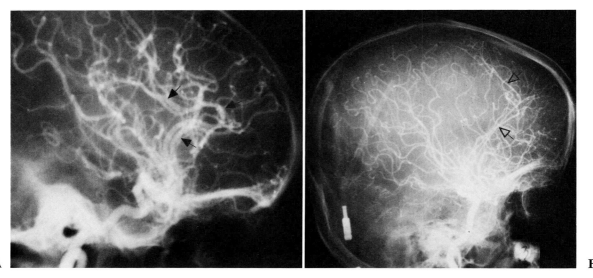

Fig. 16-44. Angiography and an absent corpus callosum. A, Markedly wavy course of the anterior cerebral artery (arrows) without its usual form around the corpus. **B,** Elevation and distortion of the anterior cerebral (arrows) with an absent corpus callosum and a large superiorly herniated third ventricle. Note the wavy course of the middle cerebral arteries, which in this patient indicates an associated polymicrogyria.

the possible congenital lack of a callosal bundle in the isolated locations, neither the sharp slitlike frontal horns nor the severe medial concavity will be seen. A mild to moderate hydrocephalus, together with greater dilatation of the occipital horns and porencephalic cysts, may accompany these findings (Fig. 16-42).

ANGIOGRAPHY. Cerebral angiography further details the morphological abnormalities of the absent corpus callosum (Holman and MacCarty, 1959; Morris, 1962; Nobler et al., 1963; Handa et al., 1969), thereby providing a clue to a possible *acquired* encephaloclastic form of absence.

At angiography, there may be evidence of peripheral arterial occlusive disease. It has been our experience and the experience of Brun and Probst (1973) that these cases of absent corpus callosum are due to some encephalomalacic process during or after the development of the corpus callosum.

Whatever the possible cause, the isolated agenesis form is associated with the following abnormalities:

1. The anterior cerebral artery initially takes a *wavy vertical course* without the normal smooth anteriorly convex curve that occurs around an intact rostrum and genu (Fig. 16-44, *A*). The latter is present, however, in the posterior partial absence. There is no clear division into the pericallosal and callosomarginal arteries, and the cortical branches extend fanlike up the medial wall of the cerebrum. The anterior cerebral branches may also be widely separated and elevated by the superiorly herniating third ventricle (Fig. 16-44, *B*). An azygous anterior

cerebral artery may uncommonly be present (Danziger et al., 1972). A sharp angle may occur anteriorly as the anterior cerebral abruptly courses posteriorly near its origin. This happens especially when the herniation of the third ventricle is more posterior than anterior (Fig. 16-44, *B*).

2. The middle cerebral arteries are usually not altered; but their *branches* may appear to be more wavy, indicating polymicrogyria with relative lack of major sulcal formation (Fig. 16-44, *B*). The middle cerebral arteries may also appear to course in a steeper orientation.

3. The veins of the *septum pellucidum* are paired and usually quite apart due to the herniated third ventricle; they drain the medial wall of the frontal horns. Due to the upward extension of the third ventricle (Fig. 16-45), the internal cerebral veins are higher and more posteriorly placed; or if the extension is considerable, the veins are split apart on each side of this herniation. The vein of Galen is straightened, for there is no splenium to give it the usual U shape (Fig. 16-45).

4. Because absence or hypoplasia of the falx is commonly associated with an absent corpus callosum, the inferior sagittal sinus may not be present.

Hydrocephalus will tend to alter the general orientation of these vessels by virtue of the mass effect of the dilated ventricles themselves. The wavy appearance of the anterior cerebral artery persists. A shunted severe hydrocephalus without agenesis of the corpus callosum will often demonstrate a remarkably similar wavy anterior cerebral artery due to the partial return

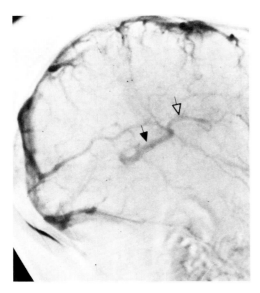

Fig. 16-45. Absent corpus callosum and the deep venous drainage. The internal cerebral vein is displaced superiorly (open arrow), and the vein of Galen is straightened and displaced posteriorly and superiorly (solid arrow).

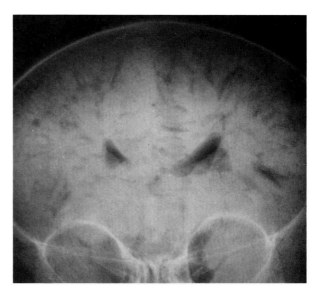

Fig. 16-46. Anterior lipoma of the corpus callosum. There is acute displacement laterally and inferiorly of the lateral ventricles. This appearance can be induced by any mass lesion in the region, be it cystic or neoplastic. Lipomas may calcify.

of the corpus callosum to its normal orientation (its having been remarkably stretched and elevated by the hydrocephalus). The anterior cerebral artery does not follow this descent.

Angiography will assist in differentiating mass lesions of the corpus callosum that may give a false impression of partial absence. Hematoma (Probst, 1974), lipoma (if not associated with absence of the corpus), and astrocytoma are such masses.

The differentiation of a large third ventricle, a midline arachnoid cyst, and a midline porencephalic cyst may be rather difficult. A porencephalic cyst and a huge third ventricle will fill on ventriculography and may be either a postinfarction porencephalic cyst or part and parcel of the early embryonic malformation (i.e., a schizencephalic cyst described by Yakovlev and Wadsworth, 1946). Disordered vascular architecture in turn will be produced. A porencephalic cyst is associated with hydrocephalus. An arachnoid cyst, however, will not; rather it will fill via lumbar pneumoencephalography and is often not associated with hydrocephalus.

Lipoma of the corpus callosum

A lipoma of the corpus callosum commonly presents in teen-agers and young adults and is very rare at any age (Chapters 2 and 11). We have had experience with only one such case, in an 8-year-old child. Agenesis of the corpus is said to be associated with 50% of lipomas (Sabourard et al., 1967). A lipoma is a congenital malformation due to defective embryogenesis and results in a masslike remnant of primitive fat in

the midline telencephalon. A dysraphic neural axis abnormality is usually an accompanying feature (Krainer, 1935).

A lipoma is a localized mass within or replacing the genu of the corpus callosum. Due to its fatty content, it may be visible on standard skull radiographs as a lucent image; and in older children it may contain a rim of calcification. Computed tomography will precisely reveal its constituents and its location. Ventriculography or pneumoencephalography will demonstrate a mass between the frontal horns and above the anterior third ventricle (Fig. 16-46) as well as the possible absence of the rest of the corpus callosum. Angiography of the anterior cerebral arteries (which may be azygous) (Danziger et al., 1972) will show the arteries to be quite dilated and their lumina distorted within the mass itself in an odd fusiform aneurysmal fashion (Wolpert et al., 1972).

Cranial meningocele and encephalocele

The cranioschisis group of disorders of closure include meningocele, encephalocele, and anencephaly (Pollock and Newton, 1971). The last is of purely pathological interest in its true form (Warkany, 1971). A cranial meningocele and an encephalocele are less common than their spinal counterpart (1 to 6) and occur predominantly in the midline occipital region with or without concomitant upper cervical meningocele. A cranial meningocele and an encephalocele occur in approximately 4 of every 10,000 births (Leck, 1966), or in 15% of all craniospinal dysraphic states with a meningocele alone or with neural herniations

(Ingraham and Swan, 1943). An occipital encephalocele is the commonest, and then, in order, the frontal, parietal, and finally the basal encephalocele.

The neuroradiological characteristics of these anomalies are described in Chapter 2. Their ventricular and angiographic characteristics merit description for two reasons. Neuroradiological investigations will provide the neurosurgeon with evidence of the presence of possible absence of brain tissue within the meningocele sac (Lorber, 1967; Guthkelch, 1970; Gilmor et al., 1972). Furthermore, such investigations will establish the possible presence of associated congenital cerebral malformations like agenesis of the corpus callosum (Pollock et al., 1968; Tandon, 1970), porencephaly, and holoprosencephaly (Suwanwela and Suwanwela, 1972).

Ventriculography will often fail to reveal brain tissue in a large craniomeningocele but will best detect abnormalities of the ventricular system such as an absent corpus callosum, porencephaly, or a heterotopia. Ventriculography also will demonstrate ventricular connections within the encephalocele as from the suprapineal recess or fourth ventricle. Hydrocephalus is commonly associated with an occipital encephalocele, the incidence increasing with age, but hydrocephalus is uncommon with meningoceles elsewhere. If a meningocele is associated with craniolacunia at birth, the likelihood of a Chiari malformation's being present is quite high. The Chiari malformation that occurs with an occipital encephalocele is the so-called type III.

Pneumoencephalography is performed on infants with a small cranial meningocele in a site other than the occipital area. Occipital meningoceles usually do not fill satisfactorily at pneumoencephalography. The transsphenoidal encephalocele, however, which fills via the chiasmatic cistern, may distend the nasopharynx and obstruct the airway unless the infant is intubated prior to the study.

Angiography best demonstrates the presence of brain tissue in the encephalocele—the tissue may be from the frontal lobe in nasal encephaloceles, the parietal lobe in parietal encephaloceles, the occipital lobe and/or cerebellum in occipital encephaloceles. The position of the brain stem within the occipital encephalocele is directly related to the surgical outcome (Gilmor et al., 1972); in one bizarre instance the brain stem and cerebellum were transposed, the cerebellum lying anterior to the brain stem.

It is often not possible to completely sort out the disordered anatomy even with the many neuroradiological studies that are available. The basilar artery is usually extremely hooked backward in occipital encephaloceles, and the proximal posterior cerebral arteries take on a most characteristic appearance of the abnormality: they angle sharply upward in a V to attain their supratentorial course.

A small parietal encephalocele that contains a nubbin of parietal lobe may have an associated gross and complex cerebral anomaly such as cerebral hypoplasia, together with unilateral dysplastic internal carotid artery and microencephaly similar to the appearance seen in alobar holoprosencephaly.

Disorders of diverticulation
Holoprosencephaly

Defective diverticulation is exemplified by the formation of a holospheric cerebrum due to failure of the primitive prosencephalon vesiculation, in part or in whole, to develop a telencephalon (cerebral hemispheres) and a diencephalon (thalamus, hypothalamus), between the fourth and eighth weeks of fetal development. Cleavage of this prosencephalon then fails to form the complex cerebral hemispheres.

The preferable term is *holoprosencephaly* (DeMyer et al., 1964) rather than *arrhinencephaly* (Kundrat, 1882); for, although the rhinic lobe may be absent, this absence does not form the cornerstone of the abnormality since the lobe is often present in holoprosencephaly (Yakovlev, 1959).

Variations of holoprosencephaly are determined by the degree of separation of the holosphere, which in its basic form is a thin pancakelike primitive cerebrum. *Alobar holoprosencephaly* has no cerebral hemispheres; rather a large central monoventricular cavity and fused thalami are present with anterior or posterior saucerlike cerebral holospheric tissue incompletely closing over the monoventricle. There is no sagittal dural fold. *Lobar (semilobar) holoprosencephaly* has partial or complete separation into cerebral lobes; however, the frontal horns are always fused. The cerebral sagittal falx is partially developed. Arrhinencephaly is the mildest form, with absence of the rhinic lobe only.

DeMyer and co-workers (1964) used the fact that prechordal mesoderm interposes itself between the primitive foregut and the potential forebrain and thereby induces the formation of neural ectoderm. The eventual morphology of these defects in the embryo may be induced by or associated with maternal diabetes mellitus (Dekaban and Magee, 1958), toxoplasmosis, or trisomy 13-15 syndrome (Warkany, 1971) in about 50% of cases. Amino acid abnormalities (Bishop et al., 1964), endocrine dysgenesis (Hintz et al., 1968), familial tendencies (DeMyer et al., 1963; Hintz et al., 1968), or intrauterine rubella (Zingesser et al., 1966) may also be determinants.

Because the face also develops from the primitive mesoderm, it is closely associated with intracranial anomalies so induced; there is thus a complete spectrum of facial and cerebral malformations (DeMyer et al., 1964; Zingesser et al., 1966) in which the face often predicts the specific type of brain anomaly. The severest facial malformations—cyclopia, ethmocephaly, cebocephaly—are rarely viable conditions (Warkany, 1971) that are associated with alobar holoprosencephaly and microcephaly. They do not usually come to neuroradiological investigation. Aberrations such as median harelip, cleft palate, hypotelorism, or trigonocephaly and lateral cleft lip, cleft palate, or trigonocephaly with hypotelorism are concomitants of alobar or lobar holoprosencephaly, often with an absent or dysplastic olfactory apparatus. In our experience, some children with trigonocephaly and hypotelorism alone may have fused frontal horns but relatively normal cerebral hemispheres. These infants probably represent the mildest form of the holoprosencephalic spectrum. Trigonocephaly per se, however, can be associated with a normal brain. Multiple extracerebral anomalies are often present in these conditions, particularly in an infant with trisomy

D 13-15 syndrome (Currarino and Silverman, 1960; Warkany, 1971), and include polydactyly, pulmonic stenosis, microphthalmia, external and inner ear malformations, diaphragmatic hernias, and spina bifida.

Neuroradiology of holoprosencephaly. Our experience consists of seven infants with alobar or lobar holoprosencephaly over an eight-year period. Previous reports of the neuroradiology of holoprosencephaly are by Wisen and co-workers (1965), Kurlander and co-workers (1966), Zingesser and co-workers (1966), and Bligh and Laurence (1967).

SKULL RADIOGRAPHY. Examination of the face of the child is an integral part of the neuroradiological consultation.

The usual skull radiographic abnormalities (Fig. 16-47) are microcephaly with varying degrees of hypoplasia of the ethmoidal, sphenoidal, and nasal structures, cleft palate, hypotelorism, trigonocephaly, or indeed a single small flat frontal plate of bone. The crista galli is absent, as often is the cribriform plate; but the latter may not be completely ossified until

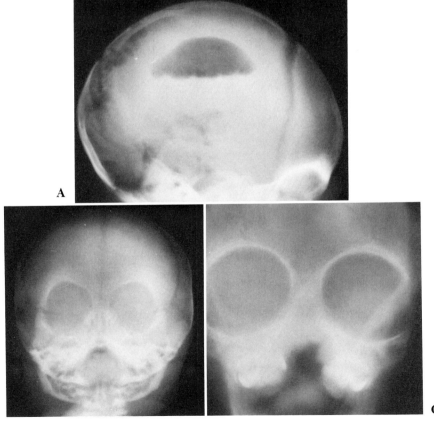

Fig. 16-47. Holoprosencephaly. A, Microcephaly. Note the air-filled single ventricle with the normal fourth ventricle inferiorly. B, Hypotelorism. C, A tomogram reveals the markedly cleft palate, hypoplasia of the ethmoids, hypotelorism, and fused metopic suture. There is no crista galli.

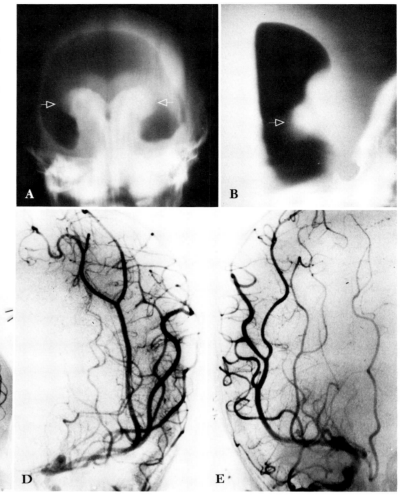

Fig. 16-48. Alobar holoprosencephaly. A and **B, A** ventriculogram reveals a single ventricle with fused thalami (arrows), best seen in the AP projection. On the lateral tomogram (**B**) the thalami (arrow) are seen to be anteriorly placed. **C,** Lateral and, **D,** AP left carotid arteriograms show a single large anteriorly placed middle cerebral artery, indicating a saucerlike cerebral mantle in the frontal region only. **E,** The AP right carotid angiogram demonstrates a similarly large anteriorly placed middle cerebral but only a small anterior cerebral artery.

after 1 year of age. Tomography is essential in the proper examination of the cribriform plate. A densely calcified and ossified anterior ridge at and/or within the falcine attachment is quite characteristic of these median anomalies (Chapter 2). Microcephaly is invariable but not extreme, and the head may be quite spherical compared with the elongated posteriorly pointed microcephaly due to intrauterine cerebral atrophy unrelated to holoprosencephaly. Axial tomography of the optic canals may show them to be abnormally small or absent.

PNEUMOENCEPHALOGRAPHY AND VENTRICULOGRAPHY. The most important feature of this malformation is a variable lack of separation of the ventricles. The term *semilobar* may be applied to the form of holoprosencephaly with separation of the occipital horns only and a single large more anterior ventricle. The *lobar* form may be considered to occur when the frontal horns alone are fused, with a separate body of the lateral ventricles, and this form has a pneumoen-

cephalographic appearance similar to that of simple absence of the septum pellucidum. To avoid further confusion, we prefer to gather most of these conditions under the name lobar.

Pneumoencephalography is performed if the head is normal or small; ventriculography if the head is large or when pneumoencephalography fails to fill the ventricles or fills only the fourth ventricle.

Alobar holoprosencephaly is a large monoventricular cavity (Fig. 16-48), often extremely difficult to differentiate from hydranencephaly. Some cortical tissue may be identified (usually anteriorly, but in some infants posteriorly). A midline falcine cleft is not present, however, contrary to hydranencephaly. Furthermore, alobar holoprosencephaly has some middle cerebral vasculature whereas hydranencephaly does not. Hydranencephaly does not have the median cleft facial complex. An infant with hydranencephaly usually presents a normal or large head, which is uncommon in alobar holoprosencephaly. A recognizable

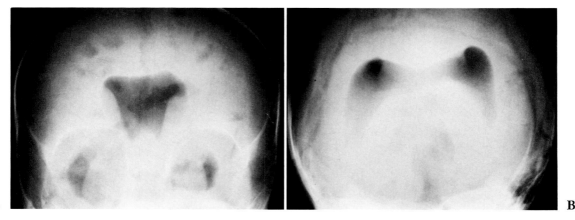

Fig. 16-49. Lobar holoprosencephaly. Fused frontal horns create a single anterior ventricle. Though the fusion extends posteriorly into the body, the occipital horns are clearly formed (**B**).

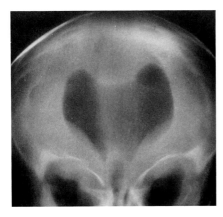

Fig. 16-50. Absent septum pellucidum. Note that the V roof of the anterior ventricles is still formed, differentiating the two ventricles from a single frontal horn.

third ventricle is usually not identified but may be represented as an ill-defined midline cavity at the base of the single ventricle. The fourth ventricle and aqueduct may be normal and patent; but if they are not and no hydrocephalus is present, choroid plexus function may be considered to be deficient.

In *lobar* or *semilobar holoprosencephaly,* pneumoencephalography will usually fill the lateral ventricles—which are often posteriorly separated. A falx is present posteriorly, and the frontal horns are fused. There is thus an attempt at cerebral hemispheric formation. Due to deficient brain substance rather than hydrocephalus, the "ventricles" may be large. We do not consider agenesis of the corpus callosum and a midline cyst (Zingesser et al., 1964) to be part of the holoprosencephalic syndrome.

Simple fused frontal horns and trigonocephaly are the minor forms of this spectrum. The single frontal horn usually contains a hypoplastic corpus callosal rostrum and a *straight* roof with rounded lateral angles (Fig. 16-49). Simple absence of the septum pellucidum may occur and is not part of the spectrum (Fig. 16-50). The two frontal horns maintain the upper V roof (often widened). Absence of the septum, commonly seen in hydrocephalus, is probably acquired.

ANGIOGRAPHY. The vascular pattern in holoprosencephaly is often difficult to define precisely. Yakovlev (1959) and Maki and Kumagai (1974) described a median (anterior) and two lateral (middle) arterial trunks that supplied a saucer-shaped holosphere in alobar holoprosencephaly (Fig. 16-48). Wisen and co-workers (1965) reported a case in which no homologues of anterior cerebral arteries were present but two lateral "middle" cerebral arteries supplied the holosphere.

The anterior cerebral artery may be paired in lobar holoprosencephaly or may start as an azygos artery (Fig. 16-51). Its course is wavy and irregular (Zingesser et al., 1966; Wolpert, 1974) and, together with the lateral arteries, appears to have no purposeful or ordered direction. Our experience, similar to the pathological experience of Wisen and co-workers (1965), has shown that one internal cerebral artery may supply most of the dysgenetic cerebral tissue and the other internal carotid artery is hypoplastic with small central branches. This may occur in both alobar and lobar holoprosencephaly but is more common in the former. The lateral arteries have no sylvian triangle, for there is no sylvian fissure. Except when a posteriorly placed holosphere cerebral remnant is present, the posterior cerebral arteries are often absent or hypoplastic. The basilar system is otherwise usually normal.

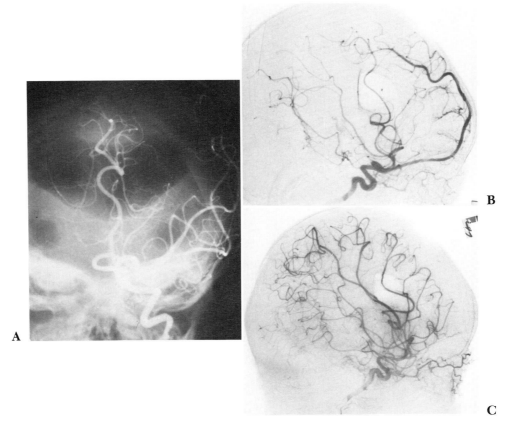

Fig. 16-51. Lobar holoprosencephaly. A and **B,** A left carotid angiogram demonstrates a dysgenetic middle cerebral artery passing laterally and not containing its regular branches. There is a single azygous anterior cerebral artery. Air can be seen in the anterior common ventricle. **C,** A left common carotid angiogram in another infant shows no filling of the anterior cerebral artery and again widely spaced abnormally formed middle cerebral arterial branches. There was marked enlargement of the ethmoidal branch of the ophthalmic artery, which fed a bulbous root of the nose. We believe this may have been a forme fruste third eye.

In minor forms of lobar holoprosencephaly, a wavy anterior cerebral artery may be present, as Kurlander and co-workers (1966) have described in a case of true arrhinencephaly with absence of the corpus callosum.

The sagittal sinus is not formed in the alobar holoprosencephaly. The presence of this sinus in the lobar form depends on the severity of the abnormality.

Septo-optic dysplasia

de Morsier (1956) described an association of hypoplasia of the optic discs with absence of the septum pellucidum and gave a detailed report of the morphology of the brain in an adult with septo-optic dysplasia. He described a thin corpus callosum and fusion of the upper bodies of the fornix and postulated an agenesis of the embryonic neuroglial anlage that bridges the origin of the corpus and the anterior commissure. Furthermore, orientation of the chiasm is rotated 90° to form an over-and-under, rather than a side-to-side, relationship of the two optic bundles and decussation. An optic ventricle with persistence of the embryonic dilated anterior third ventricle and hypoplasia of the infundibulum is also present. Growth retardation appears to be part of the syndrome (Ellenberger and Runyan, 1970; Hoyt et al., 1970). Septo-optic dysplasia is morphogenetically probably on the same basis as holoprosencephaly insofar as the prechordal mesoderm is defective.

Neuroradiology of the syndrome will confirm a diagnosis that can usually be made clinically (Brook et al., 1972). Trigonocephaly and hypotelorism may be present and indicate an overlap with the holoprosencephaly syndrome. Axial tomograms will show the optic canal to be quite small (Fig. 16-52), indicating primary optic nerve hypoplasia; the septum pellucidum is absent, and the roof of the fused frontal

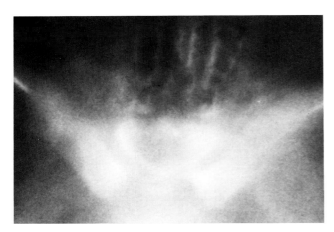

Fig. 16-52. Septo-optic dysplasia and the optic canals. Axial tomograms show the canals to be abnormally small, indicating nerve hypoplasia.

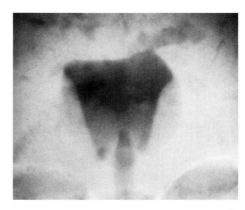

Fig. 16-53. Septo-optic dysplasia. The septum pellucidum is absent, and the roof of the frontal horns is flat—features similar to those seen in lobar holoprosencephaly.

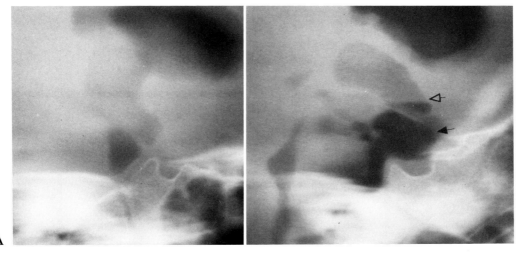

Fig. 16-54. Septo-optic dysplasia. A, Bulbous anterior third ventricle with large recesses. B, Single bulbous recess in the anterior third ventricle (open arrow) of another child with a large chiasmatic CSF cistern (solid arrow).

horns is flat with the lateral angles rounded (Fig. 16-53). This combination of features is similar to a mild form of lobar holoprosencephaly. The anterior third ventricle is characteristically bulbous and diverticulum-like anteriorly (Fig. 16-54, A) with an infundibular recess that is barely seen or situated more posteriorly than normal. The chiasmatic CSF cistern is usually large (Fig. 16-54, B). Angiography is normal except that the anterior communicating artery may be slightly higher and the septal veins will not be seen in the midline but will drain the lateral wall of the single frontal horn to merge with the thalamostriate veins to form the internal cerebral vein (Fig. 16-55).

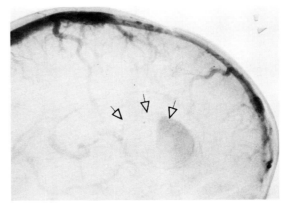

Fig. 16-55. Septo-optic dysplasia. The septal veins (arrows) are elevated and drain the lateral aspects of the fused frontal horns into an irregular internal cerebral vein.

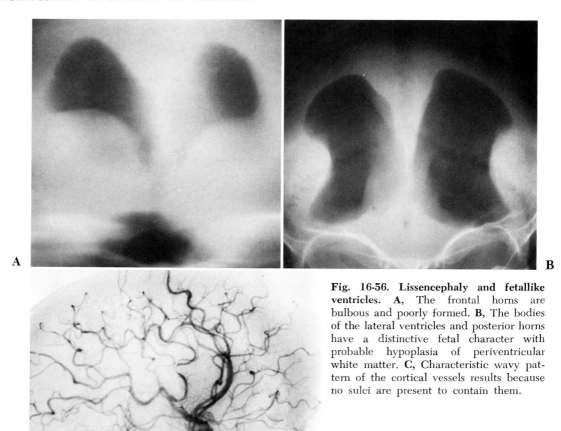

Fig. 16-56. Lissencephaly and fetallike ventricles. A, The frontal horns are bulbous and poorly formed. B, The bodies of the lateral ventricles and posterior horns have a distinctive fetal character with probable hypoplasia of periventricular white matter. C, Characteristic wavy pattern of the cortical vessels results because no sulci are present to contain them.

Miscellaneous cerebral and cerebellar malformations

Lissencephaly

In this rare congenital cerebral malformation there is a disorder of sulcation and cell migration leading to a lack of formation of the gyri; the agyric pattern of the 10-week fetus persists (Dieker et al., 1969). A nonspecific clinical appearance is present with mild microcephaly: a small chin, low-set ears, and prominent forehead and occiput. These findings are relatively nonspecific and can also occur in trisomy 17-18 (Wesenberg et al., 1966). Wesenberg and co-workers (1966) also described calcification within the upper septum pellucidum in two cases, but we did not see calcification in three infants on whom we performed neuroradiological studies. Ventriculography reveals a persistence of large fetallike ventricles (colpocephaly) due to hypoplasia of periventricular white matter (Fig. 16-56, A and B). The posterior lateral ventricles are particularly dilated, and areas of heterotopic gray matter alongside the ventricles are present. The third is moderately enlarged, and the aqueduct and fourth ventricle are usually well seen and appear to be normal.

Angiography is probably the most significant investigation. It reveals the laterally positioned middle cerebral vessels that are usually found in fetal and very premature brains. The middle cerebral branches are wavy (Fig. 16-56, C) and have no sylvian structure since a fissure is not present. The anterior cerebral artery is also wavy and has a wide sweep, reflecting the large primitive ventricles. The cerebrogram phase of angiography does not show the normal well-formed gyral pattern.

Heterotopic gray matter

Paraventricular heterotopic gray matter will sometimes occur with congenital abnormalities of the central nervous system (Bergeron, 1967, 1969)—

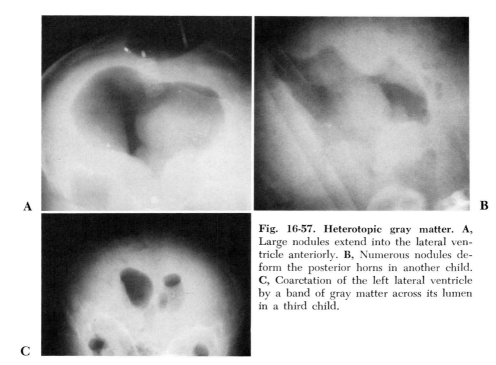

Fig. 16-57. Heterotopic gray matter. A, Large nodules extend into the lateral ventricle anteriorly. **B,** Numerous nodules deform the posterior horns in another child. **C,** Coarctation of the left lateral ventricle by a band of gray matter across its lumen in a third child.

especially with the Chiari malformation, absent corpus callosum, lissencephaly, Dandy-Walker syndrome, and encephaloceles. Small or large nodules (Fig. 16-57, *A* and *B*) project into the lateral ventricular cavity and may even cross it to partition off parts of the ventricle (Fig. 16-57, *C*). A small and relatively discrete vein may be confused with the subependymal tubers of tuberous sclerosis. The latter, however, is usually calcified (above age 5).

Cerebellar hypoplasia

We have observed certain variations in the normal shape of the cerebellum in a number of unrelated clinical instances and include these findings for a neuroradiological spectrum, acknowledging the fact that we have no morphological correlation.

Warkany (1971) described cerebellar hypoplasia in mentally retarded children or children with spastic diplegia, many of whom were siblings; in some the hypoplasia was found by chance at autopsy. Partial hypoplasia involving one cerebellar lobe for total or partial agenesis of the vermis may also occur (de Haene, 1955; Norman and Urich, 1958). Vermian atrophy in familial cerebellar ataxia, as described by Joubert and co-workers (1969), has occurred in our experience. These unusual changes are demonstrated during pneumoencephalography or ventriculography, and we believe they are probably atrophic secondary to some anoxic vascular phenomenon. The posterior fossa space is taken up with the cisterna magna.

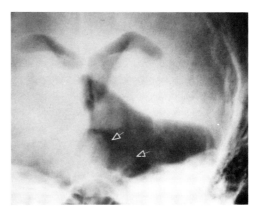

Fig. 16-58. Unilateral cerebellar hypoplasia. A pneumoencephalogram reveals a large cisterna magna on the left with severely decreased size of the left cerebral hemisphere (arrows). An angiogram showed the right cerebellar hemisphere to be normal. The etiology of this hypoplasia is unknown.

We have had experience with lateral hypoplasia of a cerebellar hemisphere (Fig. 16-58), marked hypoplasia of the entire cerebellum (Fig. 16-59), and vermian atrophy—particularly in the superior vermis. We exclude from our statistics infants with identifiable posterior fossa arachnoid cysts or the Dandy-Walker syndrome. Billings and Danziger (1973) reported a rare instance of cerebellar heterotopia that presented in a ventricle as a fourth ventricular mass in a 9-month-old boy with hydrocephalus.

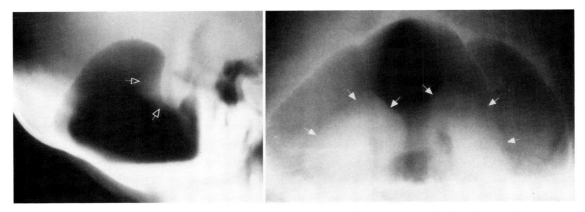

Fig. 16-59. Cerebellar hypoplasia. The cisterna magna is large. The cerebellum (arrows) is outlined and possesses both hemispheres and vermis. The fourth ventricle is normally formed with an inferior medullary velum. We do not think this a Dandy-Walker variant. No angiography was performed. The cause for the hypoplasia is unknown. There does not appear to be atrophy since the fourth ventricle is of normal size. The patient does not have hydrocephalus.

Finally, a large cisterna magna is *normal* in infants and children and therefore is not the criterion by which cerebellar hypoplasia is judged. Careful pneumotomography and angiography are the only way to assess an absolute decrease in size.

HISTOGENETIC MALFORMATIONS

Two of the malformations due to a histogenetic disorder merit separate attention: tuberous sclerosis and neurofibromatosis.

Tuberous sclerosis and neurofibromatosis are abnormal cell proliferations in which a particular cell in a given part of an organ continues to divide beyond what is normal. In neurofibromatosis and tuberous sclerosis that involve the central nervous system, the Schwann cell and the astrocyte respectively (and often more than one cellular element) multiply to create a mass lesion—usually with benign characteristics. Abnormal cell proliferation also occurs in other parts of the body. In neurofibromatosis, mesodermal cells are involved. If the exuberant cell type resembles normal nervous tissue, the neoplasm may be called a hamartoma.

Both tuberous sclerosis and neurofibromatosis involve many organ systems other than the central nervous system; and abnormalities in ectoderm, mesoderm, endothelium, and bone may occur. Due to quite distinctly separate autosomal dominant genes and variable penetrance, the disorders are hereditary in nature; the genes may affect the same embryonic layers and lead to the same pathological entity.

Neurofibromatosis, in particular, leaves few organs untainted by its particular spectrum of histogenetic disorders; and its protean manifestations throughout the central nervous system and coverings feature in the discussions of many sections of this text. We feel a need, however, to consider it as a single subject and to describe its particular effect on children.

Tuberous sclerosis

History records von Recklinghausen in 1862 as first describing a cardiac rhabdomyoma and cerebral cortical sclerotic areas in an infant. Bourneville (1880) is credited with both providing the clinical eponym and depicting the distinct pathological character of the disorder. Vogt (1908) reported the clinical triad of epilepsy, mental deficiency, and adenoma sebaceum as characteristic of tuberous sclerosis. It is now apparent, however, that the name tuberous sclerosis refers only to the cerebral lesions and not to the many manifestations in other organs of the body; but the name persists. Epiloia (a combination of the names *epilepsy* and *anoia* or "mindless") is another synonym (Lagos and Gomez, 1967).

Tuberous sclerosis is a disorder of varying expression and clinical and radiological presentation with many *formes frustes*; and the term tuberous sclerosis complex is often appropriate (Norman, 1963). Its uncommon dominant autosomal gene may be modified by an associated nondominant gene, leading to variable penetrance (Gunther and Penrose, 1935; Borberg, 1951).

Critchley and Earl (1932) considered the triad of epilepsy, mental deficiency, and adenoma sebaceum to be pathognomonic of tuberous sclerosis; and they stated that incomplete forms were rare. Lagos and Gomez (1967) showed that one of the triad may often occur without the others. Lagos and Gomez also described in great detail the history and the manifestations of the disease, together with a report of seventy-one patients (fifty-two of whom were under the age of 15 years). The incidence of any form

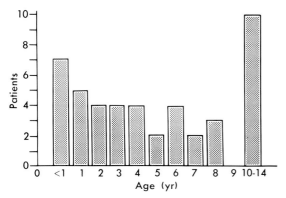

Fig. 16-60. Age and tuberous sclerosis. There were forty-five children in this study—twenty-five girls and twenty boys. (From Fitz, C. R., et al.: Radiology 110:635, 1974.)

Table 16-2. Clinical and radiographic data in the Hospital for Sick Children and Mayo Clinic series*

Presentation	HSC series (forty-five children) (%)	Mayo Clinic series (fifty-two children, nineteen adults) (%)
Clinical		
Seizures	78	93
Mental retardation	71	62
Seizures alone	13	25
Mental retardation alone	11	0
Seizures and mental retardation	8	11
Adenoma sebaceum	27	83
Hypopigmented spots	44	56
Intracranial neoplasm	11	6
Radiography		
Skull		
Intracranial calcification	48	51
Vault calcification	0	1
Neuroradiological studies		
Tubers	100	
Mass lesion	11	
Cerebral atrophy	42	
Other lesions		
Bone cyst	2	
Renal mass	11	
Cardiac mass	4	

*From Lagos, J. C., and Gomez, M. R.: Tuberous sclerosis; reappraisal of a clinical entity, Mayo Clin. Proc. **42**:26, 1967.

of tuberous sclerosis is said to be 1 in 150,000 persons (Dawson, 1954).

In our reported series of forty-five children under the age of 15, we have shown that the neuroradiological evidence of the cerebral lesions may be present with none, one, or all of the triad. Our experience now totals fifty-five children.

Distribution of lesions. Hamartomas of a fibrocellular nature, commonly benign and unencapsulated, are multifocal throughout the body and vary greatly in incidence of detection. This variation is related directly to the vigor with which investigative studies are performed. The one morphological abnormality common to all is the *tubers* within the brain. The following list of abnormalities is comprehensive for all ages (Simonton and Jamison, 1966); those peculiar to children will be considered later.

> *Brain.* Calcifications, subependymal and cortical tubers in which malignant change is uncommon
> *Skeletal system*
>   *Skull:* Calvarial sclerotic densities within the diploic space or inner table, calvarial thickening
>   *Long bones:* Metaphyseal cysts, irregular cortical thickening, increased trabeculation, small periosteal nodules
>   *Spine and pelvis:* Irregular patches of increased density
>   *Hands and feet:* Irregular cortical thickening of metatarsals, less commonly in metacarpals, pharyngeal pseudocysts with cortical pitting of phalanges
> *Skin.* Adenoma sebaceum (fibromas), shagreen patches, subungual fibromas, achromic patches (ash leaf form, in particular), subcutaneous nodules, areas of hyperpigmentation, café au lait spots
> *Viscera.* Cardiac rhabdomyoma, mixed embryonal hamartomas of kidney, duodenum, liver, thyroid, adrenal, ovary, and interstitial pulmonary tissue, retinal tumors (phakoma)

Clinical features. In our reported series of forty-five children (Fitz et al., 1974), girls (twenty-five) slightly outnumbered boys (twenty). The diagnosis was more commonly made in the young, and as early as

5 months of age (Fig. 16-60). Thibault and Manuelidis (1970) reported the occurrence at postmortem examination of cerebral tuberous sclerosis in a premature infant, and they included twelve other similar reports indicating intrauterine origin of the disease. Seizures were present in 78% of our series, 93% of the Mayo Clinic series (Table 16-2) (Lagos and Gomez, 1967).

Some degree of mental retardation was present in 71% of our series (62% of the Mayo series). Mental retardation is difficult to assess in infants, however, and its incidence is probably higher. Lagos and Gomez (1967) stated that mental retardation is not an essential presenting feature in tuberous sclerosis and that adenoma sebaceum was never a sole manifestation of the disease. Four patients in their series who were not mentally retarded had seizures. In our series, 11% had mental retardation alone, 13% seizures alone, and 8% neither; but the 8% had skin abnormalities and/or a strong family history.

Far fewer (27% of our patients, compared with 83% of the Mayo series) had adenoma sebaceum. We believe that this clinical feature is uncommon in infants and young children. Hypopigmented spots

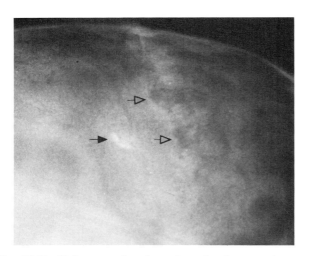

Fig. 16-61. Tuberous sclerosis and vault changes. An area of sclerosis in the vault (solid arrow) is associated with ill-defined lytic areas (open arrows).

were present in 44% of our series, but only two patients had the characteristic ash leaf–shaped macules (Fitzpatrick et al., 1968). Ultraviolet light is often necessary to detect this abnormality. Shagreen patches were uncommon.

Neuroradiology of tuberous sclerosis. Consequent to our practice of aggressively investigating by pneumoencephalography the seizures and mental retardation in children, we have discovered by neuroradiology the presence of tuberous sclerosis in twenty-two (49%) of the forty-five cases *before* such diagnosis was made clinically. The presence of intracranial tubers confirms the diagnosis of tuberous sclerosis. Dickerson (1945), Sutton and Liversedge (1951), Whitaker (1959), Green (1968), and Lagos and co-workers (1968) provided extensive accounts of the radiography of tuberous sclerosis at all ages.

SKULL RADIOGRAPHY. Lagos and co-workers (1968) reviewed the skull radiographs of twelve patients of indeterminate age with tuberous sclerosis. The finding by them and by others (Holt and Dickerson, 1952) of sclerotic zones in the calvarium (Chapter 2) has been uncommon in our experience (Fig. 16-61); we

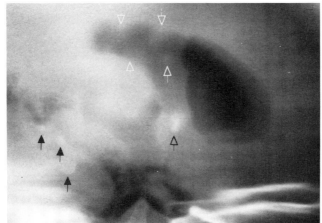

A

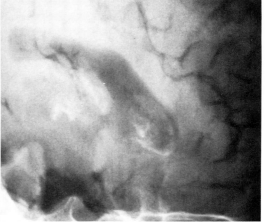

B

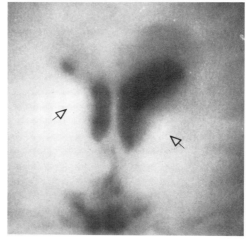

C

Fig. 16-62. Tuberous sclerosis and cacification. A, Densely calcified nodule just anterior to the foramen of Monro (open black arrow). Faintly calcified nodules are in the body of the lateral ventricle (open white arrows), and calcified nodules surround the temporal horn (solid arrows). B, Dense calcifications around the frontal horn, floor of the lateral ventricle, and lateral aspect of the third ventricle. C, Faint sand-like calcified tubers (arrows) in the region of the basal ganglia. This type of calcification is seen only by tomography.

presume that it is more common in the adult. One child in our series had additional irregular lucent areas within the vault (Fig. 16-61). In 48%, intracranial calcifications were detected and virtually all were centrally placed. The calcifications in the brain generally were related to the anterior half of the lateral ventricles and were multiple and bilateral but could also be single (Fig. 16-62, A and B). Although Lagos and co-workers (1968) reported tuberous sclerosis and cerebellar calcification, we have not identified this in children. The majority of calcifications occurred in the region of the basal ganglia but uncommonly anterior to the foramen of Monro or within the third ventricle. Rarely did the nodules occur in the temporal horns. The calcification varied from dense nodules to fine sandy aggregates often detected only during pneumotomography (Fig. 16-62, C). Cortical calcifications have not been common in our experience; Yakovlev and Corwin (1939) described five patients with cortical "brain stones" and tuberous sclerosis.

Eleven of the twenty-two children diagnosed first by neuroradiological methods had intracranial calcification. The incidence of calcification increased with age; but in infants less than 1 year of age, 14% had intracranial calcification—the youngest being 7 months of age. Calcification was present in 31% of the children under 2 years of age. Sixty percent of the older patients (10 to 14 years of age) in our group had calcification. The presence of calcification in no way indicates that an associated mental retardation is more likely to be found (Lagos and Gomez, 1967).

Periventricular calcifications in infants and children that must be distinguished from tuberous sclerosis are cytomegalic inclusion disease and toxoplasmosis (Chapter 2). Calcification of a glomus in an older child, calcification and astrocytoma near the lateral ventricles, calcification in a lateral ventricular ependymoma, and a choroid plexus papilloma are other lesions that may be confused with tuberous sclerosis.

COMPUTED TOMOGRAPHY. CT reveals the precise location of such calcifications, no matter how small, that may occur in both the periventricular and the cortical areas. We believe it is now *the* study of choice in the preliminary investigation of children suspected of having tuberous sclerosis.

PNEUMOENCEPHALOGRAPHY. Berkwitz and Rigler (1935) used the name "candle gutterings" in describing the multiple irregular, often confluent, nodular masses that impressed the air-filled lateral ventricular lumina and had been reported early in the pathological literature by Yakovlev and Guthrie (1931).

These subependymal tubers on pneumoencephalography produce discrete rounded or elongated mounds which, except in very young patients commonly contain calcification (Fig. 16-63). The nodules consist of gemnocystic giant astrocytes, spindle cells, and proliferating glial tissue; and they are covered by intact epithelium (Russell and Rubinstein, 1971). They usually occur at the basal ganglionic margins of the lateral ventricles (Fig. 16-64, A) or

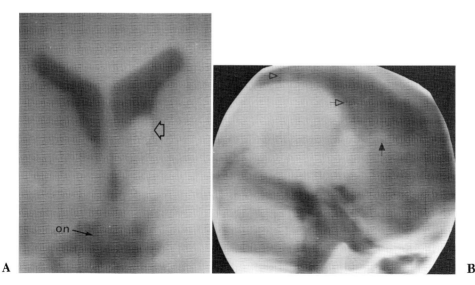

Fig. 16-63. Pneumoencephalography and tuberous sclerosis. A, A large faintly calcified tuber (arrow) in the inferolateral aspect of the left lateral ventricle, which is mildly dilated. The optic nerve (on) is also clearly seen. B, Small tubers (open arrows) that are faintly calcified project into the lumen of the lateral ventricle. The bump on the floor of the frontal horn (solid arrow) is normal.

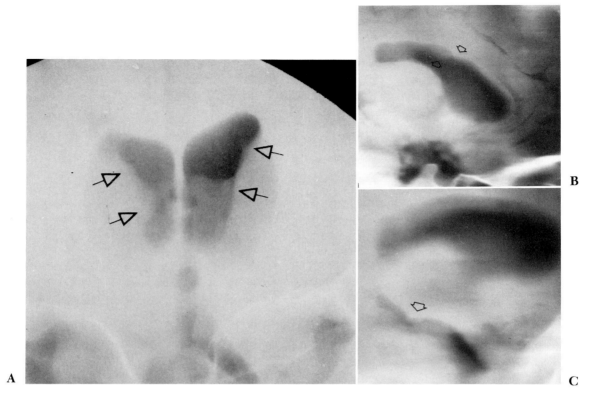

Fig. 16-64. **Classical sites of tuberous sclerosis. A,** Multiple nodules on the basal ganglionic borders of the lateral ventricles (arrows). **B,** Two discrete tubers (arrows) projecting from the roof of a lateral ventricle. **C,** A discrete tuber (arrow) projecting from the roof of the temporal horn. (**A** from Fitz, C. R., et al.: Radiology 110:635, 1974.)

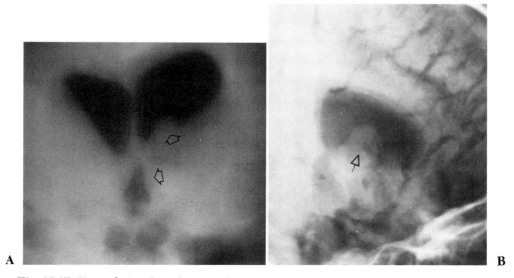

Fig. 16-65. **Unusual sites for tuberous sclerosis. A,** Extension of a left subependymal tuber of the lateral ventricle (upper arrow) down into the lateral aspect of the third ventricle (lower arrow). Note the partial obstruction of the left lateral ventricle by this extensive tuber. **B,** A large tuber projecting into the frontal horn from its floor (arrow)—a rare site. Compare this with the normal inferior frontal horn bump (Fig. 16-63, *B*).

at the lateral angles, but rarely do they project from the roof (Fig. 16-64, *B*) and they rarely occur in the temporal horns (Fig. 16-64, *C*). Nodules may involve the third ventricle usually as inferior extensions of nodules alongside the lateral ventricles (Fig. 16-65, *A*) but they do not often extend anterior to the foramen of Monro to impress the frontal horns (Fig. 16-65, *B*). They may, however, impinge on the foramen of Monro—producing varying degrees of obstruction.

These tubers were identified in all but one of our patients with tuberous sclerosis on whom pneumoencephalography or ventriculography was performed (forty-two of the forty-five). Pneumotomography in both the sagittal and the coronal planes is essential to detect these nodules, many of which may be very small. Calcification may only be seen on pneumotomography.

The *differential diagnosis* of these nodules involves, first, identifying heterotopic gray matter foci in the subependymal region (Bergeron, 1967, 1969) which may clearly simulate tuberous sclerosis (Fig. 16-57).

The heterotopic nodules are usually broad based and occur in the bodies of the lateral ventricles, but there are other associated congenital abnormalities of the brain such as an absent corpus callosum and the Chiari malformation. The nodules do not calcify. Patients with nodules do not have the clinical picture of skin lesions found in tuberous sclerosis. Due to corpus callosal fibers, corrugations of the roof of the lateral ventricles may occur but these will be multiple and small. The choroid plexus in the floor of the lateral ventricle may be quite large and nodular in infants, and the glomus may occur within the body of the lateral ventricle (Fig. 16-66). They should not be confused with tuberous sclerosis. Seizures and mental retardation are absent.

Dilatation of one or both lateral ventricles, a finding not sufficiently stressed in the past, occurred in twenty-three (55%) of our series. Four children had a large mass occluding the foramen of Monro and creating hydrocephalic ventricles (Fig. 16-65, *A*) whereas in the other nineteen the dilated ventricles were on the basis of atrophy. Unexplained preponderance of left lateral ventricular dilatation (fourteen children) of the nineteen nonobstructive cases occurred. Mild atrophy or some associated cerebral dysgenesis may account for these features.

Neoplastic mass lesions do rarely develop as part of the natural history of tuberous sclerosis (Kapp et al., 1967; Lagos and Gomez, 1967; Cooper, 1971) and occurred in four patients in our series. The lesions were near the foramen of Monro and were large (Fig. 16-67); and all produced hydrocephalus.

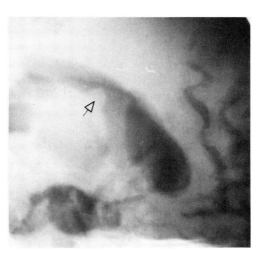

Fig. 16-66. **Normal glomus.** The glomus (arrow) in an infant may be anteriorly placed in the body of the lateral ventricle and should not be mistaken for a tuber. This finding may be related to the clinical status of the infant; if doubt exists, an angiogram should be obtained.

Their pathological identity is often inconclusive; they may be called an astrocytoma, an embryonal glioma, a spongioblastoma, or a neuroma, ependymoma, or ganglioglioma. Russell and Rubenstein (1971) termed them subependymal giant cell astrocytomas. In our experience, these neoplasms have been large with varying vascularity and have produced obstructive hydrocephalus at the foramen of Monro. They may or may not contain areas of calcification. In two cases the intracranial neoplasm was associated with a renal angiomyolipoma, and in another with a rhabdomyoma of the heart. All four cases were grouped as astrocytomas, two with glioblastoma characteristics and two of the benign giant cell type (i.e., ganglioglioma).

ANGIOGRAPHY. Hilal and co-workers (1971) described abnormal angiographic features in two children with tuberous sclerosis: occlusion of a major branch of the middle cerebral artery in one and areas of segmental stenoses and ectasia of the middle cerebral artery distribution in the other. We have not seen these rather nonspecific changes in any of our cases. Angiography is essential to the adequate evaluation of neoplastic change in the tubers. All astrocytomas and gangliogliomas that are associated with tuberous sclerosis are quite vascular (Fig. 16-67).

Extracranial abnormalities. Among our fourteen children who had an IVP, four had an embryonal hamartoma, (Fig. 16-68, *A*), an "angiomyolipoma," of one or both kidneys (Farrow et al., 1968); a rhabdomyoma of the heart (Fig. 16-68, *B*) (Elliott and McGeachy, 1962) occurred in one child, and a nonspecific femoral cyst (Fig. 16-68, *C*) in another.

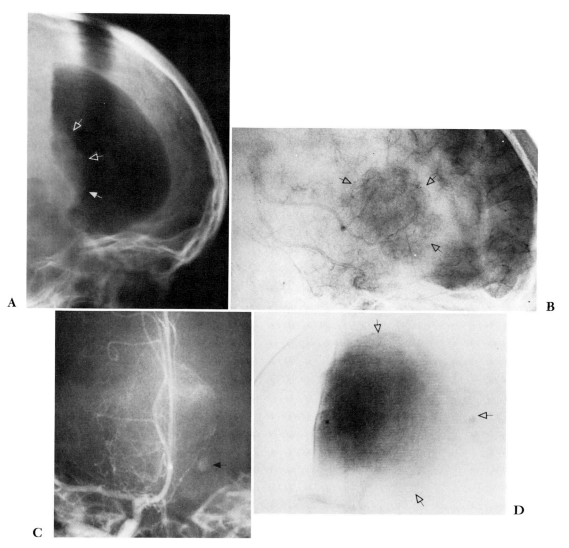

Fig. 16-67. Gangliogliomas. A, A ventriculogram in a child reveals markedly dilated ventricles and a large nodular mass (arrows) projecting into both frontal horns. **B** and **C,** A carotid angiogram on the same patient demonstrates a vascular ganglioglioma arising in the midline at the level of the foramen of Monro. Note the intense blush of the neoplasm (**B,** arrows) being drained by the septal veins into the internal cerebral vein. A calcified tuber (**C,** arrow) is alongside the ganglioglioma. **D,** A large vascular ganglioglioma (arrows) in another infant. The angiographic stain has persisted past the venous phase.

One child with a subinguinal fibroma had associated cystic changes of the phalanges. Other bony changes listed previously are rare in children, as is pulmonary involvement (Milledge et al., 1966).

Neurofibromatosis

Since von Recklinghausen's description of neuro-fibromatosis in 1882 as a hamartomatous disorder of neural crest origin, its specific spectrum of involvement in children has received scant attention (Fienman and Yakovac, 1970). It is an inherited autosomal dominant disease of neuroectodermal and mesenchy-mal origin, the latter probably secondarily induced. Spontaneous mutations explain why only 50% of patients have positive family histories. Members of the same family may exhibit various and differing manifestations of the disease. Crowe and co-workers (1956) estimated an incidence of 1 in 3,000 births. Males are more commonly affected than females (2 to 1).

The cutaneous stigmas of the disease, café au lait spots exceeding 1.5 cm in diameter and at least five in number in each child, together with cutaneous neurofibromas (fibroma molluscum) are often but

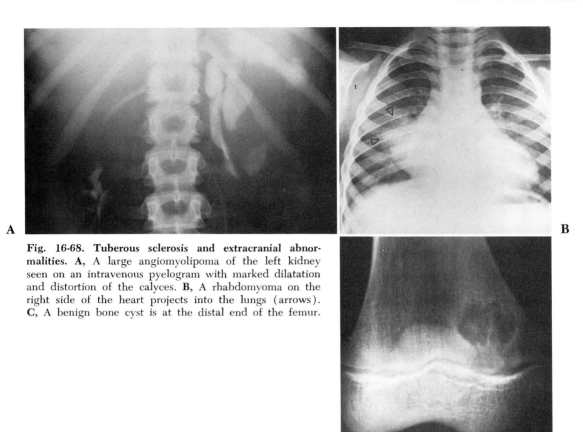

Fig. 16-68. Tuberous sclerosis and extracranial abnormalities. A, A large angiomyolipoma of the left kidney seen on an intravenous pyelogram with marked dilatation and distortion of the calyces. **B,** A rhabdomyoma on the right side of the heart projects into the lungs (arrows). **C,** A benign bone cyst is at the distal end of the femur.

not necessarily present at birth and usually by the age of 2. Children will exhibit the cutaneous manifestations of the disease and later, in adulthood, become afflicted with evidence of the more serious visual and neural manifestations and neoplasms of the central nervous system. The musculoskeletal defects involving the skull and spine and limbs are common and occur in 20% to 50% of patients of all ages (Holt and Wright, 1948; Hunt and Pugh, 1961). These include skeletal and soft tissue hemihypertrophy, acceleration of epiphyseal ossification, elephantoid hyperplasia of soft tissues, congenital bowing and pseudoarthrosis of the long bones (especially the distal tibia and fibula), and intraosseous cystic lesions. Seizures and mental retardation occur with the neurofibromatosis in approximately 10% of children (Fienman and Yakovac, 1970). Precocious or retarded sex development may also occur in children but will be due to hypertrophic or neoplastic involvement of endocrine organs. Peripheral neural fibromas may become sarcomatous. The radiographic features of this fascinating disease have been extensively reported in patients of all ages by Holt and Wright (1948), Hunt and Pugh (1961), Davidson (1966), and Meszaros and co-workers (1966).

Neuroradiology of neurofibromatosis. The manifestations of neurofibromatosis that interest the paediatric neuroradiologist occur in the skull, spine, brain, cranial nerves, and spinal cord:

Skull
    Sphenoid wing dysplasia
    Abnormal sella
    Enlarged optic canal
Brain
    Cranial nerve gliomas
Spinal cord
    Intra-axial and extra-axial neurofibromas
Spine
    Vertebral dysplasia
    Kyphoscoliosis
    Posterior vertebral body scalloping

As a general rule, the older the child the more common is the incidence of significant clinical abnormalities specific to warrant neuroradiological investigation. Furthermore, the older the child, the more likely are frank mass effects of neurofibromas or associated neural neoplasms to occur. Some features of the disease are quite rare in children, and others are as common in children as in adults.

Skull. Posterior orbital wall defects such as sphenoid wing dysplasia and sellar changes due to optic nerve lesions are the commonest abnormalities presenting in children.

The *posterior orbital wall defect,* first described by Lewald (1933) and discussed at length by Binet and co-workers (1969), is an anomaly that is a bony dysplasia with latent ossification of one or both greater wings of the sphenoid. With anterior protrusion of the ipsilateral and pulsating temporal lobe and coverings, the defect of the greater sphenoid wings creates a pulsating exophthalmos which in turn creates a pressure displacement of the lesser wings with marked upper angulation (Fig. 16-69, *A*) and

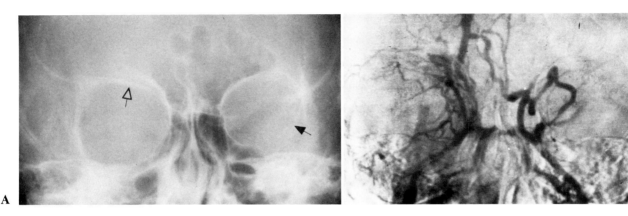

Fig. 16-69. Neurofibromatosis and sphenoid wing dysplasia. A, The right anterior clinoid and upper border of the right greater wing of the sphenoid are displaced markedly superiorly (open arrow). The superior orbital fissure is absent, and the orbit appears to lack its posterior bony wall. The orbital oblique line (solid arrow), normal on the left, has been displaced far laterally on the right and is not seen. The orbit is also slightly enlarged. **B,** An orbital venogram of the same patient shows marked displacement of the right ophthalmic veins medially and superiorly. The left veins appear to be normal.

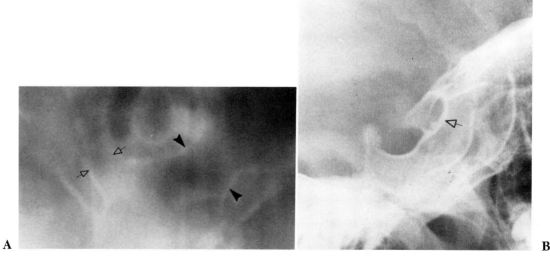

Fig. 16-70. Axial tomography and neurofibromatosis with optic glioma. A, Grossly widened left optic canal (arrowheads) and a normal right canal (arrows). A large left optic glioma involving the left side of the chiasm was confirmed at operation. **B,** Marked elongation and enlargement of the chiasmatic groove (arrow) with thinning and undercutting of the anterior clinoids and flattening of the tuberculum sellae. A glioma of the prefixed chiasm was subsequently identified. Changes similar to these but less severe may occur in neurofibromatosis without a glioma.

lateral displacement of the orbital oblique line. The margins of the middle fossa are enlarged in all directions in the inner wall of the body of the sphenoid and often gently scalloped. Angiography will reveal medial deviation of the carotid siphon, medial and downward displacement of the ophthalmic artery, slight elevation of the horizontal proximal middle cerebral artery, and forward displacement of the orbitofrontal branches and the anterior temporal–middle cerebral branches without stretching (Binet et al., 1969). Orbital venography shows upward and inward displacement of the ophthalmic veins (Fig. 16-69, B). Burrows (1963) described the presence of neurofibromatous tissue in the orbit, which is uncommon; and Peyton and Simmons (1946) and Binet and co-workers (1969) both described an associated optic nerve glioma with such dysplasia. This ap-

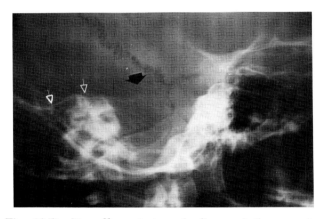

Fig. 16-71. Neurofibromatosis and glioma of the gasserian ganglion. An oblique view of the petrous bone (open arrows) reveals total destruction of the medial portion and apex of the petrous bone (solid arrow) due to a glioma of the gasserian ganglion of the fifth nerve.

pearance may simulate somewhat the appearance of a unilateral coronal synostosis (altered anterior orbital margin, elevated upper outer angle, intact greater sphenoid wing) or a middle fossa arachnoid cyst (intact supraorbital fissure); angiography and pneumoencephalography will reveal the extracerebral location in the latter.

Sellar abnormalities due to optic glioma are characteristic (Chapter 11). There is enlargement of all or part of the optic canal as seen in axial tomograms (Fig. 16-70, A) (Harwood-Nash, 1972). The chiasmatic groove is enlarged, the tuberculum sellae may be eroded and flattened (Fig. 16-70, B), the anterior clinoid thinned from side to side and up and down, and the dorsal clinoids blunted from chiasmatic and hypothalamic involvement by the glioma. These abnormalities may be unilateral or bilateral according to the extent of the glioma. An open sella with a poorly formed tuberculum sellae and a large chiasmatic sulcus may also occur in patients with neurofibromatosis without optic glioma. To exclude the more commonly associated glioma, however, optic canal axial tomography with pneumoencephalography is mandatory.

In our experience the standard radiographic views of the sella may be quite normal, as may visualization of the anterior orifice of the optic canal; and it therefore is our recommendation that axial tomography be performed on any patient with neurofibromatosis, regardless of the presence or absence of clinical signs and symptoms referrable to the optic tract. Neurofibromatosis was present in 24% of optic tract gliomas in a series we studied (Chapter 11). Such an examination will provide a basis for future examinations when clinical symptoms are more apparent.

Furthermore, an *optic nerve glioma* may be present with normal vision (Harwood-Nash, 1972). In an

A
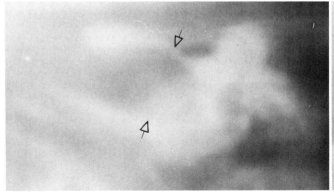
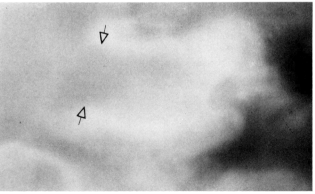
B

Fig. 16-72. Neurofibromatosis, acoustic neuromas, and internal auditory canals. On the left the canal itself is markedly expanded (**A**, arrows). On the right the orifice of the other canal is expanded (**B**, arrows). Bilateral acoustic neuromas were confirmed at operation.

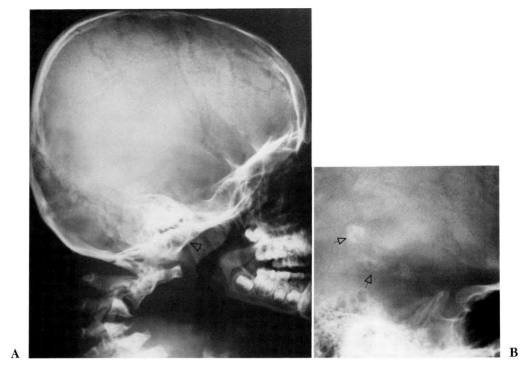

Fig. 16-73. Neurofibromatosis with macrocrania and calcification. A, A large globular head with some flattening of the chiasmatic sulcus, scalloping of the clivus (arrow), and marked vertebral dysplasia of the cervical spine are characteristic of neurofibromatosis. **B,** Calcification of the choroid plexus in the temporal horn (arrows) of another child.

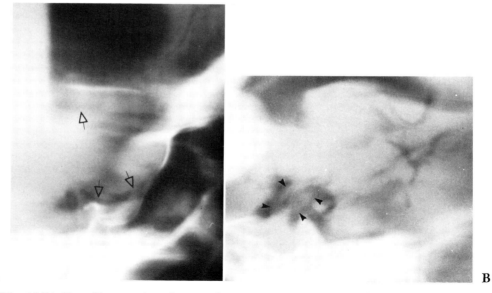

Fig. 16-74. Neurofibromatosis and optic gliomas. A, A pneumoencephalogram reveals a huge chiasmatic and hypothalamic glioma (arrows) which markedly distorts the sella with flattening of the chiasmatic groove, thinning of the anterior clinoids, and blunting of the posterior clinoids. **B,** A pneumoencephalogram in another child shows enlargement of the optic chiasm due to a glioma (arrowheads).

orbital optic glioma the posterior orbit is enlarged, as is the orbital orifice of the optic canal (Chapter 11). Standard optic foramen radiographs show only this orifice and *not* the canal itself. This orifice may therefore be quite normal in intracranial optic gliomas (Chapter 11).

Widening of other cranial nerve orifices due to neoplasms of these nerves is rare in children. One child with a glioma of the mandibular branch of the fifth nerve had a foramen ovale enlarged enough to displace the mandible. Another had a glioma of the gasserian ganglion of the fifth nerve that eroded the entire medial portion of the petrous bone (Fig. 16-71). Two children had acoustic neuromas (one bilateral, in a teen-ager) which expanded the internal auditory meatus in its canalicular portion and at its orifice (Fig. 16-72). This is the sum total of our experience with cranial nerve gliomas. Tomography is essential in the preliminary evaluation of such

neoplasms. In the absence of an acoustic neuroma, however, ectasia of the internal auditory canal may occur. Intracranial calcification developed in one optic glioma after irradiation.

Skull lucencies within the lambdoid suture inferiorly (Joffe, 1965) are a characteristic of neurofibromatosis in adults; we have not seen them in children. Davidson (1966) reported that such defects are merely a local thinning without any contiguous neurofibromatous malformation. Ovoid skull defects within the parietal bones as described by Davidson (1966) are similarly rare in children.

Macrocephaly and *macrocrania* have occurred rarely in our experience (Fig. 16-73, *A*) (Weichert et al., 1973). Calcification of the choroid plexus is also rare (Fig. 16-73, *B*).

Brain and spinal cord. More common in children than in adults with neurofibromatosis, an *optic glioma* (Fig. 16-74) occurs in approximately 10% of children with neurofibromatosis. In the forty-five children of our series, neurofibromatosis occurred in 24% of optic tract gliomas. Astrocytomas of other sites (Fig. 16-75) and ependymomas (Pearce, 1967; Russell and Rubinstein, 1971) are rarely present in children. Gliomas of the fifth nerve and a schwannoma of the fifth nerve have occurred in our experience, but acoustic neuromas in children are very uncommon (two cases in our experience, both in teen-agers, one with bilateral acoustic neuromas). Each of the acoustic neuromas was associated with marked enlargement of the internal auditory meatus. In one teen-ager, ectasia of the meninges and dura resulted in a large internal auditory canal before the neoplasm occurred. Hitselberger and Hughes (1968) described twelve patients with acoustic neuromas, three of whom were teen-agers with neurofibromatosis and bilateral acoustic neuromas. Posterior fossa contrast cisternography will reveal the acoustic neuroma if it emerges from

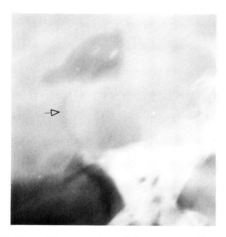

Fig. 16-75. Neurofibromatosis and brain stem glioma. A well-circumscribed neoplasm displaces the aqueduct (arrow) posteriorly.

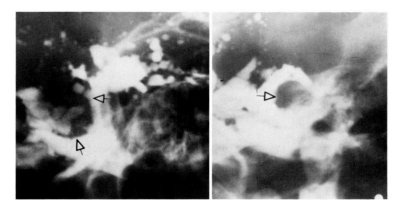

Fig. 16-76. Myelography with neurofibromatosis and bilateral acoustic neuromas. Bilateral acoustic neuromas (arrows) are demonstrated by Pantopaque posterior fossa cystography in a teen-ager. (Courtesy G. Wortzman, M.D., Toronto.)

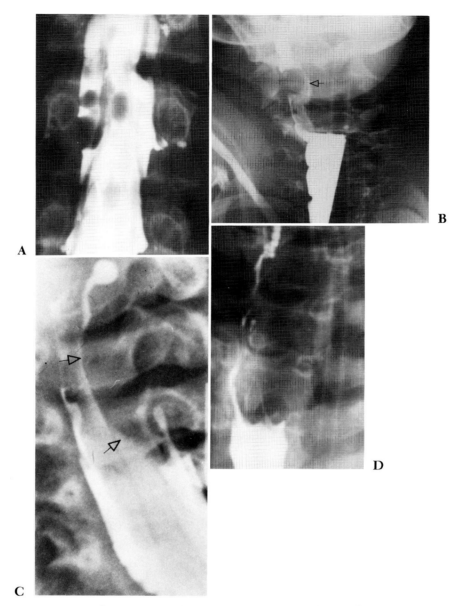

Fig. 16-77. Paraspinal and intraspinal neurofibromas. A, Multiple intradural, arising from the lumbar roots. **B,** Large plexiform, in the right side of the neck and extending into the extradural and intradural space (arrow). There is also an associated low cervical spine dysplasia. **C,** Extradural of the lower cervical spine (arrows). **D,** Large intradural and extradural, in the upper thoracic spine.

the internal auditory meatus (Fig. 16-76). These neoplasms are well demonstrated by contrast enhanced CT (Chapter 8).

Spinal root neurofibromas commonly present in children and are nearly always multiple (Fig. 16-77, *A*). They often are associated with scoliosis and severe vertebral dysplasias. The plexiform neurofibromatosis around the neck and back may continue into the extradural space (Fig. 16-77, *B*). The nerve root neoplasms arise from the nerve root sheaths and may extend into the canal as extradural masses (Fig.

16-77, *C*), rarely as intradural masses (Fig. 16-77, *D*). Astrocytomas and ependymomas of the cord are rare in children with neurofibromatosis.

Hilal and co-workers (1971) described one child with multiple cerebral vascular occlusions and neurofibromatosis (Fig. 16-78). Another child had been given radiation therapy for an optic glioma prior to the occlusive arterial disease. In the latter child the changes were probably due to radiation; but in the first child a direct relationship does appear to exist, which in our experience is extremely rare.

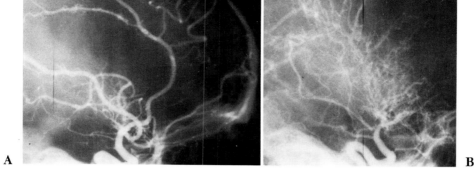

Fig. 16-78. Neurofibromatosis and cerebral artery abnormalities. Bilateral carotid arteriograms demonstrate occlusion of the anterior portion of the middle cerebral branches, with small pial vessels arising directly from the angular branch and the anterior cerebral artery (**A**). On the other side there is occlusion of the supraclinoid portion of the internal carotid artery distal to the anterior choroidal with diffuse central collaterals (**B**). (Courtesy S. Hilal, M.D., New York.)

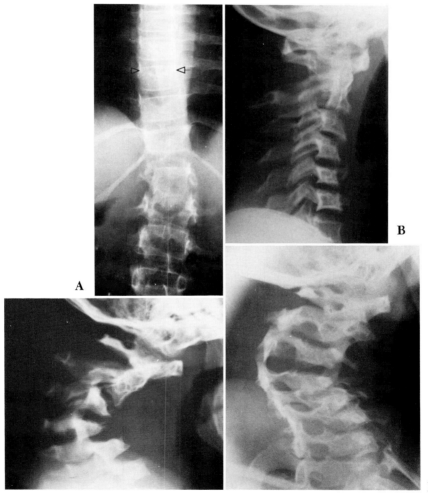

Fig. 16-79. Neurofibromatosis and vertebral dysplasia. A, Mild, of T12, L1, and L2, with a slight scoliosis convex to the left. Note the interpediculate widening of the thoracic spine (arrows) due to an associated diffuse intramedullary astrocytoma. **B,** Relatively mild, of the vertebral bodies of C2, 3, 4, 5, and 6, with a mild cervical kyphosis. **C,** Severe, of the cervical spine, with small pointed vertebral bodies and narrowed spinal canal and an acute posterior kyphosis. **D,** A kyphoscoliosis due to cervical dysplasia, including an enlarged intervertebral foramen in which a neurofibroma occurred.

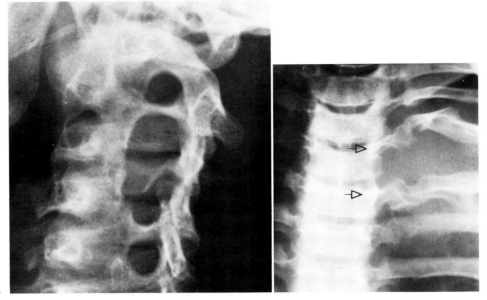

Fig. 16-80. Dumbbell spinal neurofibromas. A, Gross enlargement of the intervertebral foramina between C2 and C3. **B,** Huge paraspinal thoracic, with some sarcomatous elements intruding between the pedicles of T4 and T5 (arrows) distorting the already dysplastic associated ribs.

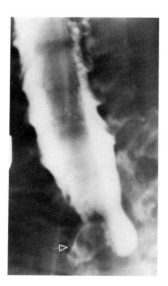

Fig. 16-81. Lateral thoracic meningocele. This may be associated with vertebral dysplasia and be small (arrow) or quite large.

Spine. One of the commonest childhood manifestations of neurofibromatosis is *scoliosis,* varying from a mild nonprogressive form without vertebral dysplasias (which is probably due to neurological muscular abnormalities or hemihypertrophy) to the grotesque form with vertebral dysplasias and angulations and distortions of the spine in any direction (usually more of a kyphosis than a scoliosis, Fig. 16-79). These changes are characteristic of neurofibromatosis (Hunt

and Pugh, 1961; Loop et al., 1965), and they occur more commonly in the thoracic and cervical spine. The neural ectodermal dysplasia (neurofibromas) and the mesodermal dysplasias (vertebral abnormalities) often geographically coexist.

Spinal root neurofibromas, often dumbbell shaped, may be associated with this dysplasia, further enlarging the intervertebral foramina (Fig. 16-80, *A*) and the interpediculate distance and distorting adjacent ribs (Fig. 16-80, *B*). Similar changes in the intervertebral foramina may occur without the vertebral dysplasias. A lateral thoracic meningocele (Sammons and Thomas, 1959; Meszaros et al., 1966) may occur at the spinal dysplastic site and is quite rare in children (Fig. 16-81). It may also enlarge the intervertebral foramina and enter the thoracic cavity, presenting as a large mass (Loop et al., 1965).

Dural ectasia, especially in the lumbar region (Fig. 16-82, *A*), leads to extensive scalloping of the posterior vertebral bodies (Fig. 16-82, *B*) and widening of the sagittal and interpediculate diameters in that area of the spinal column (Heard and Payne, 1962). This ectasia probably results from mesodermal dysplasia of the meninges; and the scalloping will often occur without a neurofibroma, intraspinal neoplasm, or meningocele. Syringomyelia may also be associated with spinal canal neoplasms. Deformity of the spinal canal may also occur in lipomas and teratodermoids within the spinal canal. In rare instances presumably due to the pulsatile effect of a distended lumbar subarachnoid space, scalloping alone may occur in

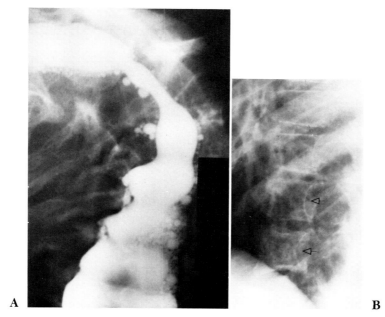

Fig. 16-82. Dural ectasia and vertebral scalloping. A, Gross, of the thoracolumbar region in a patient with severe thoracic scoliosis. **B,** Discrete, of the posterior vertebral bodies in the lower thoracic region (arrows).

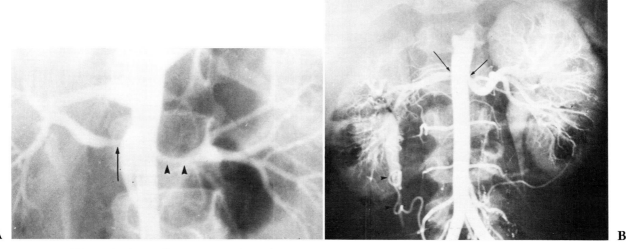

Fig. 16-83. Neurofibromatosis and renal artery stenoses. A, One child with hypertension had a long stenosis of the left (arrowheads) and a short proximal stenosis of the right (arrow) arteries. **B,** Another child had stenosis of the origin of both arteries (arrows), with a small kidney and extensive ureteral collaterals on the right side (arrowheads).

chronic extraventricular obstructive hydrocephalus.

Miscellaneous abnormalities. Renal artery stenosis and hypertension related to neurofibromatosis rarely occur in children. While performing cerebral angiography on two children with neurofibromatosis and suspect intracranial neoplasms, we obtained an angiogram of each renal artery because both children had hypertension (Fig. 16-83). One child had bilateral renal artery stenosis involving both a short and a long segment of each artery; and the other had extensive ureteral artery collaterals. These cases are similar to cases reported by Halpern and Currarino (1965), most of whose patients presented under 10 years of age.

Pheochromocytomas may be associated with neurocutaneous syndromes such as neurofibromatosis in

10% of patients of all ages (Glushein et al., 1953). We have not had experience with such an occurrence in children. Baird and co-workers (1964) described aortic coarctation in neurofibromatosis. Again, this is extremely rare.

REFERENCES

Alvord, E. C.: The pathology of hydrocephalus. In Fields, W. S., and Desmond, M. M., editors: Disorders of the developing nervous system, Springfield, Ill., 1961, Charles C Thomas, Publisher.

Baird, R. J., Evans, J. R., and Labrosse, C. L.: Coarctation of the abdominal aorta, Arch. Surg. 89:466, 1964.

Banergee, T., and Sayers, M. P.: Partial agenesis of the corpus callosum simulating a neoplasm, J. Neurosurg. 37:479, 1972.

Barry, A., Patten, B. M., and Stewart, B. I.: Possible factors in development of Arnold-Chiari malformation, J. Neurosurg. 14:285, 1957.

Benda, C. E.: The Dandy-Walker syndrome or the so-called atresia of the foramen Magendie, J. Neuropathol. Exp. Neurol. 13:14, 1954.

Bergeron, R. T.: Pneumographic demonstration of subependymal heterotopic cortical gray matter in children, Am. J. Roentgenol. Radium Ther. Nucl. Med. 101:168, 1967.

Bergeron, R. T.: Radiographic demonstration of cortical heterotopia, Acta Radiol. [Diagn.] 9:135, 1969.

Berkwitz, N. J., and Rigler, L. G.: Tuberous sclerosis diagnosed with cerebral pneumography, Arch. Neurol. Psychiatry 34:833, 1935.

Billings, K. J., and Danziger, F. S.: Cerebellar heterotopia; case report, J. Neurosurg. 38:218, 1973.

Binet, E. F., Kieffer, S. A., Martin, S. H., and Peterson, H. O.: Orbital dysplasia in neurofibromatosis, Radiology 93:829, 1969.

Bishop, K., Connolly, J. M., Carter, C. H., and Carpenter, D. G.: Holoprosencephaly; a case report with no extracranial abnormalities and normal chromosome count and karyotype, J. Pediatr. 65:406, 1964.

Blackwood, W., McMenemey, W. H., Myer, A., Norman, R. M., and Russell, D. S., editors: Greenfield's neuropathology, ed. 2, London, 1963, Edward Arnold Publishing Co., Ltd.

Blake, J. A.: The roof and lateral recesses of the fourth ventricle, considered morphologically and embryologically, J. Comp. Neurol. 10:79, 1900.

Bligh, A. S., and Laurence, K. M.: The radiological appearances in arhinencephaly, Clin. Radiol. 18:383, 1967.

Borberg, A.: Clinical and genetic investigations into tuberous sclerosis and Recklinghausen's neurofibromatosis: Contribution to elucidation of interrelationship and eugencies of the syndromes, Acta Psychiatr. Scand. 71(supp.):3, 1951.

Boulter, T. R.: The dysraphic states, Surg. Gynecol. Obstet. 124:1091, 1967.

Bourneville, D. M., 1880. In Fitz, C. R., and others, 1974.

Brocklehurst, G.: Diencephalic cysts, J. Neurosurg. 38:47, 1973.

Brocklehurst, G.: The pathogenesis of spina bifida; a study of the relationship between observation, hypothesis, and surgical incentive, Dev. Med. Child. Neurol. 13:147, 1971.

Brodal, A., and Hauglie-Hanssen, E.: Congenital hydrocephalus with defective development of the cerebellar vermis (Dandy-Walker syndrome); clinical an anatomical findings in two cases with particular reference to the so-called atresia of the foramina of Magendie and Luschka, J. Neurol. Neurosurg. Psychiatry 22:99, 1959.

Brook, C. G. D., Sanders, M. D., and Hoare, R. D.: Septo-optic dysplasia, Br. Med. J. 3:811, 1972.

Brun, A., and Probst, F.: The influence of associated cerebral lesions on the morphology of the acallosal brain; a pathological and encephalographic study, Neuroradiology 6:121, 1973.

Bucy, P. C., and Siqueira, E. B.: Malformations of the nervous system; surgical aspects. In Brenneman, J., and McQuarrie, I., editors: Practice of pediatrics, vol. 4, Hagerstown, Md., 1937, W. F. Prior Co.

Bull, J.: The corpus callosum, Clin. Radiol. 18:2, 1967.

Burrows, E. H., Bone changes in orbital neurofibromatosis, Br. J. Radiol. 36:549, 1963.

Cameron, A. H.: Arnold-Chiari malformation and other neuroanatomical malformations associated with spina bifida, J. Pathol. Bacteriol. 73:195, 1957.

Chiari, H., 1891. In Wilkins, R. H., and Brody, I. A., 1971.

Chiari, H., 1895. In Peach, B., 1965.

Chiari, H., 1896. In Wilkins, R. H., and Brody, I. A., 1971.

Cleland, J., 1883. In Peach, B., 1965.

Cooper, J. R.: Brain tumors in hereditary multiple system hamartomatosis (tuberous sclerosis), J. Neurosurg. 34:194, 1971.

Critchley, M., and Earl, C. J. C.: Tuberous sclerosis and allied conditions, Brain 55:311, 1932.

Crowe, F. W., Schull, W. J., and Neel, J. V.: Multiple neurofibromatosis, Springfield, Ill., 1956, Charles C Thomas, Publisher.

Currarino, G., and Silverman, F. N.: Orbital hypotelorism, arhinencephaly, and trigonocephaly, Radiology 74:206, 1960.

D'Agostino, A. N., Kernohan, J. W., and Brown, J. R.: The Dandy-Walker syndrome, J. Neuropathol. Exp. Neurol. 22:450, 1963.

Dandy, W. E., and Blackfan, K. D.: Internal hydrocephalus; an experimental clinical and pathological study, Am. J. Dis. Child. 8:406, 1914.

Daniel, P. M., and Strich, S.: Some observations on congenital deformity of central nervous system known as the Arnold-Chiari malformation, J. Neuropathol. Exp. Neurol. 17:255, 1958.

Danziger, J., Bloch, S., and Van Rensburg, M. J.: Agenesis of the corpus callosum associated with an azygos anterior cerebral artery, a lipoma and porencephalic cyst, S. Afr. Med. J. 46:739, 1972.

Davidoff, L. M., and Dyke, C. G.: Agenesis of the corpus callosum; report of 3 cases, Am. J. Roentgenol. Radium Ther. 32:1, 1934.

Davidson, K. C.: Cranial and intracranial lesions in neurofibromatosis, Am. J. Roentgenol. Radium Ther. Nucl. Med. 98:550, 1966.

Dawson, J.: Pulmonary tuberous sclerosis; its relationship to other forms of the disease, Q. J. Med. 23:113, 1954.

De Barros, M. C., Farias, W., Ataíde, L., and Lins, S.: Basilar impression and Arnold-Chiari malformation; a study of 66 cases, J. Neurol. Neurosurg. Psychiatry 31:596, 1968.

de Haene, A.: Agénésie partielle du vermis du cervelet à caractère familial, Acta Neurol. Belg. 55:622, 1955.

Dekaban, A. S., and Magee, K. R.: Occurrence of neurologic abnormalities in infants of diabetic mothers, Neurology 8:193, 1958.

de Morsier, G.: Études sur les dysraphies crânioencéphaliques. III. Agénésie du septum lucidum avec malformation du tractus optique; la dysplasie septo-optique, Schweiz. Arch. Neurol. Neurochir. Psychiatry 77:267, 1956.

de Morsier, G.: Median cranioencephalic dysraphias and olfactogenital dysplasia, World Neurol. 3:485, 1962.

DeMyer, W.: Classification of cerebral malformations, Birth Defects 7:78, 1971.

DeMyer, W., Zeman, W., and Palmer, C. G.: Familial alobar holoprosencephaly (arhinencephaly) with median cleft lip and palate; report of patient with 46 chromosomes, Neurology 13:913, 1963.

DeMyer, W., Zeman, W., and Palmer, C. G.: The face predicts the brain; diagnostic significance of median facial anomalies for holoprosencephaly (arhinencephaly), Pediatrics 34:256, 1964.

Dickerson, W. W.: Characteristic roentgenographic changes associated with tuberous sclerosis, Arch. Neurol. Psychiatry 53:199, 1945.

Dieker, H., Edwards, R. H., ZuRhein, G., Chou, S. M., Hartman, H. A., and Opitz, J. M.: The lissencephaly syndrome, Birth Defects 5:53, 1969.

Ebaugh, F. G., and Holt, G. W.: Neurology and psychiatry; congenital malformations of the nervous system, Am. J. Med. Sci. 246:104, 1963.

Ellenberger, C., and Runyan, T. E.: Holoprosencephaly with hypoplasia of the optic nerves, dwarfism, and agenesis of the septum pellucidium, Am. J. Ophthalmol. 70:960, 1970.

Elliott, G. B., and McGeachy, W. G.: The monster Purkinje-cell nature of so-called "congenital rhabdomyoma of heart"; a forme fruste of tuberous sclerosis, Am. Heart J. 63:636, 1962.

Elliott, G. B., and Wollin, D. W.: Defect of the corpus callosum and congenital occlusion of the fourth ventricle with tuberous sclerosis, Am. J. Roentgenol. Radium Ther. Nucl. Med. 85:701, 1961.

Emery, J. L., and Levick, R. K.: The movement of the brainstem and vessels around the brainstem in children with hydrocephalus and the Arnold-Chiari deformity, Dev. Med. Child Neurol. 11 (supp.):49, 1966.

Emery, J. L., and MacKenzie, N.: Medullo-cervical dislocation deformity (Chiari II deformity) related to neurospinal dysraphism (meningomyelocele), Brain 96:155, 1973.

Emery, J. L., and Naik, D.: Spinal cord segment lengths in children with meningomyelocoele and the "Cleland-Arnold Chiari" deformity, Br. J. Radiol. 41:287, 1968.

Farrow, G. M., Harrison, E. G., Jr., Utz, D. C., and Jones, D. R.: Renal angiomyolipoma; a clinicopathologic study of 32 cases, Cancer 22:564, 1968.

Fedrick, J., and Wilson, T. S.: Malformations of the central nervous system in Glasgow; an examination of the evidence for clustering in space and time, Br. J. Prev. Soc. Med. 25:210, 1971.

Fienman, N. L., and Yakovac, W. C.: Neurofibromatosis in childhood, J. Pediatr. 76:339, 1970.

Fitz, C. R., Harwood-Nash, D. C. F., and Thompson, J. R.: Neuroradiology of tuberous sclerosis in children, Radiology 110:635, 1974.

Fitzpatrick, T. B., Szabó, G., Hori, Y., Simone, A. A., Reid, W. B., and Greenberg, M. H.: White leaf-shaped macules; earliest visible sign of tuberous sclerosis, Arch. Dermatol. 98:1, 1968.

Friedman, M., and Cohen, P.: Agenesis of corpus callosum as a possible sequel to maternal rubella during pregnancy, Am. J. Dis. Child 73:178, 1947.

Gardner, W. J.: Anatomical features common to Arnold-Chiari malformation and Dandy-Walker malformation suggest common origin, Cleve. Clin. Q. 26:206, 1959.

Gardner, W. J., Smith, J. L., and Padget, D. H.: The relationship of Arnold-Chiari and Dandy-Walker malformations, J. Neurosurg. 36:481, 1972.

Gibson, J. B.: Congenital hydrocephalus due to atresia of the foramen of Magendie, J. Neuropathol. Exp. Neurol. 14:244, 1955.

Gilmor, R. L., Kalsbeck, J. E., Goodman, J. M., and Franken, E. A.: Angiographic assessment of occipital encephaloceles, Radiology 103:127, 1972.

Glushein, A. S., Mansuy, M. M., and Littman, D. S.: Pheochromocytoma; its relationship to the neurocutaneous syndromes, Am. J. Med. 14:318, 1953.

Gooding, C. A., Carter, A., and Hoare, R. D.: New ventriculographic aspects of the Arnold-Chiari malformation, Radiology 89:626, 1967.

Green, G. J.: The radiology of tuberose sclerosis, Clin. Radiol. 19:135, 1968.

Greenfield, J. G.: Arnold-Chiari malformation. In Blackwood, W., McMenemey, W. H., Meyer, A., Norman, R. M., and Russell, D. S., editors: Greenfield's neuropathology, ed. 2, London, 1963, Edward Arnold Publishing Co., Ltd.

Greitz, T., and Sjögren, S. E.: The posterior inferior cerebellar artery, Acta Radiol. [Diagn.] 1:284, 1963.

Gunther, M., and Penrose, L. S.: The genetics of epiloia, J. Genet. 31:413, 1935.

Guthkelch, A. N.: Occipital cranium bifidum, Arch. Dis. Child. 45:104, 1970.

Helpern, M., and Currarino, G.: Vascular lesions causing hypertension in neurofibromatosis, N. Engl. J. Med. 273:248, 1965.

Handa, J., Teraura, T., Imai, T., and Handa, H.: Agenesis of the corpus callosum associated with multiple developmental anomalies of the cerebral arteries, Radiology 92:1301, 1969.

Hart, M. N., Malamud, N., and Ellis, W. G.: The Dandy-Walker syndrome; clinicopathological study based on 28 cases, Neurology 22:771, 1972.

Harwood-Nash, D. C.: Optic gliomas and pediatric neuroradiology, Radiol. Clin. North Am. 10:83, 1972.

Harwood-Nash, D. C.: Paediatric neuroradiology, Radiol. Clin. North Am. 10:313, 1972 .

Harwood-Nash, D. C., and Fitz, C. R.: Myelography and syringohydromyelia in infancy and childhood, Radiology 113:661, 1974.

Heard, G., and Payne, E. E.: Scalloping of vertebral bodies in von Recklinghausen's disease of the nervous system (neurofibromatosis), J. Neurol. Neurosurg. Psychiatry 25:345, 1962.

Hendrick, E. B., Hoffman, H. J., and Hugenholtz, H.: Occipital encephalocoele, hydrocephalus, Klippel-Feil deformity and cleft palate—a tetrad of anomalies. In Sano, K., Ishii, S., and Le Vay, D., editors: Recent progress in neurological surgery, Proceedings of the Symposia of the Fifth International Congress of Neurological Surgery, Tokyo, Oct. 7-13, 1973, New York, 1974, American Elsevier Publishing Co., Inc.

Hilal, S. K., Solomon, G. E., Gold, A. P., and Carter, S.: Primary cerebral arterial occlusive disease in children. II. Neurocutaneous syndromes, Radiology 99:87, 1971.

Hintz, R. L., Menking, M., and Sotos, J. F.: Familial holoprosencephaly with endocrine dysgenesis, J. Pediatr. 72:81, 1968.

Hitselberger, W. E., and Hughes, R. L.: Bilateral acoustic tumors and neurofibromatosis, Arch. Otolaryngol. 88:700, 1968.

Holman, C. B., and MacCarty, C. S.: Cerebral angiography in agenesis of the corpus callosum, Radiology 72:317, 1959.

Holt, J. F., and Dickerson, W. W.: Osseous lesions of tuberous sclerosis, Radiology 58:1, 1952.

Holt, J. F., and Wright, E. M.: The radiologic features of neurofibromatosis, Radiology 51:647, 1948.

Howieson, J., and Norrell, H.: Angiographic findings in congenital infantile hydrocephalus, Acta Radiol. [Diagn.] 9: 322, 1969.

Hoyt, W. F., Kaplan, S. L., Grumbach, M. M., and Glaser, J. S.: Septo-optic dysplasia and pituitary dwarfism, Lancet 1:893, 1970.

Hunt, J. C., and Pugh, D. G.: Skeletal lesions in neurofibromatosis, Radiology 76:1, 1961.

Ingraham, F. D., and Swan, H.: Spina bifida and cranium bifidum; a survey of 546 cases, N. Engl. J. Med. 228:559, 1943.

Joffe, N.: Calvarial bone defects involving lambdoid suture in neurofibromatosis, Br. J. Radiol. 38:23, 1965.

Joubert, M., Eisenring, J. J., Robb, J. P., and Anderman, F.: Familial agenesis of the cerebellar vermis; a syndrome of episodic hyperpnea, abnormal eye movements, ataxia, and retardation, Neurology 19:813, 1969.

Juhl, J. H., and Wesenberg, R. L.: Radiological findings in congenital and acquired occlusions of the foramina of Magendie and Luschka, Radiology 86:801, 1966.

Kapp, J. P., Paulson, G. W., and Odom, G. L.: Brain tumors with tuberous sclerosis, J. Neurosurg. 26:191, 1967.

Koch, F. P., and Doyle, P. J.: Agenesis of the corpus callosum; report of eight cases in infancy, J. Pediatr. 50:345, 1957.

Krainer, L.: Die Hirn und Rückenmarkslipome, Virchow. Arch. [Pathol. Anat.] 295:107, 1935.

Kruyff, E., and Jeffs, R.: Skull abnormalities associated with the Arnold-Chiari malformation, Acta Radiol. [Diagn.] 5:9, 1966.

Kundrat, H., 1882. In Zingesser, L. H., and others, 1966.

Kurlander, G. J., DeMyer, W., Campbell, J. A., and Taybi, H.: Roentgenology of holoprosencephaly (arhinencephaly), Acta Radiol. [Diagn.] 5:25, 1966.

Lagos, J. C., and Gomez, M. R.: Tuberous sclerosis; reappraisal of a clinical entity, Mayo Clin. Proc. 42:26, 1967.

Lagos, J. C., Holman, C. B., and Gomez, M. R.: Tuberous sclerosis: Neuroroentgenologic observations, Am. J. Roentgenol. Radium Ther. Nucl. Med. 104:171, 1968.

La Torre, E., Fortuna, A., and Occhipinti, E.: Angiographic differentiation between Dandy-Walker cyst and arachnoid cyst of the posterior fossa in newborn infants and children, J. Neurosurg. 38:298, 1973.

Laurence, K. M.: The natural history of spina bifida cystica, Arch. Dis. Child. 34:41, 1964.

Leck, I.: Changes in the incidence of neural-tube defects, Lancet 2:791, 1966.

Lewald, L. T.: Congenital absence of the superior orbital wall associated with pulsating exophthalmos: report of four cases, Am. J. Roentgenol. Radium Ther. 30:756, 1933.

Lichtenstein, B. W.: Atresia and stenosis of the aqueduct of Sylvius with comments on Arnold-Chiari complex, J. Neuropathol. Exp. Neurol. 18:3, 1958.

Lichtenstein, B. W.: Distant neuroanatomic complications of spina bifida, Arch. Neurol. 47:195, 1942.

Loeser, J. D., and Alvord, E. C.: Agenesis of the corpus callosum, Brain 91:553, 1968a.

Loeser, J. D., and Alvord, E. C.: Clinicopathological correlations in agenesis of the corpus callosum, Neurology 18:745, 1968b.

Loop, J. W., Akeson, W. H., and Clawson, D. K.: Acquired thoracic abnormalities in neurofibromatosis, Am. J. Roentgenol. Radium Ther. Nucl. Med. 93:416, 1965.

Lorber, J.: The prognosis of occipital encephalocele, Dev. Med. Child Neurol. 13 (supp.):75, 1967.

Maki, Y., and Kumagai, K.: Angiographic features of alobar holoprosencephaly, Neuroradiology 6:270, 1974.

Marburg, O.: So-called agenesia of the corpus callosum (callosal defect): Anterior cerebral dysraphism, Arch. Neurol. Psychiatry 61:297, 1949.

McCoy, W. T., Simpson, D. A., and Carter, R. F.: Cerebral malformations complicating spina bifida; radiological studies, Clin. Radiol. 18:176, 1967.

McLaurin, R. L.: Parietal cephaloceles, Neurology 14:764, 1964.

Meszaros, W. T., Guzzo, F., and Schorsch, H.: Neurofibromatosis, Am. J. Roentgenol. Radium Ther. Nucl. Med. 98:557, 1966.

Milledge, R. D., Gerald, B. E., and Carter, W. J.: Pulmonary manifestations of tuberous sclerosis, Am. J. Roentgenol. Radium Ther. Nucl. Med. 98:734, 1966.

Milunsky, A., Alpert, E., and Charles, D.: Prenatal diagnosis of anencephaly, Obstet. Gynecol. 43:592, 1974.

Morris, L.: Agenesis of the corpus callosum; a new angiographic sign, Br. J. Radiol. 35:423, 1962.

Naiman, J., and Fraser, F. C.: Agenesis of the corpus callosum: a report of two cases in siblings, Arch. Neurol. Psychiatry 74:182, 1955.

Nobler, M. P., Shapiro, J. H., and Fine, D. I. M.: The cerebral angiogram in agenesis of the corpus callosum, Am. J. Roentgenol. Radium Ther. Nucl. Med. 90:522, 1963.

Norman, R. M.: Malformations of the nervous system, birth injury and diseases of early life. In Blackwood, W., McMenemey, W. H., Myer, A., Norman, R. M., and Russell, D. S., editors: Greenfield's neuropathology, ed. 2, London, 1963, Edward Arnold Publishing Co., Ltd.

Norman, R. M., and Urich, H.: Cerebellar hypoplasia associated with systemic degeneration in early life, J. Neurol. Neurosurg. Psychiatry 21:159, 1958.

Occleshaw, J. V.: The posterior inferior cerebellar arteries; some quantitative observations in posterior cranial fossa tumours and the Arnold-Chiari malformation, Clin. Radiol. 21:1, 1970.

Padget, D. H.: Development of so-called dysraphism; with embryologic evidence of clinical Arnold-Chiari and Dandy-Walker malformations, Johns Hopkins Med. J. 130:127, 1972.

Padget, D. H., and Lindenberg, R.: Inverse cerebellum morphogenetically related to Dandy-Walker and Arnold-Chiari syndromes; bizarre malformed brain with occipital encephalocele, Johns Hopkins Med. J. 131:228, 1972.

Peach, B.: Arnold-Chiari malformation with normal spine, Arch. Neurol. 10:497, 1964.

Peach, B.: The Arnold-Chiari malformation, Arch. Neurol. 12:527, 1965a.

Peach, B.: Arnold-Chiari malformation, Arch. Neurol. 12:613, 1965b.

Pearce, J.: The central nervous system pathology in multiple neurofibromatosis, Neurology 17:691, 1967.

Peyton, W. T., and Simmons, D. R.: Neurofibromatosis with defect in the wall of the orbit, Arch. Neurol. Psychiatry 55:248, 1946.

Pollock, J. A., and Newton, T. H.: Encephalocele and cranium bifidum. In Newton, T. H., and Potts, D. G., editors: Radiology of the skull and brain. Vol. 1, book 2, The skull, St. Louis, 1971, The C. V. Mosby Co.

Pollock, J. A., Newton, T. H., and Hoyt, W. F.: Transsphenoidal and transethmoidal encephaloceles; a review of clinical and roentgen features in eight cases, Radiology 90: 442, 1968.

Probst, F. P.: A defect of the anterior part of the corpus callosum simulating tumour, Neuroradiology 7:205, 1974.

Probst, F. P.: Congenital defects of the corpus callosum;

morphology and encephalographic appearances, Acta Radiol. [Diagn.] 331 (supp.):1, 1973.

Raimondi, A. J.: The angiographic evaluation of ventricular size in the hydrocephalic newborn. In Krayenbühl, H., Maspes, P. E., and Sweet, W. H., editors: Progress in neurological surgery, vol. 4, Basel, 1971, S. Karger, AG.

Raimondi, A. J., Samuelson, G., Yarzagaray, L., and Norton, T.: Atresia of the foramina of Luschka and Magendie; the Dandy-Walker cyst, J. Neurosurg. 31:202, 1969.

Rakic, P., and Yakovlev, P. I.: Development of the corpus callosum and cavum septi in man, J. Comp. Neurol. 132:45, 1968.

Russell, D. S.: Observations on the pathology of hydrocephalus, Med. Res. Counc. Rep. no. 265, 1949.

Russell, D. S., and Rubinstein, L. J.: Pathology of tumours of the nervous system, ed. 3, London, 1971, Edward Arnold Publishing Co., Ltd.

Sabourard, O., Pecker, J., Simon, P., and Chatel, M.: Lipomes du corps calleux; données angiographiques et discussion pathogénique de leur séméiologie clinique, Rev. Neurol. 117:557, 1967.

Sammons, B. P., and Thomas, D. F.: Extensive lumbar meningocele associated with neurofibromatosis, Am. J. Roentgenol. Radium Ther. Nucl. Med. 81:1021, 1959.

Simonton, J. H., and Jamison, R. C.: An outline of radiographic findings in multiple-system disease, Springfield, Ill., 1966, Charles C Thomas, Publisher.

Spillane, J. D., Pallis, C., and Jones, A. M.: Developmental abnormalities in the region of the foramen magnum, Brain 80:11, 1957.

Strandgaard, L.: The Dandy-Walker syndrome—a case with a patent foramen of the 4th ventricle demonstrated by encephalography, Br. J. Radiol. 43:734, 1970.

Sutton, D.: Radiological diagnosis of lipoma of corpus callosum, Br. J. Radiol. 22:534, 1949.

Sutton, D., and Liversedge, L. A.: Radiological and pathological aspects of tuberous sclerosis, Clin. Radiol. 2:224, 1951.

Suwanwela, C., and Suwanwela, N.: A morphological classification of sincipital encephalomeningoceles, J. Neurosurg. 36:201, 1972.

Swischuk, L. E., Meyer, G. A., and Bryan, N.: Infantile hydrocephalus and cerebral angiography; assessment and indications, Am. J. Roentgenol. Radium Ther. Nucl. Med. 115:50, 1972.

Taggart, J. K., and Walker, A. E.: Congenital atresia of the foramens of Luschka and Magendie, Arch. Neurol. Psychiatry 48:583, 1942.

Tandon, P. N.: Meningoencephaloceles, Acta Neurol. Scand. 46:369, 1970.

Teng, P., and Papatheodorou, C.: Myelographic appearance of vascular anomalies of the spinal cord, Br. J. Radiol. 37:358, 1964.

Thibault, J. H., and Manuelidis, E. E.: Tuberous sclerosis in a premature infant; report of a case and review of the literature, Neurology 20:139, 1970.

Van Epps, E. F.: Agenesis of corpus callosum with concomitant malformations including atresia of foramens of Luschka and Magendie, Am. J. Roentgenol. Radium Ther. Nucl. Med. 70:47, 1953.

Van Nouhuys, J. M., and Bruyn, G. W.: Nasopharyngeal trans-sphenoidal encephalocele, crater-like hole in the optic disc and agenesis of the corpus callosum. Pneumoencephalographic visualization in a case, Psychiatr. Neurol. Neurochir. 67:243, 1964.

Vogt, H.: Zur Pathologie und pathologischen Anatomie der verschiedenen Idiotieformen. II. Tuberöse sklerose, Monatschr. Psychiatr. Neurol. 24:106, 1908.

von Recklinghausen, F., 1862. In Cooper, J. R., 1971.

von Recklinghausen, F. E., 1882. In Davidson, K. C., 1966.

Warkany, J.: Congenital malformations; notes and comments, Chicago, 1971, Year Book Medical Publishers, Inc.

Weed, L. H.: Certain anatomical and physiological aspects of the meninges and cerebrospinal fluid, Brain 58:383, 1935.

Weichert, K. A., Dine, M. S., Benton, C., and Silverman, F. N.: Macrocranium and neurofibromatosis, Radiology 107:163, 1973.

Wesenberg, R. L., Juhl, J. H., and Daube, J. R.: Radiological finding in lissencephaly (congenital agyria), Radiology 87:436, 1966.

Whitaker, P. H.: Radiological manifestations in tuberous sclerosis, Br. J. Radiol. 32:152, 1959.

Wilkins, R. H., and Brody, I. A.: The Arnold-Chiari malformation, Arch. Neurol. 25:376, 1971.

Williams, B.: Further thoughts on the valvular action of the Arnold-Chiari malformation, Dev. Med. Child Neurol. 13 (supp. 25):105, 1971.

Wisen, M., DeMyer, W., and Campbell, R.: Unique angiographic and ventriculographic pattern of alobar holoprosencephaly (arhinencephaly), Radiology 84:945, 1965.

Wolf, B. S., Newman, C. M., and Khilnani, M. T.: The posterior inferior cerebellar artery on vertebral angiography, Am. J. Roentgenol. Radium Ther. Nucl. Med. 87:322, 1962.

Wolpert, S. M.: Vascular studies of congenital anomalies. In Newton, T. H., and Potts, D. G., editors: Radiology of the skull and brain. Vol. 2, book 4, Angiography, St. Louis, 1974, The C. V. Mosby Co.

Wolpert, S. M., Carter, B.L., and Ferris, E. J.: Lipomas of the corpus callosum: an angiographic analysis, Am. J. Roentgenol. Radium Ther. Nucl. Med. 115:92, 1972.

Wolpert, S. M., Haller, J. S., and Rabe, E. F.: The value of angiography in the Dandy-Walker syndrome and posterior fossa extra-axial cysts, Am. J. Roentgenol. Radium Ther. Nucl. Med. 109:261, 1970.

Yakovlev, P. I.: Pathoarchitectonic studies of cerebral malformations. III. Arrhinencephalies (holotelencephalies), J. Neuropathol. Exp. Neurol. 18:22, 1959.

Yakovlev, P. I., and Corwin, W.: Roentgenographic sign in cases of tuberous sclerosis of the brain (multiple "brain stones"), Arch. Neurol. Psychiatry 42:1030, 1939.

Yakovlev, P. I., and Guthrie, R. H.: Congenital ectodermoses (neurocutaneous syndromes) in epileptic patients, Arch. Neurol. Psychiatry 26:1145, 1931.

Yakovlev, P. I., and Wadsworth, R. C.: Schizencephalies; a study of congenital clefts in the cerebral mantle; clefts with fused lips, J. Neuropathol. Exp. Neurol. 5:116, 1946.

Zellweger, H.: Agenesia corporis callosi, Helv. Paediatr. Acta 7:136, 1952.

Ziegler, E.: Bösartige, familiäre frühinfantile Krampfkrankheit, teilweise Verbunden mit familiärer Balkenaplasie, Helv. Paediatr. Acta 13:169, 1958.

Zingesser, L., Schechter, M., Gonatas, N., Levy, A., and Wisoff, H.: Agenesis of the corpus callosum associated with an inter-hemispheric arachnoid cyst, Br. J. Radiol. 37:905, 1964.

Zingesser, L. H., Schechter, M. M., and Medina, A.: Angiographic and pneumoencephalographic features of holoprosencephaly, Am. J. Roentgenol. Radium Ther. Nucl. Med. 97:561, 1966.

CHAPTER 17

Normal spine

EMBRYOLOGY

Formation of the fetal vertebral column begins at approximately 3 weeks—when the paraxial bar, mesodermal tissue derived from the neural streak, begins to divide into triangular somites (Figs. 17-1 and 17-2). The division is in an axial plane, with the somites aligned rostrocaudally. A total of forty-four pairs of somites will form by the end of the 11 mm (38-day) stage, though the most rostral of these will already have further developed by the time the most caudal form. The first somite is transient (McRae, 1974). Somites 2 to 4 form the basiocciput so, unlike the remainder of the spine, the craniocervical division is at a somite division.

By the time of somite formation, the notochord

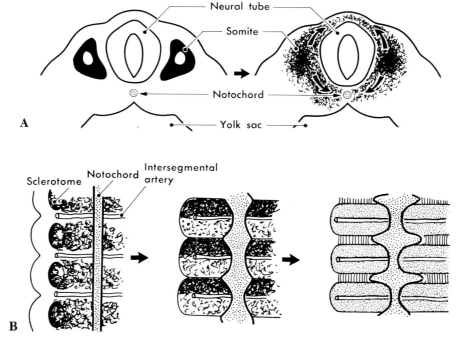

Fig. 17-1. Early embryological development. A, Section through a vertebral level. The somites form adjacent to the neural tube and then migrate medially to surround the tube and notochord, separating the notochord from both the yolk sac and the neural tube. **B,** Coronal section. The somite cells migrate to surround the notochord. The more dense caudal segment of each somite around the notochord combines with the less dense cranial segment of the somite below, forming a precursor of the vertebral body. The disk develops from the most cranial part of the caudal segment, which is now the top of the vertebral body. The nucleus pulposus develops from the widened notochord. Due to connection of the caudal segment with the cranial segment of the next most caudal somite, the intersegmental artery (previously between the somites) is now in the center of the vertebral body.

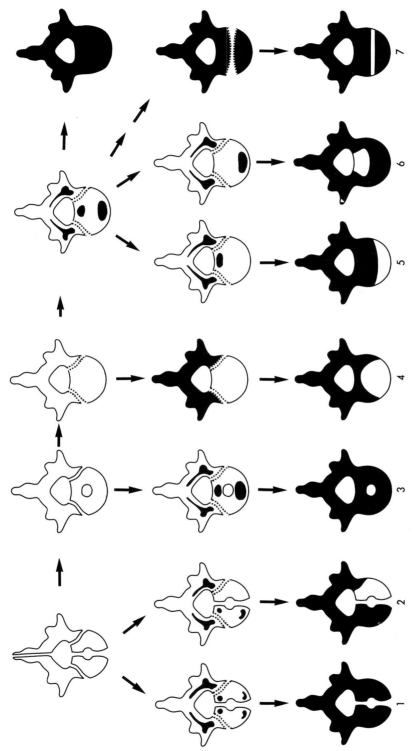

Fig. 17-2. Normal vertebral body formation and possible developmental abnormalities. Cartilaginous formation in white; osseous formation in black. Top line portrays the normal sequence. Middle line depicts intermediate stages of abnormal development. Lower line shows the final stages of abnormality. *1*, Sagittal cleft of body from nonfusion of the cartilaginous centers; *2*, hemivertebra from nonfusion of the cartilaginous centers and subsequent nondevelopment of the ossification centers on one side; *3*, notochord remnant; *4*, absent vertebral body from nondevelopment of the ossification centers; *5*, hypoplastic vertebral body from nondevelopment of the anterior ossification center; *6*, hypoplastic vertebral body from nondevelopment of the posterior ossification center; *7*, failure of fusion of the anterior and posterior ossification centers.

(arising from Henson's node) has migrated caudally between the ectoderm and endoderm and is between the neural tube and the yolk sac. The notochord is a mesodermal structure.

From the somites, cellular migrations occur. Dorsolaterally the dermatome forms and medially the myotome at each somite level. Ventrolaterally the sclerotome (spine) cells migrate and surround the notochord—forming what is referred to as the "membranous vertebral column," which separates the notochord from the neural tube and gut. As each sclerotome proliferates, it becomes more dense caudally than rostrally. The halves divide and move slightly rostrally. The intervertebral disk forms from the rostral surface of the denser caudal mass. The caudal mass also joins with the less dense rostral half of the next most caudal sclerotome.

Intersegmental arteries that were between the somites now enter the center of the forming vertebral bodies. Likewise the vertebrae, rather than remain at the same level, alternate with the myotomes.

By the middle of the sixth week (11 mm stage), the maximum forty-four somites have formed. *Chondrification centers* also appear shortly after this. There are two centers in each half of the vertebral body, initially separated by the dorsoventral sheath of the notochord, and a center for each half of the forming posterior arch (which grows around the neural tube) (Fig. 17-2). These centers are well formed in the cervical region by 7 weeks of gestation, and the lateral chondrification centers for the ribs are also being formed at this time. With the formation and joining of the chondrification centers, there is a squeezing of the notochord cells out of the vertebral bodies and into the disk spaces, where the notochord expands slightly in becoming the nucleus pulposus of the disk.

During the seventh and eighth weeks the anterior and posterior *spinal ligaments* form. Anteriorly they attach to the vertebral bodies, and posteriorly to the fibrous tissue of the disk space. Before ossification occurs, the four vertebral body chondrification centers fuse into a cartilaginous vertebral body and are joined to the cartilaginous centers of the arches, which have also fused dorsally behind the neural tube.

The *ossification centers* of the posterior arches and vertebral bodies do not appear simultaneously at the same levels. The ossification centers of the arches begin appearing in the cervical region first, during the eighth week (25 to 28 mm stage). The ossification centers of the vertebral bodies first begin in the lower thoracic and upper lumbar areas, and ossification quickly propagates cranially and caudally. The uppermost cervical and lowermost sacral bodies appear last, being radiographically visible by special techniques at about the fifth month (O'Rahilly and Meyer,

1956). Unlike the cartilaginous centers, the ossification centers appear dorsally and ventrally in the vertebral body and quickly fuse into a single center.

In the ninth week, periosteal vessels begin to invade the dorsal and ventral sides of the cartilaginous vertebral bodies and form vascular lakes. By the fifth to sixth month, the ossification centers of the vertebral body have divided the cartilaginous body into dorsal and ventral plates and the bony ossification centers have appeared everywhere but the lower sacrum and coccyx.

Variations from the pattern just described occur at the C1 and C2 vertebral bodies: the ossification center of the body of C1 forms the odontoid process of C2, and the ossification centers of the arches of C1 join anteriorly to form a ring; the C1 vertebra then has no body embryologically; in addition to or because of this, there is no disk space formed between C1 and C2. Other variations occur at different levels: the cervical and lumbar spines fuse at their costal processes to the transverse process ossification centers and prominent transverse processes result in these areas compared with the thoracic spine. Failure of fusion accounts for the development of extra ribs at C7 and L1.

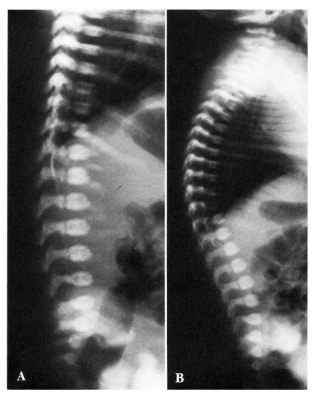

Fig. 17-3. Neonatal spines. A, Slight lumbosacral and thoracolumbar curve. **B,** More pronounced curve in the cervical, thoracic, and lumbosacral areas of another neonate.

The sacral bodies develop from central ossification centers and inferior and superior epiphyseal plates. The upper three sacral vertebrae also have lateral accessory ossification centers that later fuse with the sacral bodies but can be seen separately at birth (Fig. 17-7). The growth of the vertebral bodies and arches is thought to depend on the presence of the spinal cord. Without the cord the bony spine forms abnormally or not at all.

GENERAL DEVELOPMENT

The neonatal spine is often described as being straight. Though when viewed laterally the curvatures of the spine in the neonate are much gentler than in the older child or adult, there is still a slight cervical and lumbosacral lordosis and a slight thoracic kyphosis (Fig. 17-3). The midthoracic-to-midlumbar area is the straightest segment. With the exception of this area, a completely straight segment of spine, even in

the neonate, should be considered abnormal—particularly if seen on two consecutive examinations. Intrinsic spinal disease is not necessarily present, however; such straightening may be due to extrinsic diseases ranging from tumors to muscle spasm.

The individual vertebral bodies of the neonate tend to be ovoid but can be fairly square, especially in the thoracic area (Figs. 17-3 and 17-4). In the lateral view they will look particularly squarish, and the bone within a bone appearance will be present (Fig. 17-5). This configuration is seen primarily before the age of 6 weeks and occurs in about half of normal infants (Brill et al., 1973). It is also very common in premature infants (Martin, 1975).

At birth the vertebral bodies normally have a single fused ossification center. Each half of the posterior neural arch also has an ossified center but is cartilaginous in its attachment to the vertebral body and opposite arch, giving a normal radiographic bifid ap-

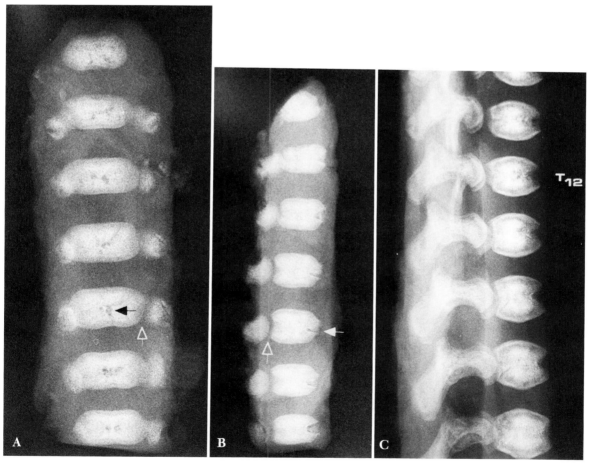

Fig. 17-4. Neonatal spines, dissected specimens. A and **B,** AP and lateral views of the thoracic spine show the vertebral bodies to be relatively square. The neurocentral synchondroses (open arrows) are readily visualized along with both anterior and posterior vascular channels (solid arrows). **C,** Lateral view of the lumbar and lower thoracic spine shows all vertebrae to be quite ovoid in another specimen.

pearance along with separation of the arch and body (Fig. 17-4).

A variation of this vertebral body configuration is the *coronal cleft* vertebra, seen mostly in the lumbar region but also occurring throughout the thoracic spine (Fig. 17-6). Though the cleft is thought to be caused by persistent notochord tissue (Cohen et al., 1956), no notochord cells are within the vertical cleft. Another possible explanation is that the separate anterior and posterior ossification centers have not completely fused. Once thought to occur almost exclusively in boys, the coronal cleft showed only a 3-to-1 male-female ratio and an incidence of 1 per 150 births in a large series of 125 cases (Fielden and Russell, 1970). There does appear to be a higher incidence of this variation in abnormal infants (Rowley, 1955; Cohen et al., 1956). The defect usually disappears in a few weeks to months, but Rowley reported one coronal cleft that remained until the child was 2 years and 9 months of age. In utero it can be seen as early as 22 weeks. The cleft causes the vertebral body to be larger than usual in the sagittal diameter.

In Fielden and Russell's (1970) large series, one or more lumbar vertebral bodies were usually affected—with L4 being involved in 64% of the cases. The thoracic spine was rarely involved, and the cervical

spine not at all. One vertebral body was affected in 37.6%, two in 17.6%, three in 18.4%, and four or more in 24.8%.

The vertebral bodies are also "cleft" by anterior and posterior *vascular channels*, which are prominent in the neonatal and infant periods (Figs. 17-3 to 17-

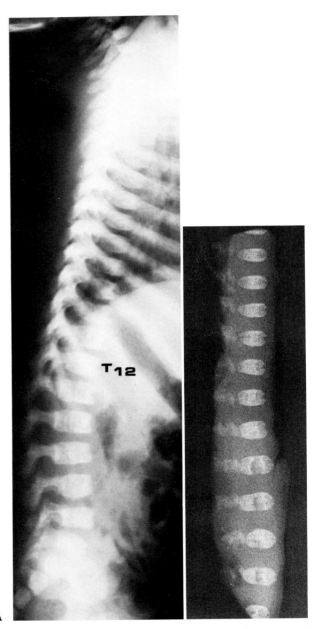

A   B

Fig. 17-6. Coronal cleft vertebrae. A, At T10, T11, and L1-L3. B, In three of the lumbar vertebral bodies. (Dissected specimen.) C, Sagittal section through two vertebral bodies showing the vertical clefts continuous with the cartilaginous end plates. Anterior vascular channels are also well seen. D, Axial section through the inferior portion of a vertebral body showing the cleft completely dividing the ventral and dorsal halves of the vertebral body.

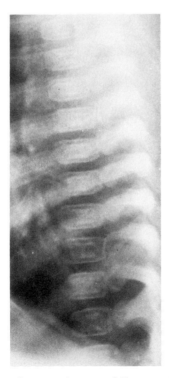

Fig. 17-5. Neonatal spine. The normal "bone within a bone" appearance of the vertebrae (which have relatively flat superior and inferior surfaces) is well shown. In older children this same pattern may accompany recovery from a severe illness.

6). The anterior channels gradually fade, persisting longest in the thoracic area. The posterior channel is visible even in adults; and though unusual in adults, the anterior channel cannot be considered abnormal when seen.

In the neonate and infant the lumbar, and especially the cervical, interpediculate distances are relatively wider than in the older child and adult. This plus visualization of the neural arch separate from the vertebral body can lead the examiner to the mistaken notion that the spinal canal is enlarged. Another minor variation of the neonatal vertebral body is its slightly shorter height anteriorly than posteriorly throughout the spine which creates a slightly wedged appearance of the bodies. The ossification centers of the sacral vertebral bodies and arches are present at birth and radiographically visible, as are the lateral secondary ossification centers (Fig. 17-7). Those of the coccyx are usually not formed at birth.

As in embryological formation, the atlas and axis are different from the remainder of the vertebral column at birth and these differences can be radiographically recognized. The anterior portion of the atlas has a separate ossification center that is present at birth in only 20.6% of normal infants (Fig. 17-8) (Tompsett and Donaldson, 1951). This ossification center is usually present by age 1. The odontoid process is attached to the body of the axis by a cartilaginous attachment and on radiographs appears to be separate (Fig. 17-8). In the AP projection the odontoid process may be vertically split in appearance. The reason for the splitting is clear, since embryologically there are two side-by-side ossification centers for the odontoid.

The changes from the neonatal period through infancy are primarily in configuration of individual vertebral bodies and the spine as a whole. Much change occurs as early as the first 6 months (Fig. 17-9). The secondary ossification center at the top of the dens usually appears by the end of the second year (Fig. 17-10). There is confusion in the literature as to the terminology of this center. We call the center the *os terminale;* and, as does Epstein (1969), we use the term *os odontoideum* to refer to an odontoid process that has not fused to its base, usually associated with a thick anterior and a thin posterior arch to the atlas.

In the first year, from the lumbar region upward,

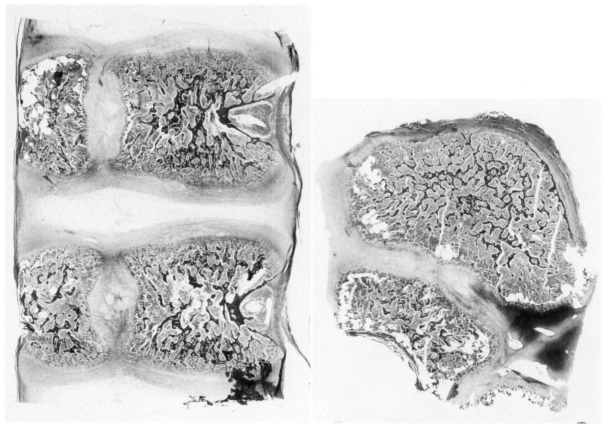

C　　　　　　　　　　　　　　　　　　　　　　　　　D

Fig. 17-6, cont'd. For legend see opposite page.

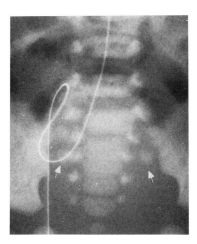

Fig. 17-7. Sacral ossification centers (arrows). These secondary centers are visible in the neonatal spine.

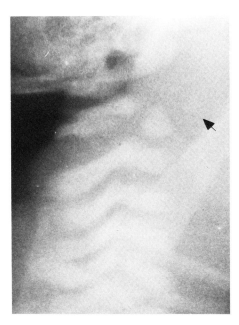

Fig. 17-8. C1 ossification center. This neonatal anterior ossification center (arrow) is small but visible. Spinous processes of the cervical vertebrae have already begun individual differentiation. A radiolucent cartilaginous segment joins the odontoid process to the body of C2.

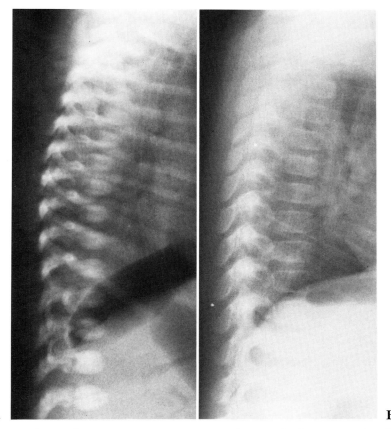

A   B

Fig. 17-9. Spinal growth. A, Neonate. **B,** Six months of age. Individual vertebral bodies have changed considerably in individual configuration and are well on their way to the adult shape. Some change in the thoracolumbar curve has occurred.

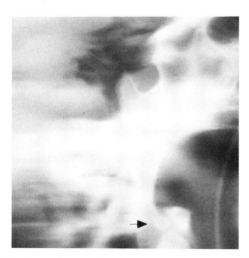

Fig. 17-10. Secondary ossification center or os terminale of the odontoid process (arrow)—lateral tomogram.

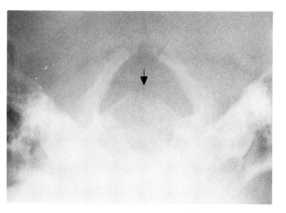

Fig. 17-11. Separate C1 ossification center (arrow). This center is posterior point of fusion of the two laminae of the atlas and is a normal variant.

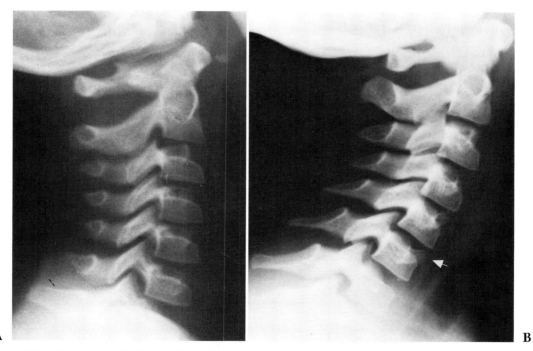

A   B

Fig. 17-12. Cervical spine. A, Four years old. **B,** Nine years old. The cervical vertebral bodies gradually develop a squared shape with a prominent anteroinferior border. In **B,** the transverse process of C6 can be seen to overlap the front of the vertebral body (arrow).

the neural arch halves begin to ossify posteriorly and fuse with each other; the cervical laminae are the last to fuse, sometimes persisting until the third year. Occasionally a separate ossification center will form at C1 (Fig. 17-11). In about 3% of individuals, nonfusion of the laminae of C1 may continue to adult-

hood (Schmorl and Junghanns, 1971). At 2 years of age, the neurocentral synchondroses of the lower sacral area fuse and the first coccygeal segment ossifies (Epstein, 1969). The curve of the spinal column also modifies during infancy. With holding up of the head, the cervical spine develops more of a lordosis. With walking, the lumbar lordosis becomes more prominent and the compensating thoracic curve between the two lordotic segments is more visible. The cervical and lumbar canals remain quite wide.

In later childhood, further changes of the spine occur. The vertebral bodies mold to their adult shape. The cervical vertebral bodies develop a prominent anterior lower border (Fig. 17-12). The lumbar vertebral bodies become slightly concave superiorly and inferiorly. The transverse processes of the cervical

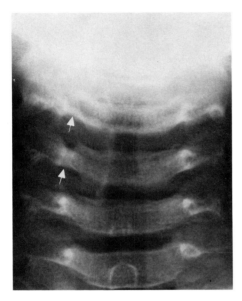

Fig. 17-13. Delayed fusion of the cervical neurocentral synchondroses. Fusion has failed to occur in two synchondroses (arrows) of a 7-year-old child. These are well corticated and should not be mistaken for a fracture.

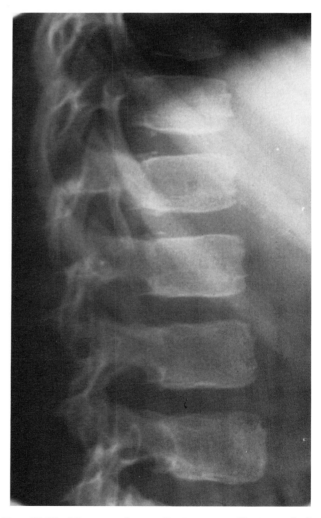

Fig. 17-15. Ring apophyses. Beginning ossification of the apophyses posteriorly, with a prominent ridge on the apophyseal edges anteriorly, has created a slightly beaked or notched appearance in the anterior borders of the vertebral bodies in this 9-year-old child.

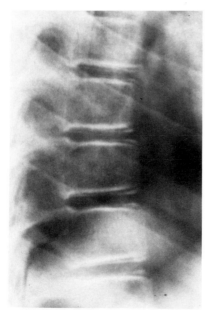

Fig. 17-14. Ring apophyses. There has been early development of ring apophyses in the thoracic spine of a 4-year-old child with no evidence of rapid growth.

vertebral bodies become larger and in a true lateral projection may overlap the anterior borders of the bodies (Fig. 17-12, B).

In the third year there is fusion of the neurocentral synchondroses of the cervical region. This tends to progress inferiorly until the lumbar area fuses, in approximately the sixth year (Caffey, 1972); the upper sacral synchondroses also fuse at that time. These fusions are sometimes delayed, and lack of fusion (Fig. 17-13) should not be mistaken for a fracture.

The ossification centers of the sacrum (one per segment) slowly appear through childhood and adolescence; S2 appears from 5 to 10 years, S3 from 10 to 15 years, and S4 maybe as late as age 20 (Epstein, 1969).

The *ring apophyses* begin to appear in the midthoracic to upper lumbar areas at about age 6 (Epstein, 1969), earlier in females than in males. Caffey (1972) reported a 2½-year-old child with visible ring apophyses. We have seen well-developed apophyses in a 4-year-old (Fig. 17-14). The "rings" are actually horseshoe shaped and are incomplete posteriorly. When they are slow to develop but the bony vertebral body continues to grow, a slightly beaked appearance of the vertebral bodies may result (Fig. 17-15). Ring apophyses are prominent throughout later childhood and completely ossify and join the vertebral bodies by age 18. They do not contribute to the longitudinal growth of the spine—which occurs superiorly and inferiorly at the cartilaginous end plates of the vertebral bodies that abut the annulus fibrosus of the disk.

Although bony fusion of the neural arches at the spinous processes has occurred throughout the spine beyond infancy, a lumbar spina bifida occulta remains in a significant number of children, especially in females (22% in girls, and 9% in boys at age 7); and by adulthood the figures have decreased to 9% and 1%, respectively (Sutow and Pryde, 1956).

The incidence of persistent spina bifida occulta in the thoracic region is higher in blacks than in whites. Levy and Freed (1973), in a survey of 5,363 chest radiographs of South African blacks, found a 2.49% incidence of cervicothoracic spina bifida occulta compared with a reported 0.02% to 0.16% incidence in whites. The authors did not study the lumbar spine, but the logical assumption is that the incidence of lumbar spina bifida would also be higher in this population.

The overall frequency of persistent spina bifida occulta, in decreasing order of frequency, is as follows: L5-S1, C1, C7-T1, lower thoracic (McRae, 1974).

During late childhood, secondary ossification cen-

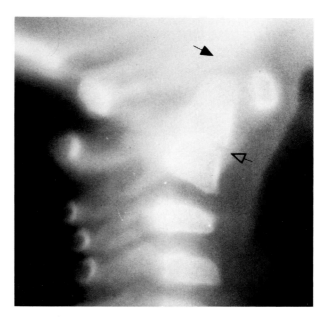

Fig. 17-16. Odontoid process. A midline tomogram of a 7-year-old child shows a typical odontoid process separated from its base by a cartilage plate (open arrow) but nearing fusion. The secondary ossification center (solid arrow) of the odontoid is barely visible.

ters appear at the tips of the spinous processes, transverse processes, and inferior articulations. The centers develop just before puberty in females and shortly after puberty in males (Caffey, 1972). They can be mistaken for fractures, especially when they become larger.

The synchondrosis between the odontoid and the body of the axis usually fuses late in childhood. Cattell and Filtzer (1965) found it unossified in 50% of 5-to-11-year-olds (Fig. 17-16). Though it normally disappears by adolescence, it occasionally persists into adulthood as a fine line. Rarely will it be seen separately in adults (Bernard et al., 1974). The secondary ossification center of the dens fuses at about age 12 (Bailey, 1952). Fusion of the lateral arch to the anterior ossification center of the axis and atlas occurs at approximately 7 years (Bailey and Kato, 1972).

During adolescence the individual vertebral bodies attain their adult shapes and configurations, with final fusion of the ring apophyses and secondary apophyses occurring during this period.

DEVELOPMENT OF THE DISK

Because the large cartilaginous end plate of the vertebral bodies is not radiographically visible, the intervertebral disk space begins radiographically as a biconcave saucer. It is also larger anteriorly than posteriorly. By late adolescence it ends as a biconvex space, which continues into adulthood. Kieffer and co-workers (1969) showed that though the nucleus pulposus is not radiographically visible at any time changes in its configuration during growth do occur. In the neonate it is ovoid, not unlike the vertebral bodies themselves. Both the annulus fibrosus and the cartilaginous end plates are fairly large. By the second decade a notch usually forms in the nucleus pulposus anteriorly, giving it the shape of a fat C. The cartilage has thinned considerably by this time and the annulus fibrosus bulges slightly convexly into the cartilage. The C shape remains, or a notch occurs posteriorly to give a sideways H appearance to the nucleus pulposus when viewed sagittally. Until degeneration occurs, this is the adult shape.

Epstein (1969) stated that vessels extend from the cartilage and vertebral body into the disk at birth and these gradually recede by adulthood. The regression points are scars, which may be weak points through which the disk can prolapse. The disk is most elastic at ages 25 to 30. At birth the nucleus pulposus has a water content of approximately 88%, and the annulus about 77%. Through childhood the water content gradually decreases in both, to 76% and 70% respectively by the third decade. The nucleus pulposus continues to lose fluid and approaches the 70% level through the remainder of life (Shmorl and Junghanns, 1971).

RANGE OF MOTION

The apophyseal joints of the spine are arthrodial (sliding) joints, and the angles of the facets change in the different areas of the spine. In the cervical area they are approximately perpendicular to the sagittal plane. In the thoracic area they have an angle of roughly 70%; and in the lumbar area they vary from 45° to a near parallel position with the sagittal plane. The disks are considered to be amphiarthrodial joints (semimoving). Due to elasticity of the ligaments around the apophyseal and disk joints, the spine of a child is particularly mobile—especially in the cervical area, which is extraordinarily mobile. Muscle spasm or other injury causing the neck to be held in a flexed position with subsequent normal sliding forward of the vertebral bodies is not infrequently mistaken for a subluxation (Fig. 17-17). Jacobson and Bleecker (1959) found that flexion occurred primarily at the C2-C3 level, with maximum angulation and glide at this point. The forward displacement of C2 on C3 in one normal case was 5 mm. Jacobson and Bleecker believe that the axis of maximum motion shifts to the C4-C5 or C5-C6 levels at age 10 or older.

Cattell and Filtzer (1965) studied 160 normal children from ages 1 to 16 years and found that thirty-two of seventy children who were younger than 8 had a motion of 3 mm or more at the C2-C3 level. In extension, twenty-two of seventy had a visible posterior

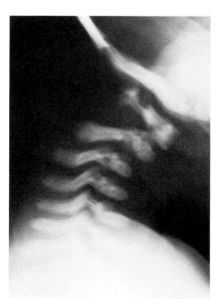

Fig. 17-17. C2-C3 pseudosubluxation. Forward flexion of the cervical spine in a small child allows considerable angulation and anterior motion at the C2-C3 space, giving a subluxed appearance. It is normal.

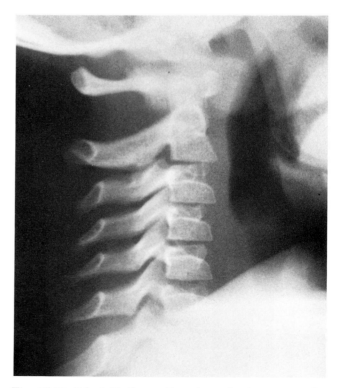

Fig. 17-18. Odontoid-atlas motion. A nearly 4 mm space between the odontoid and the anterior arch of the atlas can be seen in the flexed position. Note the normal transverse processes overlapping the disk spaces. (Five-year-old child.)

motion which was less marked. The authors stated their belief that measurement of most of the cervical spine motion was inaccurate; but they graded the motion as marked in 9%, moderate in 40%, and definite in 40%. Most of the children showing this motion were 7 years of age or younger.

Cattell and Filtzer (1965) also studied motion at the C1-odontoid level and found a range of at least 3 mm with flexion in 20% of children under age 8 (Fig. 17-18). With extension, an override (i.e., at least two thirds of the height of the anterior arch of C1 higher than the odontoid tip) occurred in 20%. Locke and co-workers (1966) studied 100 children between ages 3 and 15 and found a 4 mm maximum C1-odontoid distance. Both authors used standard 40-inch tube-film distance.

SPINAL GROWTH

Many authors have evaluated the relative and actual sizes of the spinal canals and vertebral bodies. The relatively larger width of the cervical and lumbar areas has already been noted.

The use of overlays as described by Haworth and Keillor (1962) remains a rough but rapid method of determining whether a transverse spinal diameter falls outside the average during both childhood and adulthood.

When in doubt, the examiner may refer to precise charts such as those by Simril and Thurston (1955) and Hinck and co-workers (1962, 1966). The studies of Simril and Thurston include infants but not the cervical spine, whereas those of Hinck and co-workers cover neither the infant age group nor the uppermost cervical spine.

Epstein (1969) stated that the newborn lumbar vertebral body should have a sagittal diameter of 1 cm and a canal diameter of 1.3 cm. In the cervical area the average sagittal diameter is quoted as 1 cm at 3 months and the transverse diameter somewhat larger.

Brandner (1970) compared the ratio of the greatest vertebral body height to the shortest vertebral body length in the sagittal plane of 187 children between birth and teens. He found that the ratio increases in infancy, is constant from 18 to 36 months, and rises again from ages 4 to 12. Due to longer sagittal diameters, boys have a relatively smaller index. The measurements were made only in the lower thoracic and lumbar areas.

Naik (1970), in an anatomical and radiological study, devised a useful way of accurately measuring the sagittal and transverse diameters of the cervical canal in infants. He found that the lamina is approximately square and that one may measure the distance from the back of the vertebral body to the posterior tip of the lamina, subtract the height of the most posterior portion of the lamina, and have the true sagittal diameter. He also found the pedicle and lamina to be at different planes in the AP projection because of their angulation. A transverse measurement across the canal between the points of angle change gives the maximum transverse diameter of the neural canal. The measurements of the dissected vertebrae closely match those of postmortem radiographs before dissection. Only eleven patients were examined by both methods, so the statistical accuracy of the normality of the measurements was not calculated. Shapiro found variations of up to 6.5 mm in the diameters of the same vertebral body between different infants, especially at the lowest cervical level (8-14, 5 mm); however, no cervical spine of any individual varied more than 2.5 mm from C2 to C7 in this small group.

Caffey (1972) noted that the cervical and lumbar areas are relatively longer in neonates. The cervical spine is 25% and the lumbar spine 50% of the C1-L5 length. By adulthood the cervical spine is 16.6% to 20%, and the lumbar segment 33%. Caffey gave the average total spinal length, excluding the sacrum, as 20 cm at birth, 45 cm at 2 years, 50 cm at puberty, and 60 to 75 cm at adulthood.

Kuhns and Holt (1975) measured the length of the thoracic spine in neonates of known gestational age. Besides finding longer spines in children of diabetic mothers, they discovered the knowledge of vertebral body size compared with known normals of the same gestational age to be a useful factor in estimating and comparing kidney size with vertebral body height.

In measuring the diameter of the central canal, we have found that the sagittal distance is the most sensitive to change and the easiest to measure in the cervical area. In the thoracic and lumbar areas the interpediculate distance—though not necessarily the smallest diameter in the lumbar spine—is easiest to measure.

ANATOMICAL VARIATIONS

Scalloping of the posterior aspects of the vertebral bodies, especially in the lumbar area, is seen in neurofibromatosis and expanding intraspinal lesions. Contrariwise, in childhood the posterior aspects of the vertebral bodies, especially in the upper lumbar area, may normally look somewhat scalloped (Fig. 17-19). There is unfortunately no easy guide to which one can refer for confirmation of whether such scalloping is beyond the limits of normal. Experience and comparing the asymmetry of involved vertebrae with that of adjacent vertebrae are the only recourse.

In addition to the variations in time of epiphyseal closure and ossification center closure during childhood, there are congenital variations that occur and are sometimes normal or at least asymptomatic. Because the occiput and upper cervical spine, though developing from adjacent somites, are quite different in their final forms—many variations and anomalies evolve. The outcome is a sort of push-pull contest between extra vertebral and occipital segments. Occipitalization of the C1 vertebral body is often associated with other anomalies and may be sympto-

matic. Burwood and Watt (1974), however, in examining 1,500 skull films taken for nonspinal disease, found only five patients with asymptomatic occipitalization of the atlas.

In an extensive review of occipitocervical junction anomalies, Lombardi (1961) commented that occipitalization of the atlas is a progressive evolutionary variant: the highest vertebrates showing the greatest amount of occipitalization of the embryonic cranial somites. We have noted that partial and complete occipitalization of the first cervical vertebra, even though asymptomatic, may cause asymmetry of the skull base (Fig. 17-20).

Lombardi (1961) also discussed the "third condyle," a spur attached to the inferior edge of the anterior border of the foramen magnum. In our experience this variation is most often found incidentally during tomographic studies for other reasons (e.g., pneumoencephalography) involving the base of the skull (Fig. 17-21). Lombardi discussed additional less common variations of the occipitocervical junction.

Most of the variations of the spine are reported in adults simply because children are not so frequently examined radiographically. One variation is much rarer in children than in adults: *pseudonotch* of the axis—a notch or canal on the medial aspect of the atlas arch, best seen with tomography but sometimes visible on plain films (Fig. 17-22). Scotti (1975) found the overall incidence of this variant in adults to be 49%, with a progressive increase in occurrence accompanying an increase in age. The nutrient artery normally in this area is presumed to become larger and more tortuous with aging, thereby causing a notch to form.

The ponticulus posticus, over the vertebral artery on the lamina of C1, may be seen in children as either an incomplete spur or a complete tunnel (Fig. 17-23).

Absence of the posterior arch of C1 is reported

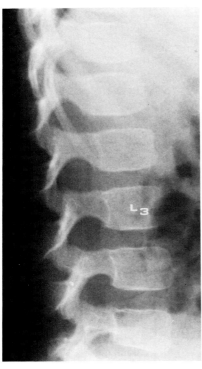

Fig. 17-19. Posterior vertebral body scalloping. Note the prominent posterior scalloping of the lumbar vertebrae, especially L3. The anterior borders of the vertebral bodies have slight normal notching. (Normal 4-year-old child.)

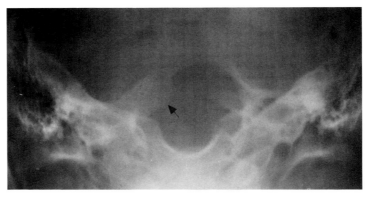

Fig. 17-20. Occipitalization of C1. Occipitalization of the right half of the posterior arch of C1 (arrow) in a 5-year-old child gives considerable asymmetry to the foramen magnum.

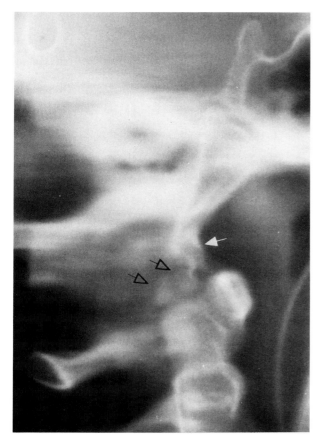

Fig. 17-21. Third condyle. Solid arrow indicates a process fused to the anterior border of the foramen magnum that was incidentally noted at pneumoencephalography. The os terminale of the odontoid process is duplicated (open arrows). The base of the odontoid process has fused.

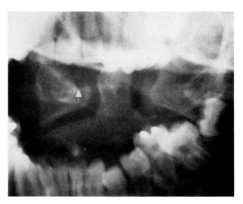

Fig. 17-22. Pseudonotch of the atlas. A radiograph of the occipitocervical junction shows the pseudonotch (arrow) of the atlas in a 13-year-old child.

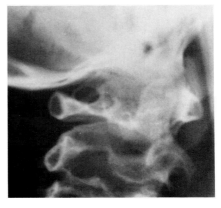

Fig. 17-23. Ponticulus posticus. The ponticulus is completely formed bilaterally in an 11-year-old child.

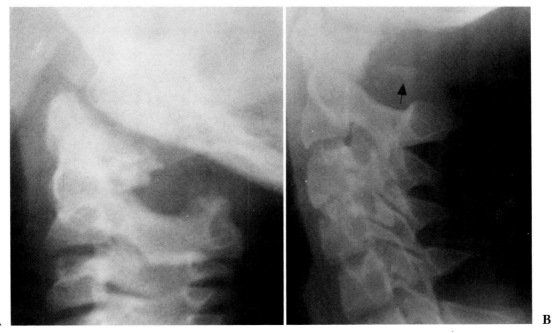

A **B**

Fig. 17-24. Absent posterior arch of the atlas. A, Complete absence of the posterior arches in a 4-year-old child. **B,** Hypoplastic development of the posterior arch (arrow) of C1 in a 14-year-old boy.

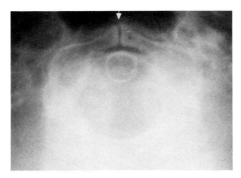

Fig. 17-25. **Absent anterior ossification center of C1.** Lack of development of the anterior ossification center caused this cleft (arrow) in the anterior aspect of the atlas in a 14-year-old boy.

rarely: twenty-four cases in the radiological literature (Dalinka et al., 1972; Logan and Stuard, 1973). We have noted three cases, the youngest patient being 4 years old (Fig. 17-24). The incidence of the variation is probably much higher than reported. It is an incidental and asymptomatic finding, probably because there is a fibrous ring (as seen in one autopsy case, Logan and Stuard, 1973) and because of the strong muscular and ligamentous attachments between the occiput and the upper cervical spine which stabilize the area. The anterior ossification center of the atlas may also fail to appear, causing an anterior cleft to occur (Fig. 17-25).

Bifurcation or duplication of the accessory ossicle of the odontoid, the os terminale, is a frequent minor variation of the C2 vertebral body (Fig. 17-21).

Absence of the pedicles of other cervical vertebrae is a rare occurrence, with a total of seventeen cases reported for the whole cervical spine (McLoughlin and

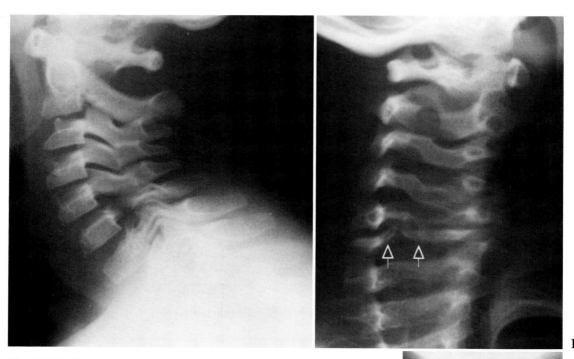

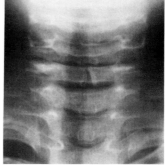

Fig. 17-26. **Absent cervical pedicles at C6. A,** A lateral projection shows a bilateral cleft which is greater on one side. There also appears to be a minor abnormality at C7. **B** and **C,** An oblique projection shows the cleft to be on the left side (**B,** arrows). Superimposed on it is the posterior spina bifida, visible in the AP (**C**). Note also (in **A** and **B**) the incomplete ponticulus posticus at C1.

Wortzman, 1972); the youngest previously reported patient was 13 years old (Oestreich and Young, 1969). We have two of our own cases (Figs. 17-26 and 17-27), the youngest patient being 6 years of age. Minor

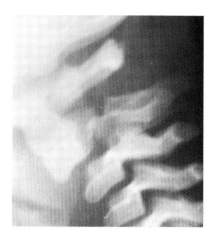

Fig. 17-27. Absent pedicles at C2.

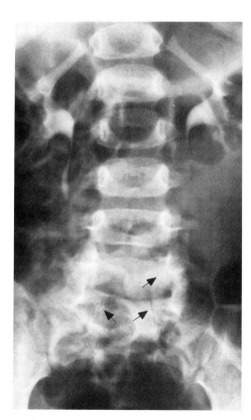

Fig. 17-28. **Thinning of the pedicles at the thoracolumbar junction.** This 2-year-old child has thin pedicles at L1 and L2. Note also the normally wide lower lumbar spine and the clearly evident lumbosacral neurocentral synchondroses (arrows).

differences in the surrounding articular processes may be seen and in one of our patients, a spina bifida was discovered posteriorly. Myelography usually shows the two nerve roots of the adjacent foramina to have migrated together more closely so they exit the spinal cord through the site of the absent pedicle. Absence of any pedicles in the thoracic spine is very rare, with only two cases reported (Tomsick et al., 1974).

Thinning of the pedicles at the thoracolumbar junction is common (Fig. 17-28), with an incidence of 7% reported in both adults and children (Benzian et al., 1971). This thinning always involves T12 or L1 and may also affect T11 or L2. We have noted that it is frequently asymmetrical, with only one side being thinned, and may be difficult to distinguish from a true localized spinal canal enlargement. Absent pedicles of the upper lumbar spine have been reported only rarely in children (Morin and Palacios, 1974). This condition must have been present throughout childhood, however, to be seen in the more commonly reported adult cases.

Lumbosacral transition variations are common, as are variations in the angle between the two areas. Sacralization of the fifth lumbar vertebra occurs when the ossification center for its transverse process becomes fused to the sacrum. These variations are often associated with symptoms in adults but are not signifi-

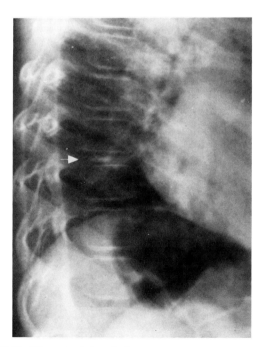

Fig. 17-29. **Thoracic disk calcification** (arrow). The only illness of this 6-year-old child was congenital heart disease, which had been repaired. Calcification was also visible on preoperative chest films back to age 13 months.

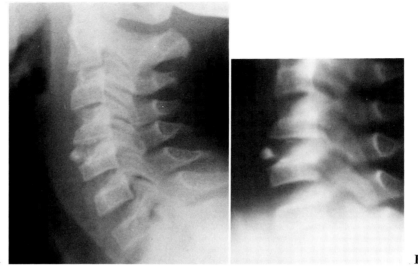

Fig. 17-30. Intervertebral disk calcification. An 8-year-old girl had neck stiffness secondary to tonsillitis. A lateral plain film (**A**) and lateral tomogram (**B**) shows calcification within the disk space and bulging anteriorly.

cant in children of our experience so will not be discussed. A good review of the subject is that by Schmorl and Junghanns (1971).

Disk calcification may be seen in children. Its origin is obscure. Most often it is accompanied by symptoms, but these may not be directly localized to the area of disk calcifications. In an extensive review of the subject, Melnick and Silverman (1963) found seven of the fifty-three reported cases incidentally; four were in infants, in whom related symptoms may have been difficult to detect. The youngest infant reported was 10 days old. All parts of the spinal column may be affected—with the lumbar area being relatively spared. We have seen eight cases (Figs. 17-29 and 17-30). In one case the child was examined because of neck stiffness and found to have tonsillitis; another was in a patient in whom congenital heart disease had been repaired. The process is quite likely abnormal since it so often regresses after discovery. It is not usually an abnormality of clinical significance, however.

REFERENCES

Bailey, D. K.: The normal cervical spine in infants and children, Radiology **59**:712, 1952.

Bailey, H. L., and Kato, F.: Paravertebral ossification of the cervical spine, South. Med. J. **65**:189, 1972.

Benzian, S. R., Mainzer, F., and Gooding, C. A.: Pediculate thinning; a normal variant at the thoracolumbar junction, Br. J. Radiol. **44**:936, 1971.

Bernard, J., Tessier, J. P., Delie, J., et al.: Trois cas d'os odontoide chez l'adulte, J. Radiol. Electrol. Med. Nucl. **55**:45, 1974.

Brandner, M. E.: Normal values of the vertebral body and intervertebral disk index during growth, Am. J. Roentgenol. Radium Ther. Nucl. Med. **110**:618, 1970.

Brill, P. W., Baker, D. H., and Ewing, M. L.: "Bone-within-bone" in the neonatal spine, Radiology **108**:363, 1973.

Burwood, R. J., and Watt, I.: Assimilation of the atlas and basilar impression; a review of 1,500 skull and cervical spine radiography, Clin. Radiol. **25**:327, 1974.

Caffey, J.: Pediatric x-ray diagnosis, ed. 6, Chicago, 1972, Year Book Medical Publishers, Inc.

Cattell, H. S., and Filtzer, D. L.: Pseudosubluxation and other normal variations in the cervical spine in children, J. Bone Joint Surg. **47-A**:1295, 1965.

Cohen, J., Currarino, G., and Neuhauser, E. B. D.: A significant variant in the ossification centers of the vertebral bodies, Am. J. Roentgenol. Radium Ther. Nucl. Med. **76**:469, 1956.

Dalinka, M. K., Rosenbaum, A. E., and Van Houten, F.: Congenital absence of the posterior arch of the atlas, Radiology **103**:581, 1972.

Epstein, B. S.: The spine; a radiological text and atlas, ed. 3, Philadelphia, 1969, Lea & Febiger.

Fielden, P., and Russell, J. G. B.: Coronal cleft vertebra, Clin. Radiol. **21**:327, 1970.

Haworth, J. B., and Keillor, G. W.: Use of transparencies in evaluating the width of the spinal canal in infants, children and adults, Radiology **79**:109, 1962.

Hinck, V. C., Clark, W. M., Jr., and Hopkins, C. E.: Normal interpediculate distances (minimum and maximum) in children and adults, Am. J. Roentgenol. Radium Ther. Nucl. Med. **97**:141, 1966.

Hinck, V. C., Hopkins, C. E., and Savara, B. S.: Sagittal diameter of the cervical spinal canal in children, Radiology **79**:97, 1962.

Jacobson, G., and Bleecker, H. H.: Pseudosubluxation of the axis in children, Am. J. Roentgenol. Radium Ther. Nucl. Med. **82**:472, 1959.

Kieffer, S. A., Stadlan, E. M., Mohandas, A., and Peterson, H. O.: Discographic-anatomical correlation of developmental changes with age in the intervertebral disc, Acta Radiol. [Diagn.] **9**:732, 1969.

Kuhns, L. R., and Holt, J. F.: Measurement of thoracic spine length on chest radiographs of newborn infants, Radiology 116:395, 1975.

Levy, J. I., and Freed, C. J.: The incidence of cervicothoracic spina bifida occulta in South American Negroes, Anatomy 114:449, 1973.

Locke, G. R., Gardner, J. I., and Van Epps, E. F.: Atlas-dens interval (ADI) in children, Am. J. Roentgenol. Radium Ther. Nucl. Med. 97:135, 1966.

Logan, W. W., and Stuard, I. D.: Absent posterior arch of the atlas, Am. J. Roentgenol. Radium Ther. Nucl. Med. 118: 431, 1973.

Lombardi, G.: The occipital vertebra, Am. J Roentgenol. Radium Ther. Nucl. Med. 86:260, 1961.

Martin, D. J.: Personal communication, 1975.

McLoughlin, D. P., and Wortzman, G.: Congenital absence of a cervical vertebral pedicle, J. Can. Assoc. Radiol. 22-23: 195, 1971-1972.

McRae, D. L.: Personal communication, 1974.

Melnick, J. C., and Silverman, F. N.: Intervertebral disk calcification in childhood, Radiology 80:399, 1963.

Morin, M. E., and Palacios, E.: The aplastic hypoplastic lumbar pedicle, Am. J. Roentgenol. Radium Ther. Nucl. Med. 122:639, 1974.

Naik, D. R.: Cervical spinal canal in normal infants, Clin. Radiol. 21:323, 1970.

Oestreich, A. E., and Young, L. W.: The absent cervical pedicle syndrome; a case in childhood, Am. J. Roentgenol. Radium Ther. Nucl. Med. 107:505, 1969.

O'Rahilly, R., and Meyer, D. B.: Roentgenographic investigation of the human skeleton during early fetal life, Am. J. Roentgenol. Radium Ther. Nucl. Med. 76:455, 1956.

Rowley, K. A.: Coronal cleft vertebra, J. Fac. Radiol. 6-7:267, 1954-1956.

Schmorl, G., and Junghanns, H.: The human spine in health and disease, ed. 2 (American), translated and edited by E. F. Besemann, New York, 1971, Grune & Stratton, Inc.

Scotti, G.: The pseudonotch of the atlas; a manifestation of the occipital vertebra or a normal variant? Neuroradiology 8:229, 1975.

Simril, W. A., and Thurston, D.: The normal interpediculate space in the spines of infants and children, Radiology 64: 340, 1955.

Sutow, W. W., and Pryde, A. W.: Incidence of spine bifida occulta in relation to age, Am. J. Dis. Child. 91:211, 1956.

Tompsett, A. C., Jr., and Donaldson, S. W.: The anterior tubercle of the first cervical vertebra and the hyoid bone; their occurrence in newborn infants, Am. J. Roentgenol. Radium Ther. Nucl. Med. 65:582, 1951.

Tomsick, T. A., Lebowitz, M. E., and Campbell, C.: The congenital absence of pedicles in the thoracic spine; report of two cases, Radiology 111:587, 1974.

Abnormal spine

PART I*

Generalized disease and the spine

Neuroradiological interest in generalized disease of the spine derives from the effect an involved vertebra or vertebrae may have on the spinal cord and its roots rather than on the genetically determined or acquired disease. Investigation and subsequent treatment depend on extracting from the plain films, tomograms, and myelograms the localized manifestations of that generalized disease. The genetic disorders of the osseous skeleton constitute a diagnostic jungle, but we shall attempt to be as concise and practical as possible.

Anyone who is interested in congenital abnormalities of skeletal development well knows there has been an increasing tendency to divide and subdivide many diseases previously lumped together. The diseases are still known variously as chondrodystrophies, osteochondrodysplasias, or simply bone dysplasias; but they have become minutely classified on the basis of an international nomenclature which is in the process of jelling. Though little doubt exists that the classification of many subgroups of a skeletal growth abnormality, apparently similar phenotypically and genotypically, will add to the almost overwhelming pool of knowledge regarding inherent errors of bone metabolism and development—elucidation probably lies in the electron microscopic examination and histochemistry of bone, not in relatively gross histology or in the radiological classification of shapes and sizes.

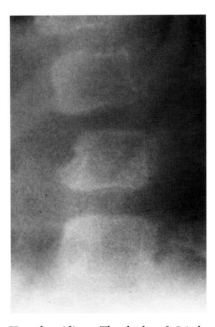

Fig. 18-1. Hypothyroidism. The body of L1 has a typical anteroinferior hook.

*Bernard J. Reilly, M.B., Ch.B., M.A., F.R.C.P.(C), Radiologist-in-Chief, Department of Radiology, The Hospital for Sick Children; Professor of Radiology, University of Toronto, Toronto, Canada.

For readers who are interested in obtaining more precise knowledge of these skeletal disorders, many books have been written (McKusick, 1972; Bailey, 1973; Spranger et al., 1974; Taybi, 1975).

To enumerate all the variations of a vertebral anomaly seen in growth disorders would be superfluous. We are concerned with only those that will produce or be associated with orthopedic, neurological, or neurosurgical disease requiring neuroradiological investigation. The spinal cord and its roots may be impinged on as a result of an intrinsic abnormality in its shape and texture or as a result of the malalignment of one or more vertebral bodies. The abnormal shape may be a primary maldevelopment or secondary to a nonspecific condition producing hypotonia. This is most apparent at a fulcral area such as the upper lumbar spine, where L1 and L2, the so-called "lazy sisters," tend to show adaptive wedging and hooking not only in the chondrodystrophies but also in Down's syndrome and hypothyroidism (Fig. 18-1).

BONE DYSPLASIAS
Achondroplasia

Achondroplasia is one of the commonest and most readily recognizable bone dysplasias. It is an inherent defect in endochondral bone formation, resulting in dwarfism and a disruption of the normal size relationship of one bone with another (Fig. 18-2). Bones which have the greatest growth potential are the most stunted. Thus the femurs are shortened relative to the tibias, and the tibias relative to the fibulas.

This analogy is applicable to the vertebral column, where thoracic and lumbar vertebrae fail to show the expected variations in size. The normal increases in vertebral body size and interpediculate distance throughout the thoracic and lumbar vertebrae are not present. The transverse diameter of L5 is little more than that of T12, and both vertebrae are smaller than they should be. The pedicles in L5 are relatively larger, however. Consequently, though the bony canal is small throughout the spine, it is relatively the smallest in the lumbar region—producing a significant stenosis of the spinal canal. Thus posterior disk herniation will produce a serious compression of the cord and nerve roots more rapidly in an achondroplastic patient than in a normal individual.

As a rule there is a marked lumbar lordosis because of the attachment of the spine at the sacral level to a small and stunted pelvis. There is usually no localized lumbar kyphosis. In a minority of cases, however, a distortion of the upper lumbar vertebrae occurs with varying degrees of anterior wedging and hypoplasia (Langer et al., 1967). As the interverte-

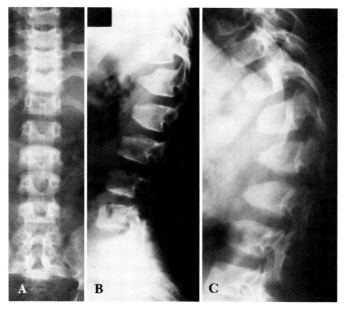

Fig. 18-2. Achondroplasia. A, An AP projection of the thoracolumbar spine shows relative uniformity in vertebral body size with enlarging pedicles but diminishing interpediculate distance and spinal stenosis within the lumbar vertebrae. **B,** A lateral projection in the same patient shows anterior wedging of L1 and to a lesser extent of L2. This deformity was not present in infancy. **C,** A lateral view in another patient reveals increasing lumbar kyphosis with anterior wedging in the bodies of T12, L1, L2, and (to a lesser extent) L3, with retrodisplacement of L1.

bral disks slide over the oblique superior and inferior surfaces of the vertebral body, there may be retrodisplacement of the affected vertebra with consequent compression of the cord. This localized deformity, which is so typical of the mucopolysaccharidoses, is fortunately rare in childhood and constitutes the exception.

There is a group of spondyloepiphyseal dysplasias which resemble achondroplasia inasmuch as short-limbed dwarfism is lumped with a more normal-looking back as *pseudoachondroplasia* (Maroteaux and Lamy, 1959). The significance of these disorders is that they may also have a small skull base with a diminished foramen magnum and stenosis of the spinal canal.

The mucopolysaccharidoses

The mucopolysaccharidoses are a heterogeneous group of disorders characterized by mucopolysaccharide excretion in the urine and abnormal mucopolysaccharide storage in the tissue. They are distinguished from one another by the varying patterns of lysosomal storage disorder.

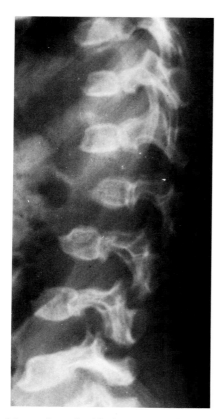

Fig. 18-3. Mucopolysaccharidosis, type IH (Hurler's disease). The visible vertebral bodies are all hooked to varying degrees. There is a gibbus with retrodisplacement of the relatively small body of L1.

All the mucopolysaccharidoses share a common denominator: abnormal bone texture and shape with characteristic involvement of the spine, particularly the upper lumbar spine (Fig. 18-3). There is a localized gibbus due to progressive retrodisplacement of either L1 or L2. The consequent cord compression may be mild or severe (Fig. 18-4).

The phenomenon of cord compression can be graphically and dramatically demonstrated during myelography by flexing the spine of the supine or decubitus patient and seeing the small bullet-nosed and retrodisplaced lumbar vertebra impinge on the column of contrast medium. At the same time, bulging but nonherniated intervertebral disks may be seen. In the majority of cases, the degree of cord compression is mild. Though each of the seven groups and subgroups of the mucopolysaccharidoses has been described as showing varying constellations of radiological signs—what really matters clinically is the degree of spinal deformity, not the precise biochemical abnormality. If there is significant retrodisplacement of a vertebral body, differentiation of Hurler's disease (MPS IH) from the Maroteaux-Lamy syndrome (MPS VIA or VIB) is of little import.

Morquio's syndrome (MPS IV)

A variety of dwarfism first described by Morquio in 1929 (Fig. 18-5) has clinical and radiological features that make it more easily distinguishable.

We shall concern ourselves only with the spinal changes. There is universal vertebra plana. Though the spine may appear to be normal in infancy—as the child stands up and begins to walk, a progressive flattening with loss of height in the vertebral bodies occurs with marked irregularity of development in the end plates and ring apophyses. The odontoid process is so dysgenetic that with extension of the head it tends to subluxate under the anterior arch of C1. Because of the cervical spine shortening such that the head appears to be sunk into the squat kyphotic chest, extension of the head is difficult. These patients protect themselves from pithing their own spinal cord on the anterior arch of C1 by their inability to extend the head upon the neck. Similar odontoid dysgenesis may be seen in other types of growth disorder such as Kniest's syndrome or metatropic dwarfism.

The mucolipidoses are a group of disorders clinically and radiologically similar to the mucopolysaccharidoses. They differ biochemically inasmuch as there is no excretion of excess mucopolysaccharides in the urine (Spranger and Wiedemann, 1970).

Miscellaneous bone dysplasias

It should be stressed that the shape of the vertebral body is in no way diagnostic of the exact type of bone

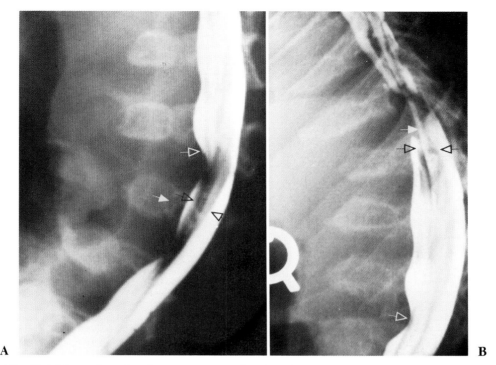

Fig. 18-4. Mucopolysaccharidosis. A, Type IH (Hurler's disease). There are large intervertebral disks bulging posteriorly (open white arrow) and compression of the spinal cord at L1(open black arrows) by the retrodisplaced vertebrae (solid arrow). **B,** Similar changes are seen in a case of the Maroteaux-Lamy syndrome (type VI).

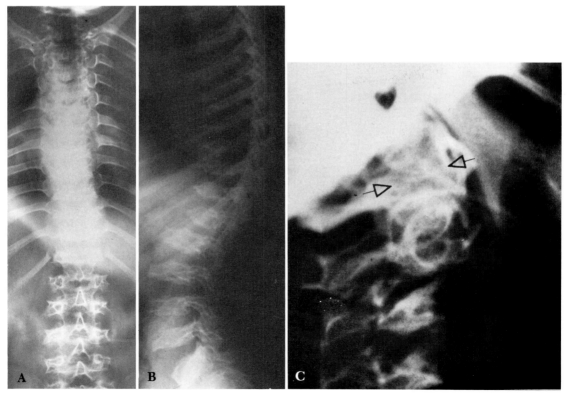

Fig. 18-5. Morquio's disease. A and **B,** There are dorsal kyphosis, lumbar lordosis, universal vertebra plana, and anterior wedging most pronounced at L1 and L2. **C,** The odontoid process (arrows) is markedly hypoplastic.

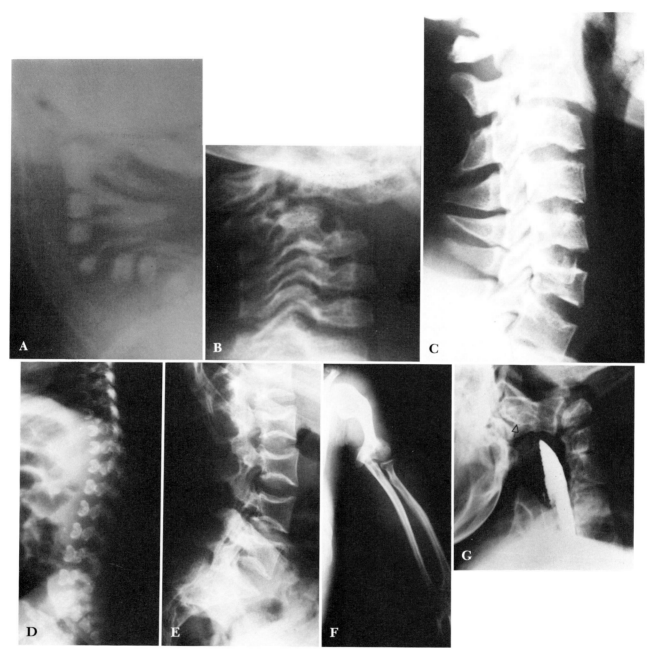

Fig. 18-6. **Assorted spondyloepiphyseal dysplasias. A,** Hypoplastic C5 with acute lordosis of the cervical spine in a case of camptomelic dwarfism. **B,** Apparent retrodisplacement of C2 and absence of the odontoid process with almost no laminar arch development in a case of spondyloepiphyseal dysplasia. **C,** Irregular enlargement of C3, C4, and C5 with growth disturbance at the end plates and ring apophyses in a case of spondyloepiphyseal dysplasia. **D to F, Two cases of Conradi's disease.** In an infant, with typical universal coronal clefting of the vertebral bodies (**D**). In an adult, with retarded central vertebral development producing a codfish vertebra appearance (**E**). The marked shortening and deformity of the humerus are typical (**F**). **G, Spondylocostal dysostosis.** There is posterior subluxation at C2-C3, with a 90° angulation. The odontoid process is horizontal (arrow). Note the incomplete segmentation at C4-C7, the absence of neural arches C1 to C5, and the complete block in the myelographic oil column.

dysplasia; also, though of importance in genetics, precise diagnosis is by and large irrelevant in the practice of neuroradiology. Some radiologists are "dwarf people" and some are not; neuroradiologists who must be pragmatic tend toward the latter rather than the former group. There are certainly assorted varieties of dwarfism which produce spectacular abnormalities, particularly in the cervical spine (Fig. 18-6), and these are of great practical significance.

SCHEUERMANN'S DISEASE

Scheuermann's disease has many synonyms—some straightforward like juvenile roundback, others more impressive like *kyphosis dorsalis juvenalis*. The descriptiveness of the title has mirrored a lack of certainty about the etiology. The term "osteochondritis" has been applied without justification. Only those cases showing clinical and radiological evidence of spondylarthritis, in which inflammatory destruction of bone occurs with subsequent extrusion of the intervertebral disk into the vertebral body above or below and which have shown histological evidence of true inflammatory disease, can be so classified.

Recently at The Hospital for Sick Children, Toronto, an adolescent diagnosed as having Scheuermann's disease required surgical correction of his spinal deformity. Histological examination of the excised bone showed not only transosseous disk protrusion but an irregular proliferation of cartilage in the region of the ring apophyses, indistinguishable

from an epiphyseal dysplasia (Bobechko, 1975). The clinical presentation of the disorder may be insidious or abrupt with increasing dorsal kyphosis and backache of variable severity. Two types of lesion have been described radiologically (Fig. 18-7):

1. Irregularity of the ring apophyses with disruption of bone growth at the end plates and consequent flattening and anterior wedging of the vertebral bodies
2. More sharply demarcated areas of what have been called transosseous disk protrusions

It might be mentioned parenthetically at this point that unexplained backache in a child is a much more ominous and important symptom than unexplained backache in an adult. As originally described, Scheuermann's disease may be localized to the middorsal spine but may involve both thoracic and lumbar spine. Backache when the spine is radiologically normal is often an indication for myelography. The role of trauma is difficult to assess in an active adolescent, particularly when superimposed on a spine which intrinsically may not be completely normal. In the case of Scheuermann's disease or juvenile diskogenic disorder (Murray and Jacobson, 1972), the examiner must decide whether he is confronting a localized phenomenon in an otherwise normal individual or whether indeed the vertebral changes are part of a more extensive growth disorder. Irregular flattening of the vertebral bodies is seen in a variety of spondyloepiphyseal dysplasias (Fig. 18-8) with a long-

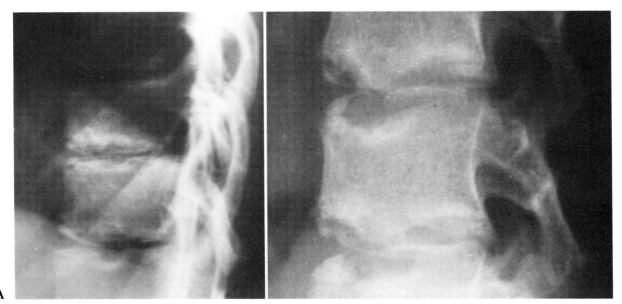

A   B

Fig. 18-7. Scheuermann's disease. A, Irregular development of the thoracic ring apophyses with disruption of bone growth at the end plates and early anterior wedging. B, More sharply demarcated areas of what have been called transosseous disk protrusion in the lumbar spine of the same patient.

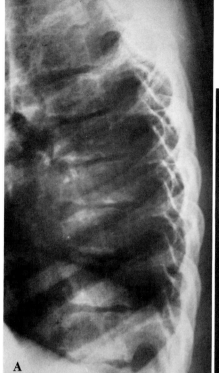

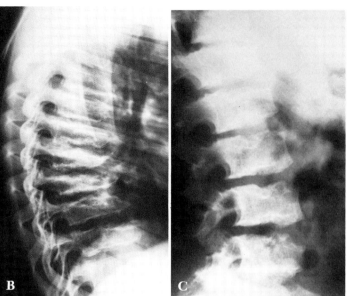

Fig. 18-8. Spondyloepiphyseal dysplasias. A and B, Two different patients showing irregularity of the adjacent vertebral body margins and dorsal kyphosis, more marked in B than in A. C, Sharply defined defects in the adjacent vertebrae of a third child.

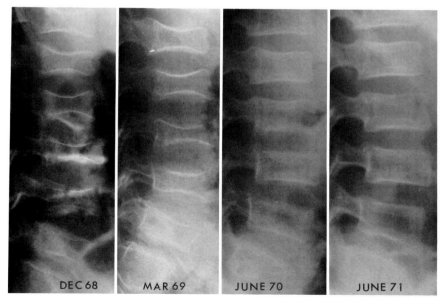

Fig. 18-9. Idiopathic juvenile osteoporosis. A series of examinations made over four years shows severe flattening of the vertebrae with progressive filling of the biconcavity by new bone. (Courtesy W. A. Cumming, M.D., Toronto.)

term outlook, particularly genetic, quite different from the outlook of the ordinary case of Scheuermann's disease. If there is any question that the spinal changes are part of a more widespread genetically determined disease, a complete skeletal survey is mandatory.

OSTEOPOROSIS

The practical problem in osteoporosis, no matter what the etiology, is central compression collapse of the vertebral bodies with decrease in the vertical height of the spine. It may be seen in osteogenesis imperfecta, idiopathic juvenile osteoporosis, scurvy, or endocrine abnormalities such as Cushing's disease; it may be secondary to treatment with steroids or part of a malignant process such as leukemia or neuroblastoma. The cord is unlikely to be compromised unless there is a sagging accentuation of lumbar lordosis with elongation of the pars interarticularis of L5 and spondylolisthesis of L5 on S1 with an intact arch causing compression of the cauda equina (Newman, 1963).

In both scurvy and idiopathic juvenile osteoporosis there may be such a spectacular loss of height that the vertebral bodies resemble biconcave intervertebral disks. There is usually no neurological problem, however; and with regression of the disease, a dramatic return to normality takes place (Fig. 18-9).

LEUKEMIA

Infiltration of the spine with compression collapse is common in leukemia and occasionally will be the

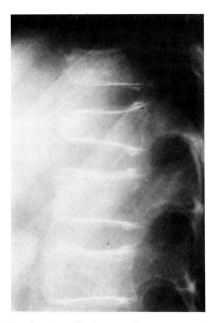

Fig. 18-10. Leukemia. All the vertebrae are washed out and porotic. There is compression collapse of the upper two.

first skeletal manifestation (Fig. 18-10). The mechanical sequelae (e.g., an extradural mass effect with or without involvement of the meninges) may be responsible for irritation of the spinal cord and nerve root.

HISTIOCYTOSIS X

This nonmalignant but potentially lethal disease, whose prognosis depends on the number of systems involved rather than on the degree of bone destruction at any site, may produce single or multiple areas of compression collapse (Fig. 18-11). Formerly known as Calve's vertebra plana, the disease is usually considered to be fairly certain evidence of eosinophilic granulomatous infiltration until proved otherwise (Kieffer et al., 1969). It has a characteristic appearance. The disk above and below the dense waferlike compressed vertebral body may remain the same or even become somewhat wider—indicating that, though there is loss of bone, more nonosseous tissue may lie between the intervertebral disks than is apparent. As the process heals, a surprising degree of recovery in vertebral body height may occur. The disease may spread into the neural arch and epidural space or into the paravertebral soft tissues. If vertebral body compression collapse is diagnosed as part of a generalized skeletal involvement, the diagnosis presents little problem; but an isolated lesion may mimic primary or metastatic malignancy, necessitating biopsy.

ANGIOMATOSIS

This is the name given a disease of protean manifestation and uncertain etiology. It is often characterized by remissions and relapses difficult to relate directly to treatment (Reilly et al., 1972). The vertebral bodies and other parts of the skeleton are replaced by endothelium-lined spaces containing either lymph or blood (Fig. 18-12). We have seen lymphatic spaces outlined at lymphography in affected vertebral bodies that have undergone irregular asymmetrical collapse. Since any interference may accelerate the speed at which dissolution of bone occurs, surgical treatment by bone grafting is not usually advised. In the case illustrated, radiation treatment to the upper thoracic spine was associated with regression of the lytic processes both locally in the irradiated area and also in other remote sites.

RADIATION DAMAGE

In the irradiation of abdominal malignancies, particularly neuroblastoma and Wilms' tumor, it is inevitable that the growing spine will be affected with cessation of growth at the end plates and failure of development of the ring apophyses (Fig. 18-13).

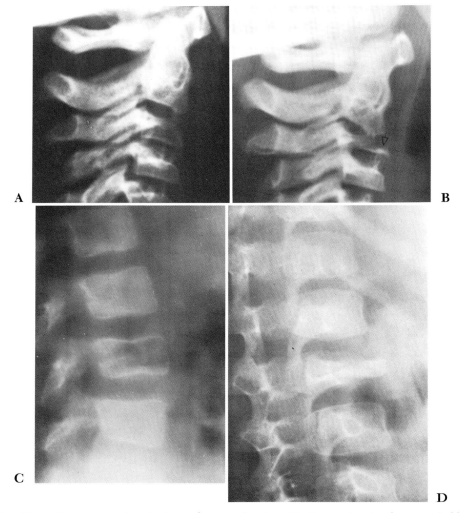

Fig. 18-11. Histiocytosis X. A, Normal cervical spine. B, Progression to dense waferlike compression collapse of C3 (arrow) in the same patient. C, Extensive infiltration of the body of L2 with early compression collapse. D, Increasing compression collapse in the same patient.

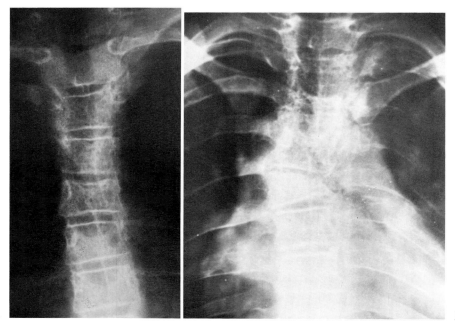

Fig. 18-12. Angiomatosis. A, The initial examination showed early compression collapse of the left half of T4. The bubbly texture of the upper vertebral bodies is apparent. B, There is a localized scoliosis at T4-T5; but after radiation therapy, the texture of these involved vertebrae has improved.

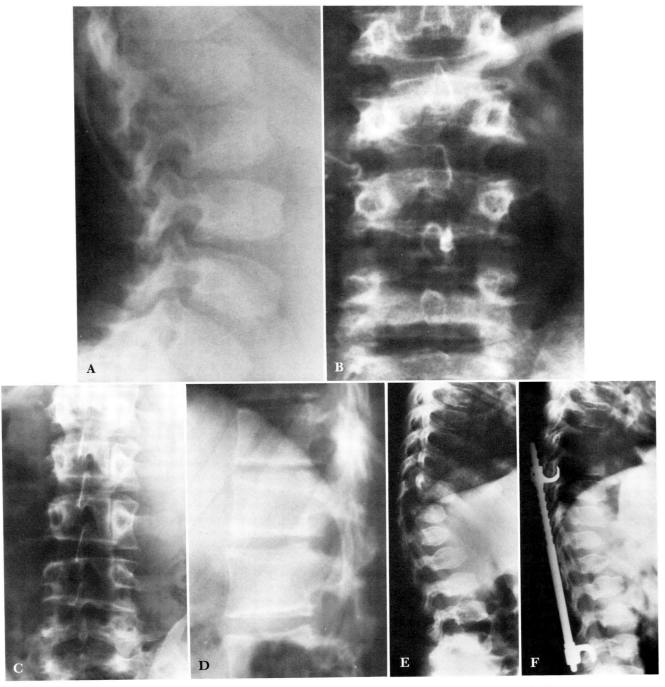

Fig. 18-13. Effects of radiation therapy. A and **B,** Symmetrical stunting of growth in the lumbar vertebrae after therapy for neuroblastoma. The appearances are reminiscent of a spondyloepiphyseal dysplasia. **C** and **D,** Asymmetrical growth disturbance after therapy for a right-sided Wilms' tumor. **E** and **F,** Severe lumbar gibbus before and after surgical stabilization.

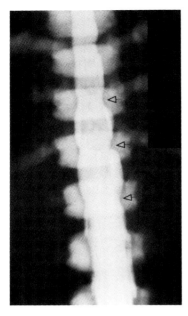

Fig. 18-14. Osteopetrosis. A myelogram illustrates the irregular narrowing of the spinal canal (arrows) due to increased volume of the abnormal bone.

Nowadays, the treatment ports are so arranged that the effect on the spine is symmetrical. If only half the spine is included in the field of treatment, growth disruption will be asymmetrical and intractable scoliosis will result. A marked lumbar gibbus with retrodisplacement of L1 may also develop. The main reason for including these illustrations is to show how closely this acquired growth defect may mimic the congenital diseases already described.

OSTEOPETROSIS

In osteopetrosis the skeleton is composed of an abnormal bony and cartilaginous matrix containing large amounts of hydroxyapatite. As the optic canals and basal foramina of the skull are encroached on by abnormal bone, so is the spinal canal (Fig. 18-14); however, for the unfortunate child who suffers from this dreadful disease, the segmental canal stenosis is but one of many problems.

PART II
Abnormalities localized to the spine

Vertebral abnormalities in infants and children may be isolated to the spine itself or be part of a generalized congenital or systemic disorder (Part I). Such abnormalities may have a direct effect on the spinal cord and its nerve roots.

The neuroradiology of the vertebral column is concerned more with abnormalities that compromise the neural axis. Be that as it may, many abnormalities are disorders of development, growth, and alignment; others are congenital or acquired dysplasias of the vertebral column; still others derive from trauma, infection, or neoplasia.

Many congenital abnormalities or minor variations of normal development will have no neural involvement and therefore *relatively* insignificant neuroradiological connotations. Other seemingly benign abnormalities or variations may appear to the general radiologist to be equally insignificant yet may be the indicator of a specific underlying present or potential neural abnormality. Still other vertebral abnormalities occurring in children with a marked and obvious neural skeletal disorder will be apparent to all observers.

We consider it valid therefore to provide in general terms only the spectrum of vertebral abnormalities pertinent or peculiar to the paediatric patient *that may have neuroradiological connotations.* Treatises such as those by Schmorl and Junghanns (1959) and Epstein (1969) provide an overall discussion of abnormalities of the spine, be they common in children and/or in adults.

ABNORMAL ORIENTATION OF THE VERTEBRAL COLUMN

There are two important aphorisms relating to the radiographic diagnosis of abnormalities: (1) Know the normal and its variations; and (2) assess the general structure under scrutiny before becoming absorbed in details, no matter how dramatic these may be.

Scoliosis and kyphosis, or a combination of the two, are important general alterations of spinal form.

Scoliosis

Scoliosis is a lateral curvature of the spine consisting of a primary curve (produced by a deforming factor or force) and a secondary curve (due to compensatory muscular action to align the head and the pelvis). Spinal components are upper lordosis, rotation, lateral curvature (scoliosis), counterrotation, and lower lordosis (Roaf, 1966). A nonstructural scoliosis is correctable by right or left bending; a structural scoliosis is not correctable.

Nonstructural scoliosis

A reversible scoliosis is often produced by extra-axial causes—muscle spasm due to thoracic and abdominal or indeed vertebral pain, leg length discrepancies, or simple postural attitudes. Before extensive neuroradiological investigations ensue, how-

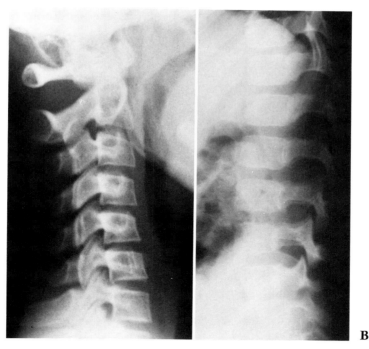

Fig. 18-20. Straight spine. A, Relatively immobile, in the cervical region, due to surrounding muscle spasm from trauma. **B,** Straight, in the lumbar region with widening of the sagittal diameter of the canal and an associated large intraspinal ependymoma.

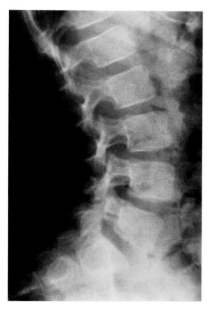

Fig. 18-21. Accentuated lumbar lordosis. Uncommonly will this occur, as in a child with a diffuse ependymoma of the cauda equina.

kyphosis will occur at the site of multiple laminectomies.

An adolescent kyphos (Scheuermann-Schmorl disease, Caffey, 1972) occurring commonly in the lower thoracic and upper lumbar vertebrae is usually relatively mild. Herniation of the nucleus pulposus due to injury of or congenital defects in the intervertebral disk is probably the cause (Begg, 1954). Loss of the nuclear material leads to greater pressure anteriorly than posteriorly because support of the articular facets is lost and anterior wedging of the vertebra results.

Unless a dysraphic spine is also present, kyphosis without a scoliosis is not commonly associated with intraspinal mass lesions (Tachdjian and Matson, 1965).

Straight spine

Decrease of a cervical or lumbar lordosis in a nondysraphic spine may be due to muscle spasm commonly (Fig. 18-20, A); but more importantly, it may be due to an intraspinal mass lesion (Fig. 18-20, B). Decreased flexibility of the spine is also often associated with this straightening (Chapter 20). In an otherwise normal spine in a child who has walked, lack of the lumbar lordosis without muscle spasm is a significant abnormality and indicates the possibility of an intraspinal mass lesion. A low-fixed conus or a tethered cord will cause the child to straighten a lumbar lordosis to relieve as much tension on the cord and roots as possible. Straightening of a cervical lordosis in the absence of infection or trauma is similarly an ominous sign of an intraspinal mass lesion.

Prior to toddling, an infant will have a relatively straight lumbar spine. This is not abnormal.

Accentuation of the lordosis of the lumbar spine is *uncommonly* seen in intraspinal mass lesions but can occur with such abnormalities as a dermoid or an ependymoma of the cauda equina (Fig. 18-21). Accentuated lumbar lordosis is also seen in such generalized diseases as achondroplasia.

SPECIFIC VERTEBRAL ABNORMALITIES
Congenital abnormalities of the vertebrae

A basic and relatively simplistic understanding of the embryology of the vertebral column is necessary. Further details may be obtained from Schmorl and Junghanns (1959), Epstein (1969), James and Lassman (1972), and Gray (1973).

Between the embryonic amniotic cavity and the yolk sac lies the embryonic disk with the primitive ectoderm dorsally alongside the amniotic cavity and the endoderm ventrally alongside the yolk sac. A caudal primitive streak forms in ectoderm, and a pit appears at the primitive knot (Hensen's node); craniad growth forms the notochord between the ectoderm and the endoderm layers. Further migration of the more lateral cells of the primitive streak occurs, and these cells differentiate into mesoderm parallel with the notochord. At the second week of gestation, segmentation of this mesoderm into primitive muscles (myotomes) and primitive vertebrae (sclerotomes) takes place. At the third week a more cranial differentiation of ectoderm forms the neural plate dorsal to the notochord, which plate forms the neural tube.

The neural tube begins to form in the midportion and progresses craniad and caudad; it will develop the brain and spinal cord. At 12 weeks the spinal cord and spinal canal are of equal length; at 25 weeks the conus is at the S1 level. The craniad move of the conus results in caudad formation of the differentiated neural tube into the filum terminale, whose length increases with the movement of the conus. At birth the conus is at the L3 level; and with the relatively greater growth of the vertebral column, the conus moves to the L2 vertebral level by 2 to 4 months (Barson, 1970; James and Lassman, 1972) and remains at approximately the L2 level or slightly higher from then onward.

From the ninth week, the notochord is progressively compressed into the intervertebral disk to form a nucleus pulposus.

Concomitant with these developments, the *cartilaginous anlagen* of the vertebral bodies themselves begin to form at the fourth week, one cartilaginous center on each side of the notochord compressing the notochord into the disk spaces. *Two primitive cartilaginous centers* are formed laterally to a ventrodorsal prechordal cleft in the sagittal plane (Fig. 18-22). Though theoretically possible, a persistent notochord never occurs.

Ossification centers form dorsally and ventrally in each cartilaginous center. A single dorsal and a single ventral ossification center then follow and ultimately fuse into a single vertebral body ossification center. The posterolateral angles of the vertebral bodies result from a projection of the vertebral arch from the body to the neurocentral synchondrosis.

Thus minor developmental anomalies of the vertebrae can be easily understood (Fig. 18-22).

1. *Absent vertebral body.* Lack of ossification of cartilaginous centers in toto. This rarely occurs as an isolated event but is often part of a generalized dysraphic defect.
2. *Sagittal cleft vertebra or butterfly vertebra.* Lack of consolidation of the two cartilaginous centers and independent ossification of each center side by side. Ossification of each cartilaginous center may vary in symmetry.
3. *Hemivertebra.* Lack of ossification of one lateral cartilaginous center. A rudimentary hemivertebra with a normally ossified hemivertebral portion on the other side may also occur.
4. *Anterior or posterior hemivertebra.* Failure of formation of the dorsal or ventral ossification centers respectively.
5. *Coronal cleft vertebra.* Failure of fusion of the dorsal and ventral ossification centers with a remnant cartilaginous coronal cleft.

Such vertebral body anomalies may occur in isolation or may be multiple, but more often than not they are associated with complex vertebral arch anomalies and create complex dysraphic spines.

Spina bifida is a congenital developmental anomaly whereby there exists a defect of fusion of the posterior arches of one or more vertebrae. The midportion of the arch is normally cartilaginous (Fig. 18-23) in infants and young children and does not represent spina bifida.

We prefer the term *spinal dysraphia* (Barson, 1970), which implies splaying of the pedicles and laminae associated with nonfusion and varying defects and disorganization of spinal elements. Such dysraphia may be *occult*, with no overlying cutaneous abnormalities, or *manifest*, with overlying

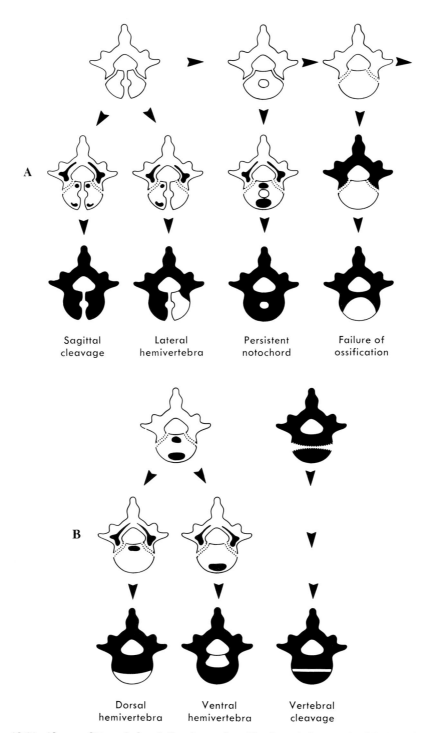

Sagittal cleavage   Lateral hemivertebra   Persistent notochord   Failure of ossification

Dorsal hemivertebra   Ventral hemivertebra   Vertebral cleavage

Fig. 18-22. Abnormalities of chondrification and ossification of the vertebral bodies. (Modified from Schmorl, G., and Junghanns, H.: The human spine in health and disease. (Translated from fourth German edition, S. P. Wilk and L. S. Goin, editors), New York, 1959, Grune & Stratton, Inc.)

cutaneous abnormalities (hairy patch, lipoma, vascular nevus, sinus, abnormal pigmented patch). Spinal dysraphia commonly includes abnormalites of segmentation as between vertebral laminae, pediculate fusion, and vertebral body ossification defects (Fig. 18-24).

Till (1968) includes in the term spinal dysraphia such entities as diastematomyelia, neurenteric fistulae, dermoid cysts, congenital sinus tracks, and lipoma formation.

Spina bifida cystica is spinal dysraphia associated

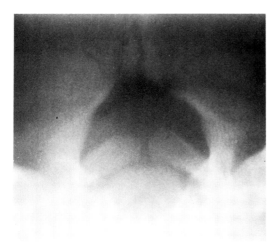

Fig. 18-23. Pseudo–spina bifida. A lack of ossification of the midportion of the spinous process as in this C1 vertebra commonly occurs in infants. The cartilage is soon ossified. This is not a spina bifida occulta.

with protrusion of thecal membranes out of the canal either with or without spinal cord and nerves. Such defects are termed myelomeningoceles or meningoceles respectively.

Defects in vertebral segmentation, such as block vertebrae, may occur alone or with posterior arch defects to form a dysraphic spine. Block vertebrae occur, in which there is a fusion of one or more vertebrae without a visible intervertebral disk or merely a rudimentary disk (Fig. 18-25). Contrary to the acquired fused defects due to disk abnormalities, however, there is no loss of segmental height. Vertical fusion of parts of or a whole vertebral arch may also take place.

These dysraphic anomalies are often associated with sclerotome abnormalities, like absent or deformed ribs, and with cardiopulmonary or gastrointestinal anomalies. Paramount are those associated dural arachnoid and neural anomalies that occur with spinal dysraphia and the formation of congenital space-occupying lesions such as dermoids, teratomas, and lipomas. All the foregoing abnormalities are related inasmuch as some intrauterine catastrophe occurred during the development of the tissues and organs within the embryo—affecting ectoderm, mesoderm, and endoderm. The resultant structural and visceral growth abnormalities ensue.

Minor anomalies

The significance of spinal dysraphia in neuroradiology is that the structural vertebral abnormalities may

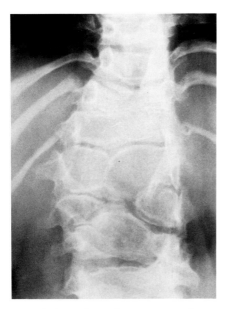

Fig. 18-24. Spinal dysraphia. There is a conglomerate of lack of fusion of the posterior arches and intersegmental bars along with sagittal cleft vertebrae and hemivertebrae.

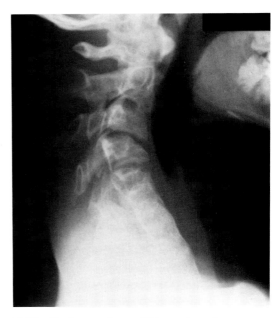

Fig. 18-25. Block vertebrae. This patient has a congenital lack of segmentation of the lower cervical and upper thoracic vertebrae. Rudimentary disk spaces are seen.

affect the normal cord or they may be a marker for significant underlying spinal cord maldevelopment or congenital intraspinal mass lesions.

A minor spinal abnormality may be associated with a significant neural abnormality. A severe spinal abnormality, however, will not necessarily be associated with an underlying neural abnormality or mass lesion but rather with some dural dysplasia. In our experience, anomalies of the cord and/or roots or a develop-

mental mass lesion have been nearly always associated with spinal dysraphia. To detect and remove a congenital mass lesion or prevent by surgery further neurological deterioration, an aggressive neurosurgical and neuroradiological approach is indicated toward spinal dysraphia. Clinical abnormalities may result purely from structural deformities of the spine and/or cord that are amenable to neurosurgical correction, such as transsection of a fixed filum terminale

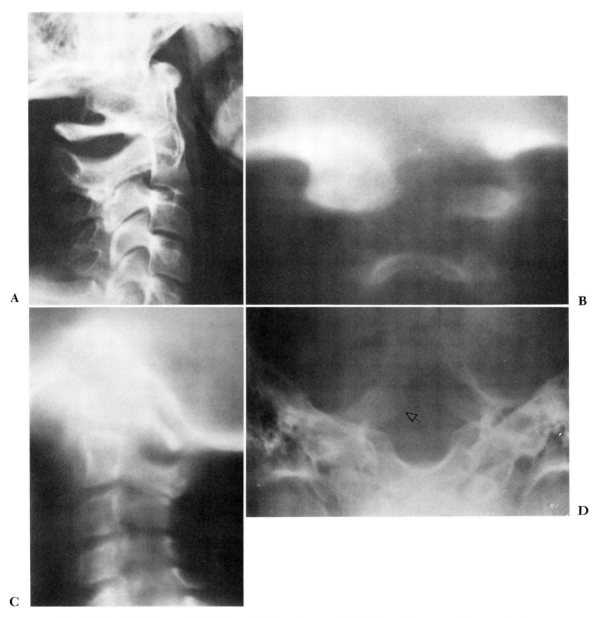

Fig. 18-26. Occipitocervical fusions. A, Assimilation of both lateral masses of C1 with the occiput. **B,** An AP tomogram demonstrates unilateral assimiliation of the right lateral condyle of C1 with the occiput. **C,** Assimilation of the body of C1 and occiput, absence of the odontoid, and basilar invagination. **D,** Lack of ossification of the midportion of the posterior arch of C1 and assimilation of the right posterior arch with the occipital bone, creating a projecting bony mass (arrow) into the spinal canal.

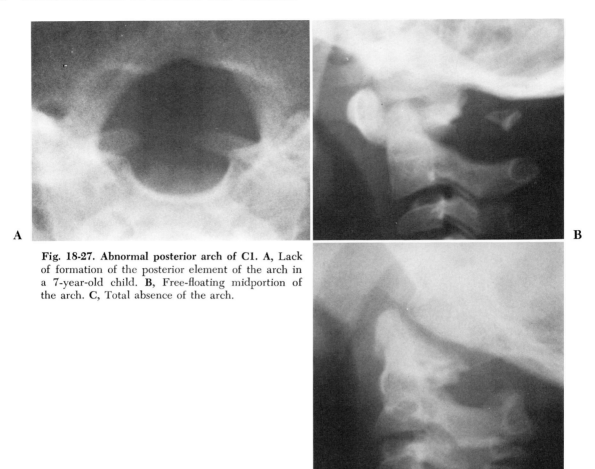

Fig. 18-27. Abnormal posterior arch of C1. A, Lack of formation of the posterior element of the arch in a 7-year-old child. **B,** Free-floating midportion of the arch. **C,** Total absence of the arch.

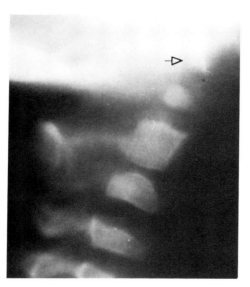

Fig. 18-28. An occipital vertebra. There is total absence of C1. A small occipital vertebra (arrow) articulates with the dens of C2.

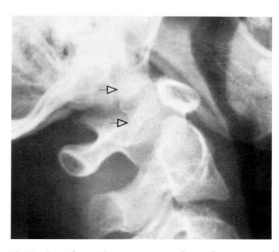

Fig. 18-29. Os odontoideum. Arrows show the os completely separate from the body of C2 and slightly retrosubluxated.

or dissection of lipomatous tissue from embedded lumbar and sacral roots or freeing of a low-fixed conus.

Mention will be made of anomalies which may connote underlying abnormalities of the neural axis and/or coverings. Schmorl and Junghanns (1959) and Epstein (1969) provide exhaustive descriptions of all types of congenital spinal anomalies, and the reader is referred to these monographs. We shall consider first the relatively minor but no less important anomalies of the spine that are usually localized in specific areas or that involve only a few segments of the spine. Severe and complex spinal dysraphia merits separate attention; such complex anomalies are often composites of many relatively minor and often isolated anomalies as detailed next.

Cervico-occipital junction anomalies

Unilateral or bilateral fusion of the occipital condyles and lateral masses of the atlas or fusion between the posterior arch of the atlas and the occiput may occur in varying degrees (Fig. 18-26, A and B) and be associated with basilar invagination (Fig. 18-26, C). The foramen magnum may be compromised insofar as its diameter and shape are altered (Fig. 18-26, D) (Kruyff, 1965), which may lead to bony pressure on the cervicomedullary junction in later life (McRae, 1960)—the so-called foramen magnum syndrome. Asymmetry of the occipital condyles and/or lateral masses without assimilation may also occur. Incomplete formation of C1 (Fig. 18-27) such as absence of the posterior arch of the atlas or lack of fusion of the posterior arch with a lateral mass is uncommon as an isolated anomaly and is not usually associated with neurological abnormalities in children. Surprisingly little instability results. In the accurate delinea-tion of these anomalies of the cervico-occipital junction, tomography in both anterioposterior and lateral planes is essential.

Persistence of an occipital vertebra, the caudalmost of the three primitive somites forming the clivus (Fig. 18-28), is extremely rare (Wollin, 1963). A small condyle called the os occipitale may occur in the anterior of the foramen magnum and represents the body of this vertebra. It may articulate with the dens of C2. Anomalies of the odontoid process are complex (Chapter 17) and are best summarized by Greenberg (1968).

The ossiculum terminale derived from the fourth occipital sclerotome is the ossicle of the tip of the odontoid that usually fuses with the odontoid itself, at about 6 years of age, whereas the os odontoideum is due to a lack of fusion of the upper two thirds of the odontoid with its base (Fig. 18-29). The latter must not be misdiagnosed as a traumatic sequela. Due to the chronic atlantoaxial dislocation, neurological symptoms may occur in adulthood (McRae, 1960). Instability and excessive movement at the C1-C2 level may result. As an isolated anomaly, total absence of the odontoid is quite rare (Schultz et al., 1956; Gwinn and Smith, 1962). Marked odontoidal abnormalities are common in the Klippel-Feil syndrome (Fig. 18-30). A small hypoplastic odontoid per se is uncommon.

Basilar invagination, whereby the abnormal upward convexity of the base of the skull in the occipital condyles (McRae, 1960) leads to an abnormally high position of the tip of the odontoid relative to the base of the skull, is uncommon in children either as a congenital anomaly or due to acquired diseases such as rickets, osteomalacia, cleidocranial dysostosis, and hypophosphatasia (Fig. 18-31).

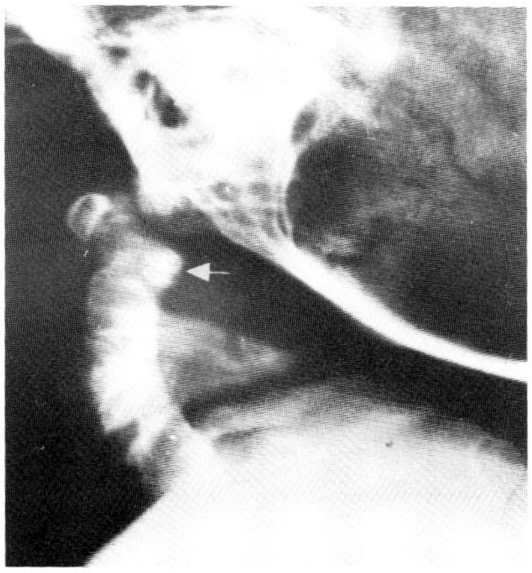

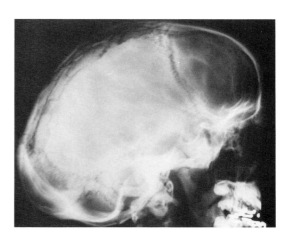

Fig. 18-30. Hypoplastic odontoid and the Klippel-Feil syndrome. The posterior arch of C1 is absent. The odontoid (arrow) is small.

Fig. 18-31. Basilar invagination. In a child with hypophosphatasia tarda. The associated sagittal synostosis has been treated by cranial morcellation around the suture.

Cervical vertebral anomalies

Congenital absence or lack of fusion of the posterior or anterior arches of the atlas is uncommon. Posterior spina bifida of C1 is said to occur in 5% of adults (McRae, 1960). The cartilaginous cleft of the posterior arch of the upper cervical vertebra, which usually fuses after the first year of life, is not a spina bifida (Fig. 18-23). A separate midline ossicle anteriorly and posteriorly (Fig. 18-32) may occur and subsequently fuses with the arch. This is a normal phenomenon.

Although rare, an absent cervical pedicle as an isolated anomaly (Fig. 18-33) (Oestreich and Young, 1969; McLoughlin and Wortzman, 1972) is often associated with minor neurological symptoms and pain. At myelography, a dural deformity here may produce a concavity simulating an extradural tumor. Careful oblique views and tomography are essential in the investigation of such an absent pedicle. A congenital cleft between the posterior arch and the body is another uncommon anomaly (Fig. 18-34).

Congenital fusion of the cervical vertebrae, usually associated with absence or anomalies of the posterior arch, may be isolated or part of the Klippel-Feil syndrome. The latter abnormality is a congenital fusion of part or all of the cervical spine with or without a reduction in the normal number of vertebrae (Fig. 18-35). A short neck and low hairline with limited movement of the neck are present (Shoul and Ritvo, 1952). A Sprengel's shoulder (Fig. 18-35, B) and/or an omovertebral bone (Fig. 18-36), in which a high-positioned scapula with a connecting bone to an upper transverse process of a cervical vertebra occurs, may (rarely) join the Klippel-Feil syndrome. Associated renal anomalies (Ramsely and Bliznak, 1971) or petrous bone maldevelopment (Palant and Carter, 1972) may also occur. Significant neural anomalies associated with this syndrome are occipital encephaloceles, Chiari malformation, and subsequent hydrocephalus with aqueductal stenosis. This combination is more common in girls.

Other cervical vertebral body anomalies—such as an isolated lateral hemivertebra—are usually innocuous. An isolated congenital absence of a body of a cervical vertebra is rare and has occurred only once in our experience. An occult bifid posterior arch of C6 or C7 (Fig. 18-37) can occur as a localized entity; and underlying anomalies that may be associated with

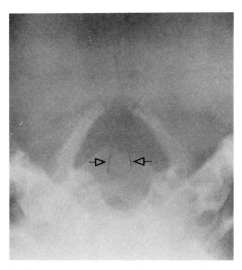

Fig. 18-32. **Posterior spinous ossicle of C1.** This is a normal ossification variant (arrows) and completely fuses by the age of 4 or 5.

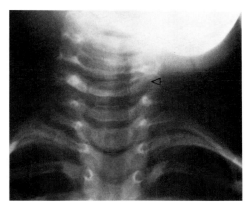

Fig. 18-33. **Congenital absence of a cervical pedicle.** The left pedicle of C5 (arrow) is missing. There are bilateral cervical ribs.

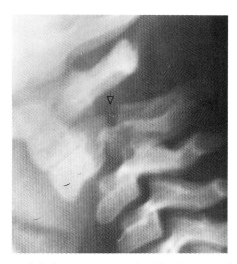

Fig. 18-34. **Cleft between a vertebral body and arch.** A congenital lack of fusion of the arch of C2 to the body is present bilaterally (arrow).

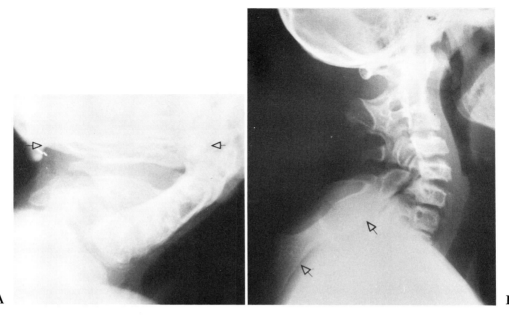

Fig. 18-35. Klippel-Feil syndrome. A, Fusion of at least the upper three or four cervical vertebrae. A cervical vertebra is probably missing. There also is partial fusion of some of the laminae, and the foramen magnum (arrows) is wide. A Chiari malformation was also present. **B,** Fusion of the posterior arches of C2, C3, and C4 with fusions of the bodies of C2 and C3. Note the high scapula (arrows), which is fused to the posterior arches of the lower cervical spine.

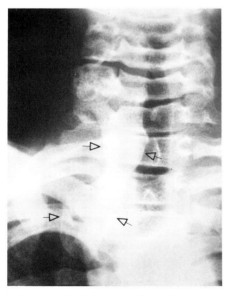

Fig. 18-36. Omovertebral bone. A large bone (arrows) connects the medial border of a high right scapula with the transverse processes of C6 and C7.

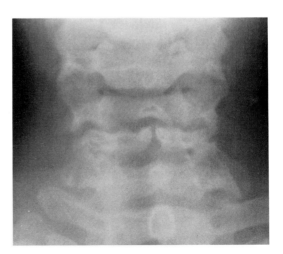

Fig. 18-37. Occult bifid cervical spine. An isolated bifid C6 spine is present with no underlying spinal cord. There was no thecal abnormality on myelography or any cutaneous abnormality.

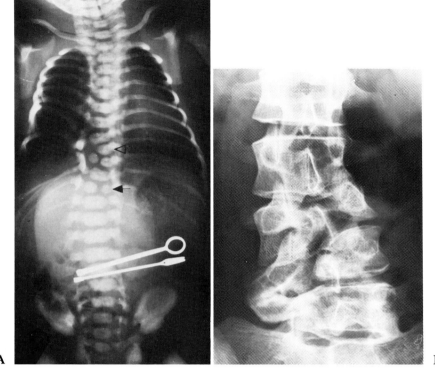

A B

Fig. 18-38. Hemivertebrae. A, Large lumbar meningocele with a true lateral hemivertebra (open arrow). The other half is absent. Caudally can be seen a sagittal cleft vertebra with a hypoplastic left hemivertebra (solid arrow). B, Gross hemivertebral disorganization of the lumbar spine. This child had an associated intraspinal lipoma.

such a bifid spine in the upper cervical level are an intraspinal lipoma or a syringomyelocele. A neurenteric cyst is associated with more severe and complex *anterior* dysraphic anomalies (Chapter 20) though often with a posterior component as well. A transpinal canal may persist in some patients (Chapter 20). A cervical diastematomyelia is extremely rare, occurring only once in our experience.

Hemivertebra

A hemivertebra is an isolated minor anomaly usually of the thoracic or lumbar spine that may be quite innocuous; but if it develops in the lumbar region it may signal an underlying lipoma, dermoid, or teratoma, or it may be associated with a low-fixed cord. A true lateral hemivertebra may occur with aplasia of its partner or be associated with a small hypoplastic other half. The hemivertebra usually involves the lateral cartilaginous center defect; however, due to dysplasia of an ossification vertebral center defect, rarely a dorsal or a ventral hemivertebra will occur. Hemivertebrae often are multiple, producing bizarre spinal forms, and often are part of a more severe dysraphia (Fig. 18-38).

Although rare, a discrete malformed dorsal or

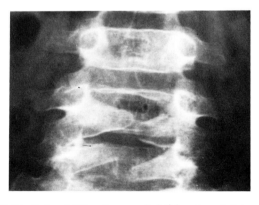

Fig. 18-39. Spina bifida. An occult bifid spine at L4 and L5 shows the characteristic butt-end twisted appearance. In the absence of cutaneous abnormalities, such bifid spines are usually innocuous.

ventral hemivertebra may result in compression of either of the hemivertebrae with a resultant kyphosis (Fig. 18-18).

Bifid spine

An isolated bifid spine in a thoracic or lumbar region other than L5 is uncommon. There is a familial

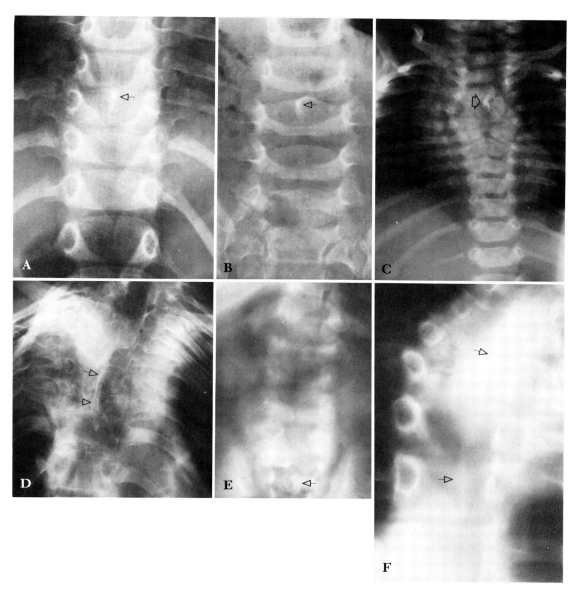

Fig. 18-40. Sites of a diastematomyelic spur. A, Lower thoracic (arrow). **B,** Upper lumbar (arrow). **C,** Upper thoracic (arrow). Note the associated cleft vertebral bodies. A neurenteric canal and small cyst were also present. **D,** A long bony bar in the upper thoracic (arrows) region associated with block vertebra. **E,** Sacral spur (arrow) on tomogram and associated with multiple lumbar anomalies. **F,** A tomogram demonstrates thin paired spurs (arrows).

tendency inasmuch as the incidence of spina bifida, particularly at the L5-S1 level, within the family of a patient who has a spina bifida is three and a half times what it is in the general population (Hoffman, 1968). The incidence of such occult spina bifida may vary from 5% to 36% (Smith, 1965; Epstein, 1969). In childhood, a simple cleft in the midline spinous process is merely unossified cartilage (Fig. 18-23). Such clefts should ossify within the first 18 months to 2 years of life. Some delay in this ossification may occur, as noted by Sutow and Pryde (1956). A de-

crease in radiographic incidence occurred from as late as 7 years of age to adulthood.

In our experience, a bifid spinous process is always asymmetrical and appears to be slightly twisted (Fig. 18-39). The unfused ends are often wide and asymmetrical. Though most of these defects are innocuous—a cutaneous hairy patch, lipoma, angioma, or dimple overlying the bifid spine, an associated neurological symptom, or a lack of peripheral nerve, bladder, or bowel control should lead to careful clinical and myelographic investigation. A lipoma, dermoid, teratoma, tight filum terminale, or low-fixed conus may all be associated with a lumbar or sacral spina bifida, especially if the interpediculate distance is widened or posterior vertebral body scalloping or pediculate thinning is an associated finding (Chapter 20).

Diastematomyelia

Diastematomyelia, whereby the cord or filum terminale is split in the sagittal plane by a fibrous,

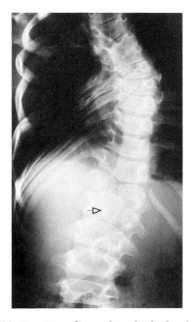

Fig. 18-41. Diastematomyelia and multiple local and distant congenital anomalies. Note the segmental upper body defects, absent ribs, sagittal cleft, butterfly vertebra T12, small bony spur (arrow), and posterior arch fusion defects inferiorly with thoracic scoliosis.

cartilaginous, or bony spur or a combination of the three, is *always* associated with some form of additional congenital spinal anomaly—be it in the vertebral body, the arch, or both. The diastematomyelic spur is common in the lower thoracic (Fig. 18-40, A) and upper lumbar (Fig. 18-40, B) regions but is rarely seen in the upper thoracic (Fig. 18-40, C and D), cervical, or sacral (Fig. 18-40, E) regions; rarely is there a double spur (Fig. 18-40, F). Especially widening of the interpediculate distances but also butterfly vertebrae, hemivertebrae, partial or complete vertebral fusion, narrow vertebral bodies, spina bifida, and anterior or posterior intervertebral fusion defects occur (in varying combinations and degree, Fig. 18-41). Fusion of the posterior arches of contiguous laminae and spines, together with bifid spines, were the anomalies most often seen, followed in incidence by various forms of vertebral body segmentation defects. A combination of these anomalies, however, was frequently observed (Harwood-Nash and Fitz, 1976).

It is more common for a diastematomyelia to occur with a relatively minor vertebral anomalous complex than with a gross spinal dysraphia. Standard spinal radiographs may clearly show this bony spur; but if a complex posterior arch block fusion is present, the spur may be difficult to differentiate from other anomalies. Furthermore, such posterior anomalies may create the appearance of a bony spur.

Prior to the myelographic investigation of diastematomyelia (Chapter 19), tomography in the anteroposterior and lateral projections is useful to determine, first, the presence and, second, the direction and extent of the ossified septum (Fig. 18-42). A fibrous or cartilaginous septum may be present alone or with an ossified part of the spur. A forward and upward projection of the spur is more common than

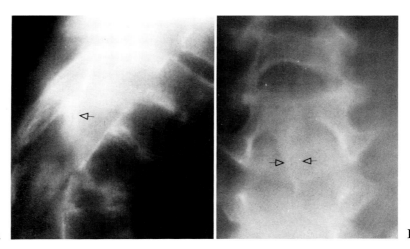

A   B

Fig. 18-42. Tomography and the bony spur. A, A sagittal tomogram demonstrates the caudally coursing bony spur (arrow). **B,** An AP tomogram reveals the pencil point shape (arrows).

a direct dorsoventral or a downward-forward direction. Hilal and co-workers (1974) state that an upward direction of the spur is associated with the maximally dysraphic spine rostral to the spur and vice versa.

The bony spur is usually wider posteriorly (Fig. 18-42, *A*), often exists only posteriorly, and may or may

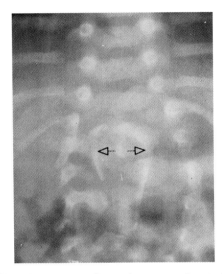

Fig. 18-43. Diastematomyelia and attempted spinal duplication. A large spur occurring in the lumbar region ossified at the periphery (arrows). It represents an attempted spinal duplication. Only two sets of roots (laterally placed) were present, indicating no spinal cord duplication.

not fuse with the posterior vertebral body or posterior fused laminae. We agree with Hilal and co-workers (1974) that the spur appears to be a separate ossification unit. It may represent a mild dysraphic attempt at the formation of an additional midline pedicular structure, probably representing an attempt at spinal duplication (Fig. 18-43).

Myelography, either positive contrast or air, will demonstrate the spur and the split cord (Fig. 18-44). Detection of such a spur prior to surgical straightening of an associated congenital scoliosis is obviously important. Furthermore, a diastematomyelic spur may also (uncommonly) be associated with an intraspinal lipoma or even a neurenteric cyst, together with an anterior neurenteric canal (Fig. 18-40, *C*).

Cleft vertebra

Cleft vertebrae may have a coronal or sagittal cleft in an otherwise normally shaped body; or they may be associated with varying forms of hypoplasia and inner wedging of the lateral halves with a sagittal cleft, the so-called "butterfly" vertebrae, or rarely inner wedging of the dorsal and ventral halves. Partial fusion may occur, giving a small interposed waist of ossified bone between the lateral or dorsal and ventral ossification centers.

Coronal cleft vertebrae (Epstein, 1969; Fielden and Russell, 1970) are uncommon and occur in neonates, predominantly boys (10 to 1); they disappear by 6 months of age (Fig. 18-45). Their genesis has been

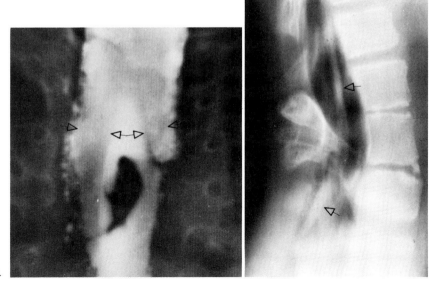

Fig. 18-44. Myelography and diastematomyelia. A, An oil myelogram demonstrates a midline cartilaginous defect, widening of the interpediculate distances, and a split cord (arrows). **B,** An air myelogram with sagittal tomography reveals the vertebral body defects and trifoil bony spur around which the split cord (arrows) passes. (Courtesy Dr. R. Hoare, London.)

detailed earlier in this chapter. They are commonly associated with chondrodysplasia congenita (Conradi's syndrome) (Fig. 18-46), and the abnormality of the vertebral body may be so severe as to cause the dorsal hemivertebra to fail to form (Fig. 18-46). Coronal cleft vertebrae are rarely associated with other malformations of the central nervous system such as a meningocele but can be associated with an imperforate anus or congenital heart disease.

Sagittal cleft vertebrae are rare (Fig. 18-47), and the cartilaginous slit in the mid–spinous process of a vertebra must not be confused with a sagittal cleft vertebra when the slit is superimposed over the vertebral body on an AP radiograph of the spine (Fig. 18-48). If present, the sagittal clefts disappear after 6 months of age. More severe aberrations of ossification result in paired lateral butterfly vertebrae, singly or multiply (Fig. 18-48).

We do not believe that a possible persistence of a notochord has any part in this anomaly. Histology

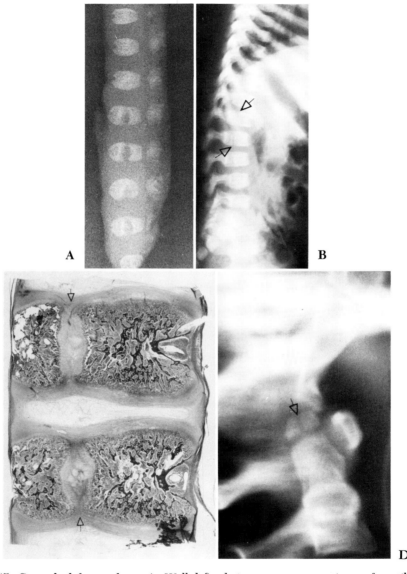

Fig. 18-45. Coronal cleft vertebrae. A, Well-defined, in an autopsy specimen of a stillborn fetus otherwise normal. These were in the lumbar region. B, Persistent (arrows), in a 3-month-old baby boy as an incidental finding. These disappeared at the age of 6 months. C, Persistent cartilaginous (arrows), in a pathological sagittal section of another stillborn fetus. D, With a persistent os terminale (arrow), between the dorsal and ventral ossification centers. This indicates that the os terminale is a remnant of a vertebral body. The os articulates with the tip of the clivus, also probably a remnant of an occipital vertebra. (C courtesy G. Culham, M.D., Toronto.)

reveals cartilaginous clefts only. Wollin and Elliot (1961), however, do report two children in whom notochordal remnants were found. The question of a cause-and-effect relationship is moot.

Defect in segmentation

Defects in segmentation result from faulty metameric segmentation (List, 1969); or, as Gardner (1973) points out, fusion occurs in the fetus only *after* the sclerotomes are formed but *before* the

cartilage is formed. Simple lumbarization of S1, or sacralization of L5, may be associated with slight loss of normal lumbar lordosis; but both are innocuous anomalies. An extra vertebra from oversegmentation rarely occurs. Extra isolated hemivertebrae may develop from two separate ossification centers and will form discrete vertically oriented quarter-vertebrae (Fig. 18-49).

The intersegmental fusion at two or more levels may occur between the laminae, pedicles, vertebral bodies, or a combination of the three. If vertebrae are fused, the term *block vertebrae* is used (Fig. 18-50). The remnant disk space may or may not be visible in part or in whole, but the vertebral bodies are of normal or increased height (Epstein, 1969). If decreased height is observed, an acquired secondary fusion must be considered.

Anteroposterior vertebral body narrowing and posterior vertebral body scalloping may occur (Fig. 18-50, A). This scalloping is usually related to associated dural dysplasia and a wide dural sac, and less commonly to a congenital intraspinal mass lesion. Loss of the normal lordotic curves of the lumbar and cervical areas also is seen.

Block vertebrae are common in the lumbar, less common in the cervical, and rare in the thoracic regions. Hemivertebrae may be associated above or below the block vertebrae and uncommonly does a spondylolisthesis (Fig. 18-50, A) or disk prolapse

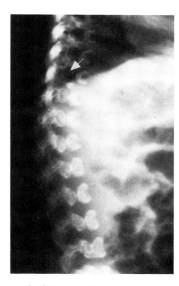

Fig. 18-46. Coronal cleft vertebra and Conradi's disease. Persistent coronal clefts have resulted from markedly dysplastic dorsal and ventral ossification centers. Note in the thoracic level the complete absence of development of the dorsal ossification center (arrow).

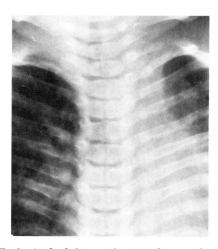

Fig. 18-47. Sagittal cleft vertebra. A discrete linear sagittal cleft is present throughout most of the thoracic vertebrae. This is most uncommon.

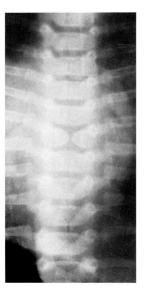

Fig. 18-48. Lateral paired butterfly vertebrae and pseudosagittal clefts. Paired lateral butterfly vertebrae of T6 leave a characteristic inner bullet-nose appearance. Superimposed "clefts" are seen above and below these but lie across the disk spaces as well and represent the cartilaginous clefts of the midportion of the spinous processes.

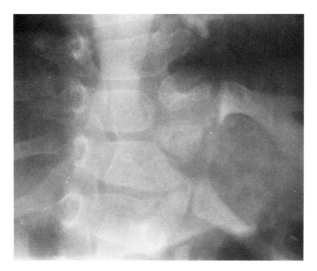

Fig. 18-49. Oversegmentation. Two vertically oriented quarter-vertebrae have developed from the left lateral cartilaginous anlage.

occur at the junction with the normal spine. These block vertebrae may indicate underlying myelodysplasia, intraspinal congenital mass lesions, or diastematomyelia (Fig. 18-44, *B*).

Defects of segmentation of the cervical region are commonly referred to as the Klippel-Feil syndrome—a lesion thought by Gardner (1973) to be due to overdistension of the cervical central canal in the fetus, causing coalescence of the sclerotomes, widening of the canal, bifid spines, and shortening of the primitive cervical canal. The common association of Klippel-Feil with an occipital encephalocele and a Chiari malformation tends to lend credence to this proposal.

Juvenile spondylarthritis, vertebral trauma, and infections may all lead to acquired vertebral body fusions, but all have loss of disk height and often loss of vertebral height.

Unusually large pediculate bony masses may form, probably due to some segmental cartilaginous anlage malformation (Fig. 18-51).

Posterior slipping of a vertebral body

A backward-sliding single vertebral body causes a significant intraspinal mass (Fig. 18-52, *A*) (Chapter 20). It is due to a defect of the arch (either absent

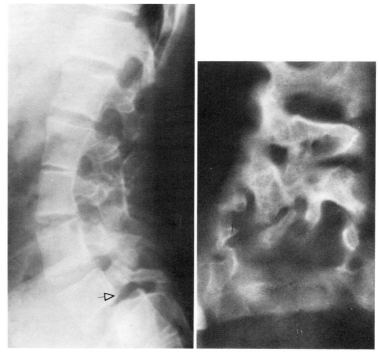

A   B

Fig. 18-50. Block vertebrae. A, A segmentation defect resulting in congenital fusion of the L2 and L3 vertebrae. Total vertebral heights equal those of adjacent pairs of vertebra. Note the scalloping, widened lumbar canal, posterior arch dysraphia, and spondylolisthesis of L5 on S1 (arrow). **B,** An AP tomogram shows intersegmental fusion of the posterior arch elements of the lumbar vertebrae.

pedicles or absent laminae) whereby the vertebral body has no posterior support. With forward spinal flexion, the floating body tends to slip backward. Often the vertebral body itself is hypoplastic or is a hemivertebra. Rarely is the body itself absent, with only a pedicle; and the contribution of the pedicle to the body posterior to the neurocentral junction then produces a posterior slippage which compresses the spinal canal. Mild to moderate kyphosis may result. Concomitant congenital transverse spinal stenosis (Fig. 18-52, *B*) is frequent and contributes to the spinal cord compression. Tomography and myelogra-

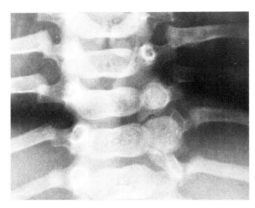

Fig. 18-51. Pediculate segmental ossification anomaly. Large overgrown pedicles may develop on a congenital basis, each associated with a normal transverse process and a rib in the thoracic spine. These pedicles are not fused to their vertebral bodies.

phy are essential in the delineation of this anomaly and effect. Early surgical treatment will prevent severe spinal cord compression. The lumbar region is by far the most commonly involved area.

Spondylolysis and spondylolisthesis

Spondylolysis and spondylolisthesis may be solely traumatic in origin.

We believe, however, that the majority of childhood *spondylolysis* has a congenital basis. This defect is probably a dysplasia in the pars interarticularis of the posterior arch, and it occurs unilaterally or bilaterally (80% of cases). A linear cleft (Fig. 18-53, *A*) or a breach with thinned bony margins of the pars (Fig. 18-53, *B*) may be seen. Wiltse (1962) proposes that the stress and strain of the upright position of man on top of an underlying dysplasia will produce a spondylolysis within the pars interarticularis. Yet such defects are also seen in infants, who have not been in the upright position. Can the birth process contribute to this defect? He claims that the stress alone is unlikely to produce such a breach. Furthermore, strong familial tendencies have been reported (Baker and McHollick, 1956). These authors report an incidence of spondylolysis in 5% of asymptomatic 6-year-old children.

Spondylolisthesis, a forward slipping to a varying degree of one vertebra relative to its inferior neighbor (rarely vice versa—retrospondylolisthesis), is usually associated with a spondylolysis (Fig. 18-53, *B*). The degree of slipping is graded according to whether the

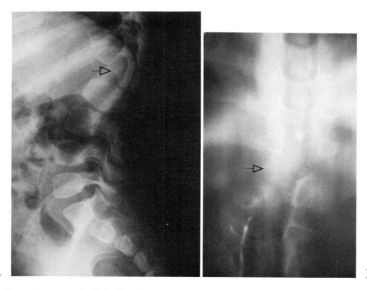

A   B

Fig. 18-52. Posterior vertebral body slipping. A, Of L1 (arrow), due to congenitally absent pedicles and creating a considerable kyphos and spinal canal mass lesion. **B,** An air myelogram with tomography demonstrates the severe spinal stenosis (arrow) at a similar level of posterior slipping in another child.

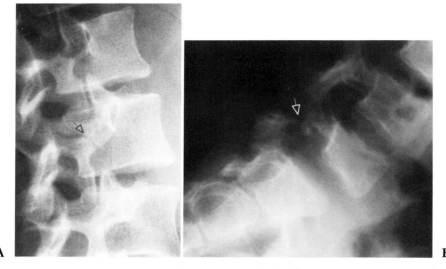

Fig. 18-53. Spondylolysis. A, An oblique view of the lumbar spine demonstrates a linear cleft in the pars interarticularis (arrow). No spondylolisthesis is present. **B,** Bilateral spondylolysis of L5 (arrow) is associated with marked thinning of the pars and a moderate spondylolisthesis.

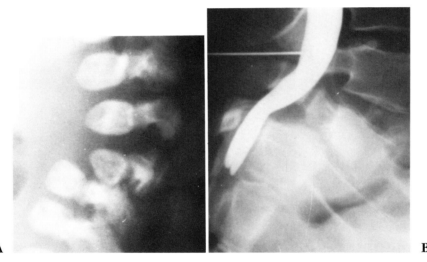

Fig. 18-54. Spondylolisthesis. A, Marked, of L2 slipping posteriorly on L3 (retrospondylolisthesis) associated with a severe lumbar spinal dysraphia of the posterior arches. **B,** Assumed congenital spondylolisthesis of L5 on S1 with marked sclerosis of L5.

slip is one third of a vertebral body's anteroposterior diameter (grade I) and so on to a complete slip (grade IV). Nonspondylolytic spondylolisthesis rarely occurs and is a congenital elongation of the intact neural arch resulting in narrowing of the spinal canal as the *entire* vertebral body slips forward. In spondylolisthesis with spondylolysis, just the vertebral body slips forward.

Less than 50% of either spondylolisthesis or spondylolysis is symptomatic; one quarter is related to trauma; 12% of symptomatic cases are in patients under 12 years of age, and the usual symptom is pain; in older children, sciatic pain is common (McKee et al., 1971). Symptoms generally are identified before 5 years of age, and the youngest reported patient with nondysraphic spondylolisthesis is 10 months of age (McRae and Decker, 1966). Spondylolisthesis may also occur in spinal dysraphia (Fig. 18-54, *A*).

Myelography will demonstrate a varying distortion of the dural sac (Fig. 18-54, *B*) and lumbar roots; more so if there is some associated slipping of the posterior arch, which may occur if the articular

bral body, or posterior slipping of a malformed vertebra (Fig. 18-52, A).

The severe spinal dysraphic complex may be at one or more regions of the spine and may even involve separately the cervicothoracic and lumbosacral regions. Thoracic defects (Fig. 18-15, B and C) are more often associated with scoliosis, absent or fused ribs, and hemivertebrae. High thoracic and cervical defects also are often associated with vertebral fusion defects and rarely with a neurenteric cyst (Chapter 20).

Anterior sacral meningoceles occur with absence or hypoplasia of all or half of the sacrum and produce a characteristic hook-shaped sacral remnant (Fig. 18-60, A). The meningocele (Fig. 18-60, B) often presents in the pelvic cavity (Kaufmann, 1967). Associated intraspinal lipomas and low-fixed cords also occur (Fig. 18-60, C).

Sacral agenesis with or without associated agenesis of the lower lumbar vertebra may produce a cloverleaf-like pinched pelvis (Fig. 18-61) (Herling, 1964). The defect is always associated with severe lower spinal and sacral root abnormalities. Sacral agenesis may be associated with absent sacral roots (Smith, 1965).

Attempted duplication of the vertebral column with the spinal cord is rare (Fig. 18-62). This total spinal dysraphia or rachischisis may have a combined

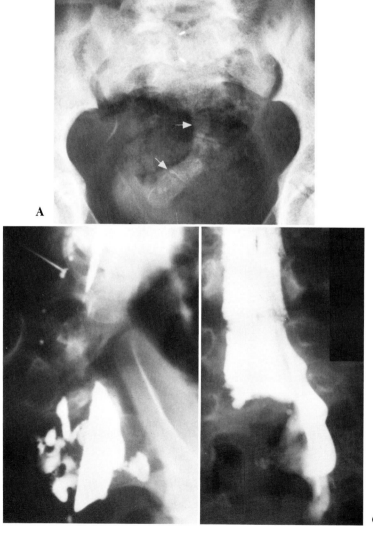

Fig. 18-60. Anterior sacral meningocele. A, Sacral hypoplasia with the characteristic hook-shaped appearance (arrows). B, Absent sacrum with a large anterior lipomeningocele protruding into the pelvis as seen at myelography (lateral view). C, Absence of the sacrum with a large intraspinal lipoma into which a low-fixed cord has entered (AP view).

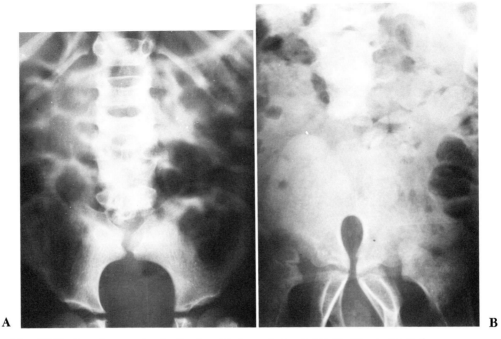

A   B

Fig. 18-61. Sacral agenesis. A, Total, with hypoplasia of L5. **B,** Classical trifoil appearance, with absent L4 and L5 and fusion of the iliac bones.

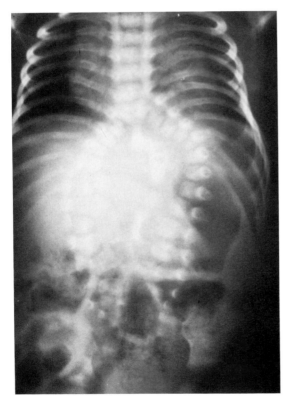

Fig. 18-62. Duplication of the vertebral column. This attempted duplication of the lower thoracolumbar spine, a central collection of disorganized bone, is surrounded by hemivertebrae and accessory hemivertebrae. (Courtesy Dr. Reuda Franco, Mexico City.)

anterior and posterior meningocele (Dodds, 1941; Rosselet, 1955). Teratogenic deformities may accompany this defect, such as a posteriorly placed extra hand (Swischuk, 1973). Neurenteric cysts or intestinal herniations into the defect may also occur (Dénes et al., 1967).

Sacrococcygeal teratomas are considered to be separate from spinal dysraphia and are really a regional teratoma that happens to involve the lower spine (Fig. 18-63). These are common in females, and they often calcify (Eklöf, 1965) or contain bone. They may present posteriorly but usually extend anteriorly into the pelvis (Gwinn et al., 1955).

MYELOGRAPHY. Positive contrast or air myelography may be performed to determine the level of the cord prior to its proposed surgical release or to detect possible associated intraspinal congenital mass lesions (e.g., a lipoma, teratoma, or hydromelia) that may be amenable to surgery. The diastematomyelic spur and split cord are well shown by either method. Both *prone* and *supine* positive contrast myelography are essential to visualize the entire cord, roots, and dural defect. The dural sac is nearly always widely ectatic at the site of the dysraphia (Fig. 18-64) and often has bulbous herniations which scallop the posterior vertebral bodies.

An intrasacral meningocele may fill at the time of the myelogram. We generally leave 2 ml of contrast in the subarachnoid space after the myelogram and obtain 24-to-48-hour radiographs of the spine to de-

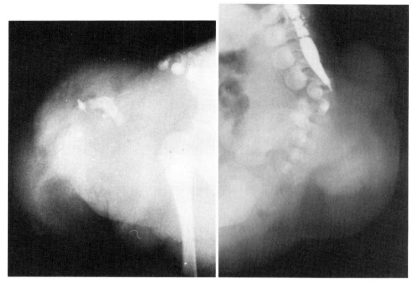

A   B

Fig. 18-63. Sacrococcygeal teratoma. A, This is not spinal dysraphia; rather it is a teratogenic malformation containing well-formed bony structures. B, A large dysraphic lipomeningocele of the lower lumbar spine and sacrum. Note the upper sacral prolapsed vertebra.

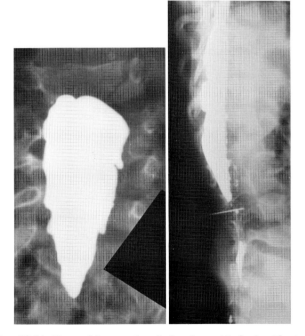

Fig. 18-64. Dysraphic ectasia of the dura. Marked widening and irregularity of the spinal subarachnoid space are associated with dysraphia as seen on an AP and lateral myelographic projection.

tect such possible meningoceles. The connection of the meningocele with the main subarachnoid space is often via a thin passage (Fig. 18-65, A) that does not fill initially (Young and Bruwer, 1969). The cord may be low fixed and extend into a sacral meningocele (Fig. 18-65, B). The sacral canal is always widened and the posterior sacral bodies scalloped.

Rarely will contrast extend up a dermal sinus that opens directly into the subarachnoid space (Fig. 18-66).

ACQUIRED SPINAL LESIONS
Spinal trauma

Injuries to the spine are not common in children. The supple active child seems to survive activities and injuries that, to the adult, would surely result in vertebral damage.

The infant's spine possesses considerable ligamentous laxity, permitting normal movements to occur that appear unusual at radiography (Sullivan et al., 1958). The normal movement between the anterior border of the odontoid and the posterior border of the arch of C1 may be as much as 4 mm, and the second cervical vertebra may move forward on the third (Fig. 18-67) or the third on the fourth a similar distance. This is called pseudosubluxation but is, in reality, quite normal and can occur in children up to approximately 6 years of age (Jacobson and Bleeker, 1959; Cattell and Filtzer, 1965). The congenital anomalies and the normal synchondroses of the dens must also be understood (Chapter 17), for fractures rarely occur in children at this site (Greenberg, 1968).

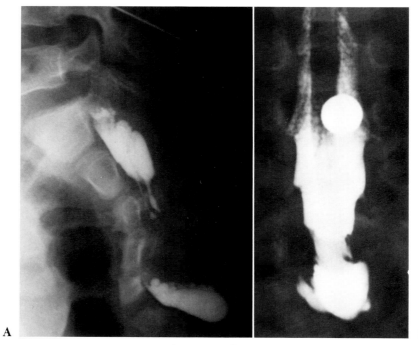

Fig. 18-65. Sacral meningoceles. A, A large distended upper sacral meningocele connects with a lower coccygeal meningocele via a thin channel. **B,** A low-fixed cord passes into the sacral meningocele in another child.

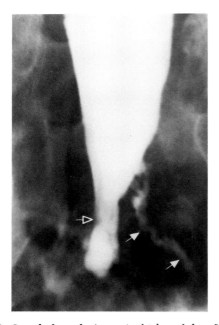

Fig. 18-66. Sacral dermal sinus. A thickened low-fixed filum (open arrow) with a large dysraphic ectatic subarachnoid space. Contrast passes up a dermal sinus (solid arrows).

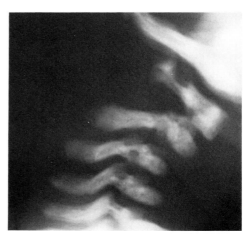

Fig. 18-67. Cervical pseudosubluxation in an infant. Forward movement of C2 on C3 is a normal phenomenon in infancy and is due to normally lax ligaments.

Tomography in both lateral and AP projections is strongly recommended to define precisely the presence of such fractures (Fig. 18-71) and possible bony displacements or fragments in the spinal canal. Spondylolisthesis may result from bilateral arch fractures (Fig. 18-72).

Ligamentous rupture may lead to spinal instability, especially in the cervical region, and such ruptures may be followed by calcification (Fig. 18-73).

The atlas may be fixed in rotation on the axis, providing a torticollis. Atlantoaxial asymmetry in the anteroposterior position produced by such rotation is not counteracted by turning of the head (Fig. 18-74) as occurs in muscular torticollis.

The disks above and/or below block vertebrae are particularly vulnerable to trauma. Posttraumatic spondylotic bars often result (Fig. 18-75) or even (rarely) a traumatic spondylolisthesis.

Myelography will again determine whether cord damage or intraspinal hematomas are present or whether root avulsions with tearing of the arachnoid and dura have occurred (Fig. 18-76).

Due to no particular cause, *calcified disks* at one or many levels, commonly in the cervical and thoracic regions (Fig. 18-77), may occur in children (Silverman, 1954) and may spontaneously disappear; some result from previous trauma. They may also herniate and be seen within the spinal canal as a calcified density. Alkaptonuria and vitamin D intoxication may cause calcified disks. Rarely is an inflammatory cause implicated.

Inflammatory spinal lesions

Inflammatory lesions of the spine are very uncommon in children.

Spondylarthritis of the spine is a nonspecific inflammatory disease in infants and young children (Fig. 18-78) (Moës, 1964). Frequently no organism will be isolated or rarely *Staphylococcus aureus*. Pain, fever, and scoliosis are commonly present. Progressive disk space narrowing with loss of adjacent vertebral margins occurs over a few months. The vertebral demineralization may recover and remineralize, and the disk space return to normal after 6 or more months. No paravertebral mass is present. The differential diagnosis of tuberculosis, osteochondritis, and Scheuermann's disease of the spine is often difficult.

Brucella or typhoid or pyogenic osteomyelitis of the spine is uncommon. *E. coli* osteomyelitis may occur in infants after *E. coli* septicemia. Tuberculosis of the spine (Fig. 18-79) is now rare, but destruction of the disk space initially occurs and the adjacent vertebral bodies are often destroyed anteriorly—such destruction spreading to the epiphyses and the central portion of the vertebral body. A local tuberculous abscess may occur in the paravertebral space and may calcify and extend down as a psoas abscess. Vertebral collapse and a kyphos inevitably follow. Epstein (1969) provides a detailed account of the historical, clinical, and radiographic features of this disease.

Eosinophilic granuloma of the spine, which may be inflammatory, is the commonest destructive lesion in children (Fig. 18-80) and must always be con-

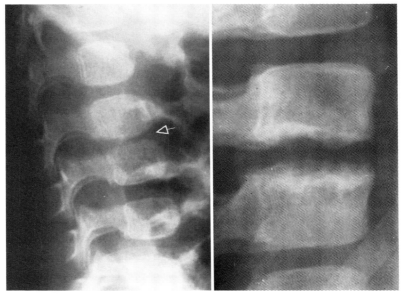

Fig. 18-78. Spondylarthritis. A, Between L2 and L3, with disk-space narrowing and ill-defined adjacent vertebral margins (arrow). **B,** Chronic stage in another child, with similar disk-space narrowing and a more sclerotic vertebral reaction.

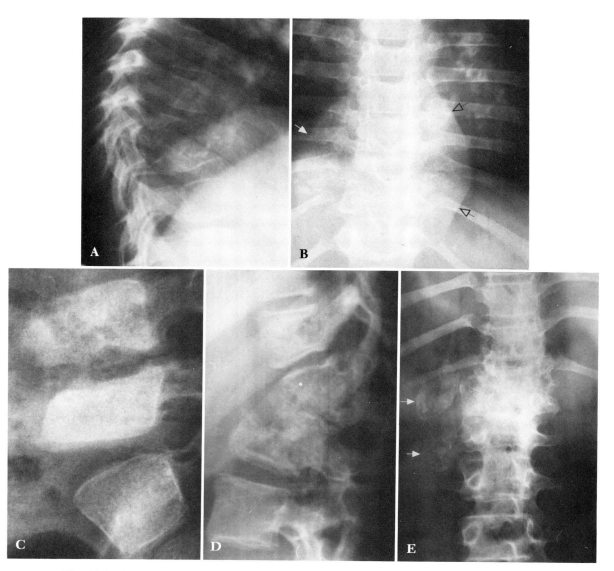

Fig. 18-79. Many faces of tuberculosis of the spine. A and **B,** Lateral and AP radiographs of a mild kyphos at T10 and T11 show marked destruction of both vertebral bodies on the adjacent aspects with a distinct paraspinal tuberculous abscess (**B,** arrows). **C,** Tuberculosis of L4 and L5 with disk-space narrowing, irregularity with sclerosis of L5, and irregular lytic lesions with sclerotic areas of L4 and not much compression of the vertebral bodies. **D,** Gross compression of T12 and L1 with a kyphos and posterior slipping of the destroyed vertebrae. There are also disk-space narrowing of the L1-L2 area and lysis with sclerosis of the relatively intact L2. **E,** Marked destruction of L1 and L2 with sideways subluxation and calcified psoas abscess (arrows).

sidered initially as the likely diagnosis in any disease of the vertebra, the body in particular (Part I).

Neoplasms of the spine

Primary neoplasms of the spine in children are rare. Giant cell tumors, aneurysmal bone cysts (Fig. 18-81), osteoblastomas, or osteoid osteomas rarely occur.

Osteoid osteomas probably are the commonest of this group and occur in older children (Fig. 18-82). The osteoid osteoma usually involves a pedicle ex-

tending into the lamina and body (MacLellan and Wilson, 1967). It may be large and is called a giant osteoid osteoma or osteoblastoma. It presents with scoliosis and pain (especially at night, often relieved by aspirin) and it creates dense frequently enlarged areas of the involved vertebral bodies. Tomography may reveal a contained lucent nidus.

Acquired spondylolysis or facet osteoarthritis (Fig. 18-83) can produce a radiographic picture similar to this (Wilkinson and Hall, 1974).

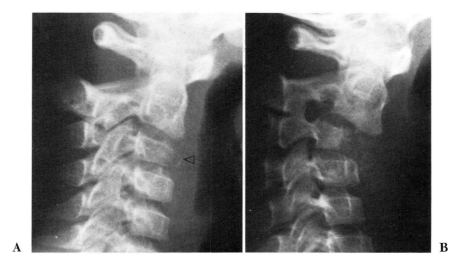

Fig. 18-80. Eosinophilic granuloma. A cervical radiograph (**A**) taken 3 months prior to **B** demonstrates subtle destruction of the anterior border of C3 (arrow). Subsequently this vertebra went on to gross destruction, with forward subluxation of C2 on C3 and kyphosis (**B**). Pathology revealed an unusual form of histiocytosis X.

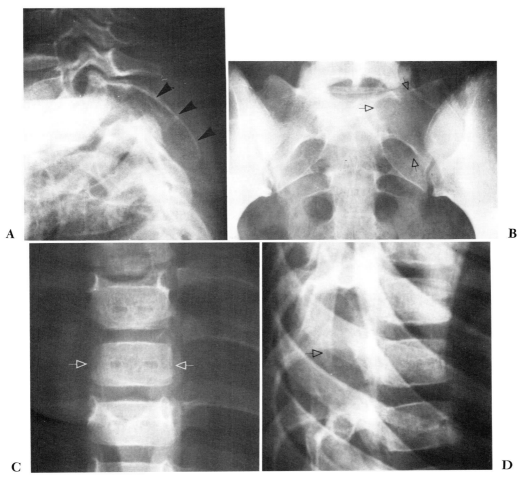

Fig. 18-81. Aneurysmal bone cyst. A, Typical shell-like expanding lesion of the spine of T1 (arrowheads). **B,** Large, of the left ala of the sacrum (arrows). **C** and **D,** Of the entire arch of T9 (arrows) with complete destruction of these elements. The vertebral body itself is spared.

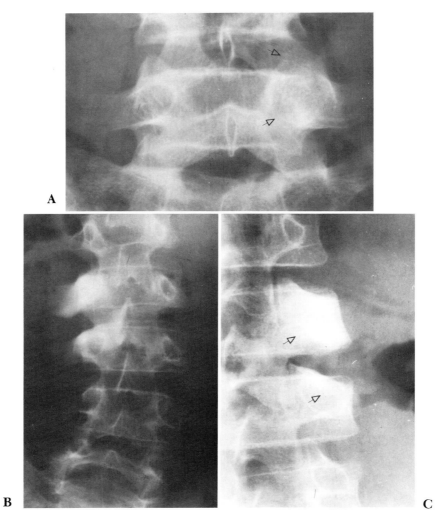

Fig. 18-82. Osteoid osteomas. A, Subtle sclerosis and mere enlargement of a pedicle and lamina (arrows) may be the only signs of this lesion. **B** and **C,** Adjacent pedicles may be involved, and the pain may produce a scoliosis (as seen in this child with osteoid osteoma involving the right pedicles of L2 and L3). The oblique projection (**C**) better shows the osteoid osteoma (arrows).

Fig. 18-83. Spondylolysis and sclerosis. Spondylolysis and facet osteoarthritis can produce in the region of the pedicle and laminae a sclerosis (arrows) that may be difficult to differentiate from an osteoid osteoma except at biopsy.

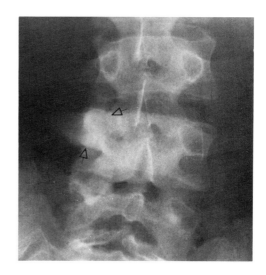

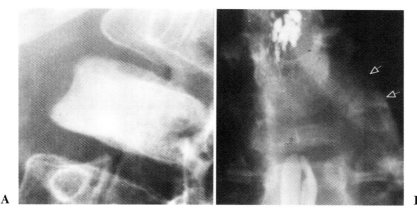

Fig. 18-84. Ewing's tumor of the spine. A, Densely sclerotic vertebral body at L1. B, Collapse of T9 and T10, due to a secondary Ewing's sarcoma. A myelogram demonstrates the extradural block together with a paravertebral soft tissue mass (arrows).

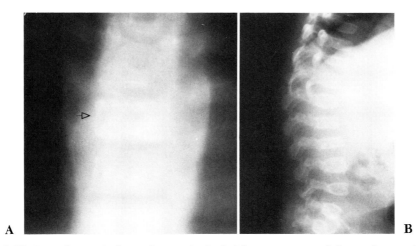

Fig. 18-85. Secondary spinal neoplasms. A, A rhabdomyosarcoma of the neck spreading to involve T6 (arrow) with lytic and sclerotic destruction and a marked paravertebral soft tissue mass. B, An abdominal neuroblastoma involving most of the lumbar vertebrae by continuity with lysis, sclerosis, and narrowing of the contiguous vertebrae.

A Ewing's tumor (Fig. 18-84) (Coley et al., 1948) and an osteogenic sarcoma rarely involve the spine primarily.

A number of secondary neoplasms such as a rhabdomyosarcoma of soft tissue (Fig. 18-85, A), a rare carcinoma of the adrenal, and a teratoma may involve the spine and its canal (Chapter 20).

Neuroblastoma (Fig. 18-85, B) and retroperitoneal sarcoma may involve the spine by contiguity (Chapter 20).

Systemic neoplasia such as leukemia and lymphoma may create multiple destructive lesions of the vertebral bodies. In neoplasia the spine disk space is usually spared.

Chordoma of the sacrum is especially rare in children (Dahlin and MacCarty, 1952; Littman, 1953).

All such secondary neoplasms may extend into the spinal canal and many will have an associated paraspinal soft tissue mass. Kyphosis may result from the vertebral body destruction.

A chondroma and a chrondrosarcoma are equally rare, and an osteochrondroma may extend into the spinal canal to produce a significant mass lesion (Chapter 20).

Eosinophilic granuloma, presumably a nonneoplastic lesion, again is the commonest destructive vertebral lesion in children.

Miscellaneous lesions

Prolonged bed rest due to severe systemic illness with subsequent recovery may produce a bone-within-a-bone appearance in the vertebral bodies simulating

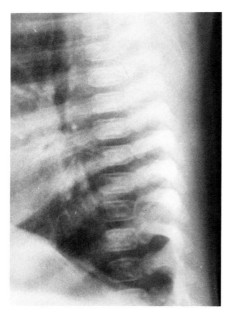

Fig. 18-86. Bone within a bone effect. This infant had prolonged bed rest due to congenital heart disease. Within months after surgical correction of the cardiac lesion, the demineralized vertebral bodies demonstrated reossification—producing the bone within a bone appearance.

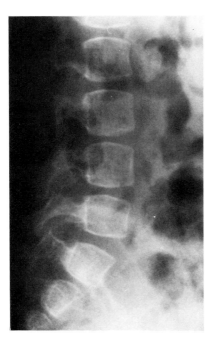

Fig. 18-87. Elongated vertebral bodies. Prolonged bed rest results in elongated vertebral bodies due to lack of weight bearing.

neoplastic infiltration (Fig. 18-86). However, prolonged bed rest can produce unusually tall vertebral bodies due to the lack of weight bearing (Fig. 18-87).

REFERENCES

Alexander, E., Jr.: Significance of the small lumbar spinal canal: Cauda equina compression syndromes due to spondylosis. V. Achondroplasia, J. Neurosurg. 31:513, 1969.

Alter, M.: Anencephalus, hydrocephalus, and spina bifida, Arch. Neurol. Psychiatry 7:411, 1962.

Arkin, A. M., Pack, G. T., Ransohoff, N. S., and Simon, N.: Radiation-induced scoliosis, J. Bone Joint Surg. 32-A:401, 1950.

Bailey, J. A., II: Disproportionate short stature, diagnosis and management, Philadelphia, 1973, W. B. Saunders Co.

Baker, D. R., and McHollick, W.: Spondylochisis and spondylolisthesis in children, J. Bone Joint Surg. 38-A:933, 1956.

Banna, M., Pearce, G. W., and Uldall, R.: Scoliosis: a rare manifestation of intrinsic tumours of the spinal cord in children, J. Neurol. Neurosurg. Psychiatry 34:637, 1971.

Barry, A., Patten, B. M., and Stewart, B. H.: Possible factors in the development of the Arnold-Chiari malformation, J. Neurosurg. 14:285, 1957.

Barson, A. J.: Radiological studies of spina bifida cystica; the phenomenon of congenital lumbar kyphosis, Br. J. Radiol. 38:294, 1965.

Barson, A. J.: Spina bifida: the significance of the level and extent of the defect to the morphogenesis, Dev. Med. Child Neurol. 12:129, 1970.

Begg, A. C.: Nuclear herniations of the intervertebral disc; their radiological manifestations and significance, J. Bone Joint Surg. 36-B:180, 1954.

Bobechko, W. P.: Personal communication, 1975.

Caffey, J.: Pediatric x-ray diagnosis, vol. 2, ed. 6, Chicago, 1972, Year Book Medical Publishers, Inc.

Cattell, H. S., and Filtzer, D. L.: Pseudosubluxation and other variations in the cervical spine in children, J. Bone Joint Surg. 47-A:1295, 1965.

Cobb, J. R.: Study of scoliosis. In Blount, W. P., and Banks, S. W., editors: Instructional course lectures, vol. 5, Ann Arbor, 1948, J. W. Edwards.

Coley, B. L., Higinbotham, N. L., and Bowden, L.: Endothelioma of bone, Ann. Surg. 128:533, 1948.

Cowell, H. R., Nelson, H., and MacEwen, G. D.: Familial patterns in idiopathic scoliosis, Exhibit of the American Medical Association, 117th Annual Convention, June, 1968.

Dahlin, D. C., and MacCarty, C. S.: Chordoma, Cancer 5:1170, 1952.

Dénes, J., Honti, J., and Léb, J.: Dorsal herniation of the gut; a rare manifestation of the split notochord syndrome, J. Pediatr. Surg. 2:359, 1967.

Dodds, G. S.: Anterior and posterior rachischisis, Am. J. Pathol. 17:861, 1941.

Doran, P. A., and Guthkelch, A. N.: Studies in spina bifida cystica. I. General survey and reassessment of the problem, J. Neurol. Neurosurg. Psychiatry 24:331, 1961.

Eklöf, O.: Roentgenologic findings in sacrococcygeal teratoma, Acta Radiol. [Diagn.] 3:41, 1965.

Emery, J. L.: The back lesions, lipomas, and dermoids. In American Academy of Orthopaedic Surgeons: Symposium on myelomeningocele, St. Louis, 1972, The C. V. Mosby Co.

Emery, J. L., and Lendon, R. G.: Neurospinal dysraphism syndrome. In American Academy of Orthopaedic Surgeons: Symposium on myelomeningocele, St. Louis, 1972, The C. V. Mosby Co.

Epstein, B. S.: The spine; a radiological text and atlas, ed. 3, Philadelphia, 1969, Lea & Febiger.

Farkas, A.: Pathogenesis of idiopathic scoliosis, J. Bone Joint Surg. 36-A:617, 1954.

Farkas, A.: Basic factors in development of scoliosis, Bull. Hosp. Joint Dis. 28:131, 1967.

Fielden, P., and Russell, J. G. B.: Coronally cleft vertebra, Clin. Radiol. 21:327, 1970.

Fineman, S., Borrelli, F. J., Rubinstein, B. M., Epstein, H., and Jacobson, H. G.: The cervical spine; transformation of the normal lordotic pattern into a linear pattern in the neutral posture, J. Bone Joint Surg. 45-A:1179, 1963.

Fitz, C. R., and Harwood-Nash, D. C.: The tethered conus, Am. J. Roentgenol. Radium Ther. Nucl. Med. 125:515, 1975.

Franken, E. A.: Spinal cord injury in the newborn infant, Pediatr. Radiol. 3:101, 1975.

Frieberger, R. H., Wilson, P. D., and Nicholas, J. A.: Acquired absence of the odontoid process, J. Bone Joint Surg. 47-A: 1231, 1965.

Gardner, W. J.: Myelomeningocele, the result of rupture of the embryonic neural tube, Cleve. Clin. Q. 27:88, 1960.

Gardner, W. J.: Anomalies of the craniovertebral junction. In Youmans, J. R., editor: Neurological surgery, vol. 1, Philadelphia, 1973, W. B. Saunders Co.

Gold, L. H. A., Kieffer, S. A., and Peterson, H. O.: Lipomatous invasion of the spinal cord associated with spinal dysraphism; myelographic evaluation, Am. J. Roentgenol. Radium Ther. Nucl. Med. 107:479, 1969.

Gray, H.: Anatomy of the human body (R. Warwick and P. L. Williams, editors), ed. 35, London, 1973, Longmanns, Ltd.

Greenberg, A. D.: Atlanto-axial dislocations, Brain 91:655, 1968.

Gwinn, J. L., Dockerty, M. B., and Kennedy, R. L. J.: Presacral teratomas in infancy and childhood, Pediatrics 16:239, 1955.

Gwinn, J. L., and Smith, J. L.: Acquired and congenital absence of the odontoid process, Am. J. Roentgenol. Radium Ther. Nucl. Med. 88:424, 1962.

Harwood-Nash, D. C., and Fitz, C. R.: Myelography and syringohydromyelia in infancy and childhood, Radiology 113:661, 1974.

Harwood-Nash, D. C., and Fitz, C. R.: Neuroradiological techniques and indications in infancy and childhood. In Kaufmann, H. J., editor: Progress in pediatric radiology. Vol. 5. Skull, spine, and contents, Basel, 1976, S. Karger, AG.

Herlinger, H.: Radiological investigation of a case of sacrococcygeal agenesis, Br. J. Radiol. 37:376, 1964.

Hilal, S. K., and Keim, H. A.: Selective spinal angiography in adolescent scoliosis, Radiology 102:349, 1972.

Hilal, S. K., Marton, D., and Pollack, E.: Diastematomyelia in children Radiographic study of 34 cases, Radiology 112:609, 1974.

Hoffman, H.: Spina bifida, Mod. Med. 23:61, 1968.

Jacobson, G., and Bleeker, H. H.: Pseudosubluxation of the axis in children, Am. J. Roentgenol. Radium Ther. Nucl. Med. 82:472, 1959.

James, C. C. M., and Lassman, L. P.: Spinal dysraphism; spina bifida occulta, London, 1972, Butterworth & Co., Ltd.

Kalter, H. G.: Teratology of the central nervous system, Chicago, 1968, University of Chicago Press.

Kaufmann, H. J.: Anterior sacral meningocele, Ann. Radiol. 10:121, 1967.

Keim, H. A., and Greene, A. F.: Diastematomyelia and scoliosis, J. Bone Joint Surg. 55-A:1425, 1973.

Kieffer, S. A., Nesbett, M. E., and D'Angio, G. J.: Vertebra plana due to histiocytosis X; serial studies, Acta Radiol. [Diagn.] 8:241, 1969.

Knuttson, F.: Vertebral genesis of idiopathic scoliosis in children Acta Radiol. [Diagn.] 4:395, 1966.

Kruyff, E.: Occipital dysplasia in infants, Radiology 85:501, 1965.

Langer, L. O., Jr., Baumann, T. A., and Gorlin, R. J.: Achondroplasia, Am. J. Roentgenol. Radium Ther. Nucl. Med. 100:12, 1967.

Leigh, T. F., and Rogers, J. V., Jr.: Anterior sacral meningocele, Am. J. Roentgenol. Radium Ther. Nucl. Med. 71:808, 1954.

Leventhal, H. R.: Birth injuries of the spinal cord, J. Pediat. 56:447, 1960.

List, C. F.: Developmental anomalies of the craniovertebral border. In Kahn, E., Crosby, E., and Schneider, T., editors: Correlative neurosurgery, ed. 2, Springfield, Ill., 1969, Charles C Thomas, Publisher.

Littman, L.: Sacrococcygeal chordoma, Ann. Surg. 137:80, 1953.

Lloyd-Roberts, G. C., and Pilcher, N. F.: Structural idiopathic scoliosis in infancy. Study of the natural history in one hundred patients, J. Bone Joint Surg. 47-B:529, 1965.

Lorber, J.: The family history of spina bifida cystica, Pediatrics 35:589, 1965.

Lorber, J., and Levick, K.: Spina bifida cystica; incidence of spina bifida occulta in parents and in controls, Arch. Dis. Child. 42:171, 1967.

MacLellan, D. I., and Wilson, F. C., Jr.: Osteoid osteoma of the spine, J. Bone Joint Surg. 49-A:111, 1967.

Maroteaux, P., and Lamy, M.: Les formes pseudo-achondroplastiques des dysplasies spondylo-epiphysaires, Presse Med. 67:383, 1959.

McKee, B. W., Alexander, W. J., and Dunbar, J. S.: Spondylolysis and spondylolisthesis in children; a review, J. Can. Assoc. Radiol. 22:100, 1971.

McKusick, V. A.: Heritable disorders of connective tissue, ed. 4, St. Louis, 1972, The C. V. Mosby Co.

McLoughlin, D. P., and Wortzman, G.: Congenital absence of a cervical vertebral pedicle, J. Can. Assoc. Radiol. 23:195, 1972.

McRae, D. L.: The significance of abnormalities of the cervical spine: Caldwell lecture, 1959, Am. J. Roentgenol. Radium Ther. Nucl. Med. 84:3, 1960.

McRae, D. L., and Decker, K., editors: Clinical neuroradiology, New York, 1966, McGraw-Hill Book Co., Inc.

Moës, C. A. F.: Spondylarthritis in childhood, Am. J. Roentgenol. Radium Ther. Nucl. Med. 91:578, 1964.

Morgagni, J. B., 1769. In Warkany, J., 1971.

Murphy, D. P.: Congenital malformations; a study of parental characteristics with special reference to the reproductive process, ed. 2, Philadelphia, 1947, J. B. Lippincott Co.

Murray, R. O., and Jacobson, H. G.: The radiology of skeletal disorders: exercises in diagnosis, 2 vols., New York, 1973, Longman, Inc.

Neuhauser, E. B. D., Wittenborg, M. H., Berman, C. Z., and Cohen, J.: Irradiation effects of roentgen therapy on growing spine, Radiology 59:637, 1952.

Newman, P. H.: The etiology of spondylolisthesis, J. Bone Joint Surg. 45-B:39, 1963.

Oestreich, A. E., and Young, L. W.: The absent cervical pedicle syndrome; a case in childhood, Am. J. Roentgenol. Radium Ther. Nucl. Med. 107:505, 1969.

Padget, D. H.: Spina bifida and embryonic neuroschisis—a

causal relationship; definition of postnatal conformations involving a bifid spine, Johns Hopkins Med. J. **128**:232, 1968.

Padget, D. H.: Development of so-called dysraphism; with embryologic evidence of clinical Arnold-Chiari and Dandy-Walker malformations, Johns Hopkins Med. J. **130**:127, 1972.

Palant, D. I., and Carter, B. L.: Klippel-Feil syndrome and deafness; a study with polytomography, Am. J. Dis. Child. **123**:218, 1972.

Patten, B. M.: Embryological stages in the establishing of myeloschisis with spina bifida, Am. J. Anat. **93**:365, 1953.

Perovic, M. N., Kopits, S. E., and Thompson, R. C.: Radiological evaluation of the spinal cord in congenital atlantoaxial dislocation, Radiology **109**:713, 1973.

Ramsey, J., and Bliznak, J.: Klippel-Feil syndrome with renal agenesis and other anomalies, Am. J. Roentgenol. Radium Ther. Nucl. Med. **113**:460, 1971.

Rand, R. W., and Crandall, P. H.: Central spinal cord syndrome in hyperextension injuries of the cervical spine, J. Bone Joint Surg. **44-A**:1415, 1962.

Reilly, B. J., Davidson, J. W., and Bain, H.: Lymphangiectasis of the skeleton; a case report, Radiology **103**:385, 1972.

Roaf, R.: Scoliosis, Baltimore, 1966, The Williams & Wilkins Co.

Roberson, G. H., Llewellyn, H. J., and Taveras, J. M.: The narrow lumbar spinal canal syndrome, Radiology **107**:89, 1973.

Rose, R. S., and Smith, J. P.: Hydronephrosis in infants with meningomyelocele: its early recognition, J. Urol. **90**:129, 1963.

Rosselet, P. J.: A rare case of rachischisis with multiple malformations, Am. J. Roentgenol. Radium Ther. Nucl. Med. **73**:235, 1955.

Schatzker, J., and Pennal, G. F.: Spinal stenosis, a cause of cauda equina compression, J. Bone Joint Surg. **50-B**:606, 1968.

Schmorl, G., and Junghanns, H.: The human spine in health and disease. (Translated from fourth German edition, S. P. Wilk and L. S. Goin, editors), New York, 1959, Grune & Stratton, Inc.

Schultz, E. H., Jr., Levy, R. W., and Russo, P. E.: Agenesis of the odontoid process, Radiology **67**:102, 1956.

Selig, S., and Arnheim, E.: Scoliosis following empyema, Arch. Surg. **39**:789, 1939.

Shoul, M. L., and Ritvo, M.: Clinical and roentgenographic manifestations of the Klippel-Feil syndrome, Am. J. Roentgenol. Radium Ther. Nucl. Med. **68**:369, 1952.

Silverman, F. N.: Calcification of the intervertebral discs in childhood, Radiology **62**:801, 1954.

Smith, E. D.: Spina bifida and the total care of spinal myelo-meningocele, Springfield, Ill., 1965, Charles C Thomas, Publisher.

Spranger, J. W., Langer, L. O., Jr., Wiedemann, H-R: Bone dysplasias; an atlas of constitutional disorders of skeletal development, Philadelphia, 1974, W. B. Saunders Co.

Spranger, J. W., and Wiedemann, H. R.: The genetic mucolipidoses, Humangenetik **9**:113, 1970.

Stern, W. E., and Rand, R. W.: Birth injuries to the spinal cord; a report of 2 cases and review of the literature, Am. J. Obstet. Gynecol. **78**:498, 1959.

Sullivan, C. R., Bruwer, A. J., and Harris, L. E.: Hypermobility of the cervical spine in children; a pitfall in the diagnosis of cervical dislocation, Am. J. Surg. **95**:636, 1958.

Sutow, W. W., and Pryde, A. W.: Incidence of spina bifida occulta in relation to age, Am. J. Dis. Child. **91**:211, 1956.

Swischuk, L. E.: Radiology of the newborn and young infant, Baltimore, 1973, The Williams & Wilkins Co.

Tachdjian, M. O., and Matson, D. D.: Orthopaedic aspects of intraspinal tumors in infants and children, J. Bone Joint Surg. **47-A**:223, 1965.

Taybi, H.: Radiology of syndromes, Chicago, 1975, Year Book Medical Publishers, Inc.

Till, K.: Spinal dysraphism; a study of congenital malformations of the back, Dev. Med. Child Neurol. **10**:470, 1968.

von Recklinghausen, 1886. In Warkany, J., 1971.

Warkany, J.: Congenital malformations; notes and comments. II. Iniencephaly, Chicago, 1971, Year Book Medical Publishers, Inc.

Wilkinson, R. H., and Hall, J. E.: The sclerotic pedicle; tumor or pseudotumor? Radiology **111**:683, 1974.

Wilson, C. B.: Significance of the small lumbar spinal canal: cauda equina compression syndromes due to spondylosis. III. Intermittent claudication, J. Neurosurg. **31**:499, 1969.

Wiltse, L. L.: The etiology of spondylolisthesis, J. Bone Joint Surg. **44-A**:539, 1962.

Winter, R. B., Moe, J. H., and Eilers, V. E.: Congenital scoliosis; a study of two hundred and thirty-four patients, treated and untreated, J. Bone Joint Surg. **50-A**:1, 1968.

Wollin, D. G.: The os odontoideum, J. Bone Joint Surg. **45-A**:1459, 1963.

Wollin, D. G., and Elliott, G. B.: Coronal cleft vertebrae and persistent notochordal derivatives of infancy, J. Can. Assoc. Radiol. **12**:78, 1961.

Young, I. S., and Bruwer, A. J.: The occult intrasacral meningocele, Am. J. Roentgenol. Radium Ther. Nucl. Med. **105**:390, 1969.

Young, L. W., Oestreich, A. E., and Goldstein, L. A.: Roentgenology in scoliosis: contribution to evaluation and management, Am. J. Roentgenol. Radium Ther. Nucl. Med. **108**:778, 1970.

tumor and inflammation, the arteries can be distended and enlarged at myelography.

Lumbar area

Although the anterior spinal artery usually ends at the conus tip, this termination may be difficult to

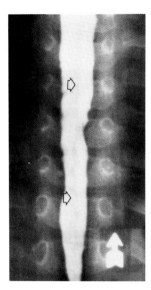

Fig. 19-17. Anterior spinal artery. The artery (arrows) becomes wider and more serpiginous in the lower thoracic cord. (From Harwood-Nash, D. C.: Semin. Roentgenol., vol. 7, no. 3, 1972.)

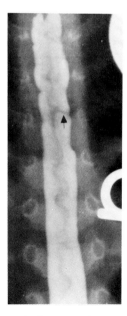

Fig. 19-18. Anterior spinal artery. A typical artery of Adamkievicz (arrow) joins the anterior spinal artery at the T9 level. The anterior spinal is more serpentine than most but normal.

see at myelography because the conus rises to the dorsal aspect of the spinal canal and is usually outside the oil column. In a study of cadaver sections, Dommisse (1974) also showed that the anterior spinal artery may actually continue beyond the ending of the conus medullaris.

The vertebral level at which the conus ends has not been extensively studied in anatomical dissections of children. In his study of normal fetuses, Barson (1970b) suggested that the conus ends at the adult level (T12-L1) at birth. Other authors believe there is some migration between birth and adulthood. Our own experience suggests a lower level for the conus tip in infancy and early childhood (Fig. 19-19). We accept as the *lowest* normal conus tip the mid-L3 level at birth, L2-L3 at age 5, and mid-L2 at age 12. By oil myelography, this can be seen only in the

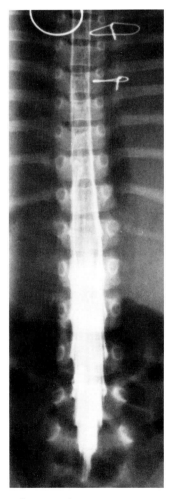

Fig. 19-19. Normal conus. A postmortem water-soluble myelogram in an infant who died of nonneurological disease shows the conus tip at the L1-L2 interspace. (From Fitz, C. R., and Harwood-Nash, D. C.: Am. J. Roentgenol. Radium Ther. Nucl. Med. **125:**515, 1975.)

supine position (as previously noted). Because of its dorsal location, the filum also is seen only in the supine position. In comparison with the thoracic cord, the normal conus is seen to widen (Fig. 19-19)—visible on lateral and especially supine AP views. The nerve roots are noted to be nearly parallel with the conus. A nerve root will occasionally be directly against the filum terminale, making assessment of the width of the filum difficult.

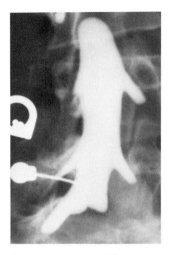

Fig. 19-20. Lumbar nerve roots. These are very prominent in an oblique prone view of a 13-year-old girl.

The subarachnoid space is said to vary considerably with hyperventilation, with breathing of 10% CO_2, and with various physiological maneuvers. Since we examine children under general anesthesia, these variations are considerably muted. The lumbar nerve root sleeves can be quite prominent (Fig. 19-20)—a finding also present in some adults.

Complications

The local complications of myelography are well known and primarily related to needle placement. Because any needle puncture of the subarachnoid space will often cause CSF leakage, even for several days after the needle is withdrawn, we avoid myelography within 1 week of any lumbar puncture. This both avoids unsuccessful attempts due to a collapsed subarachnoid space from leakage and prevents the misdiagnosis of a defect due to remaining pockets of CSF as a subdural mass.

Extra-arachnoid injection of contrast material may occur even when free flow of CSF is present and needle placement appears to be excellent. If the injection is done under fluoroscopy, the incidence of extra-arachnoid injection of oily contrast material will be minimized. Leakage of CSF or contrast material through the needle puncture site can occur even when the needle is properly positioned and can take place while the needle remains in the subarachnoid space or after it is withdrawn.

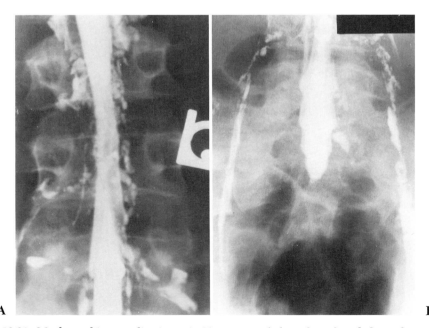

A   B

Fig. 19-21. Myelographic complications. A, Narrowing of the subarachnoid dye column over a two-interspace level from subdural and extradural leakage of CSF and Pantopaque. **B,** Marked extravasation of contrast material extradurally down the sciatic nerve sheaths in spite of an initial completely intra-arachnoidal injection of oil in another patient.

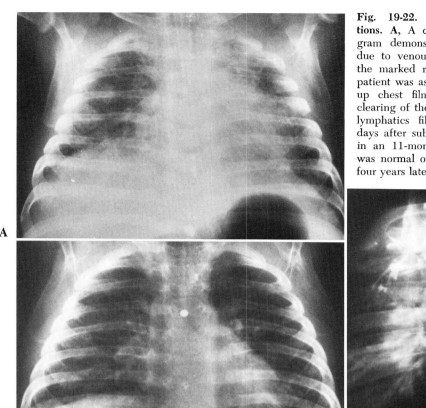

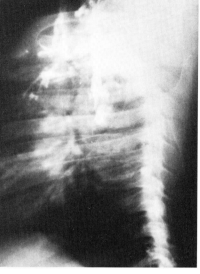

Fig. 19-22. Myelographic complications. A, A chest film after a myelogram demonstrates pulmonary edema due to venous oil emboli. In spite of the marked radiographic changes, the patient was asymptomatic. B, A follow-up chest film 24 hours later shows clearing of the edema. C, Peribronchial lymphatics filled with Pantopaque 4 days after subdural-extradural injection in an 11-month-old infant. The chest was normal on subsequent radiographs four years later.

Fig. 19-23. Myelographic complications. A, AP and, B, lateral views of the abdomen after myelography show a patent lumboperitoneal shunt (arrow) and oil in the peritoneal cavity.

The results of leakage may vary from a small *diskogenic-like* defect to a subdural encirclement of the cord (Fig. 19-21, *A*), rather dramatic leakage extradurally down the sciatic nerve roots (Fig. 19-21, *B*), and systemic complications of intravasation into veins and lymphatics (Fig. 19-22). The venous intravasation can sometimes be controlled by positional change. When a patent lumboperitoneal shunt is present, contrast material may also escape into the peritoneal cavity (Fig. 19-23).

The postmyelographic headache and nausea are accepted frequent complications of myelography. They seem to occur less in children; but since we do most of our procedures under general anesthesia, it is difficult to say what the modifying effect of the anesthetic is.

The question of long-term inflammatory reactions to oily contrast material is unresolved. There is general agreement that blood and Pantopaque will cause a significant inflammatory reaction (Howland and Curry, 1966), but what Pantopaque alone does is less clear.

Reports of reactions to uncomplicated myelography (Mason and Raaf, 1962; Mayher et al., 1971) indicate that inflammatory response to Pantopaque does occur which may be severe enough (rarely) to cause death. Probably the reaction is allergic, though Ferry and coworkers (1973) reported mild CSF cellular and protein changes in many patients with disk disease or disk symptoms. Rare occurrence of cerebral vasospasm (Mayher et al., 1971) and visual loss (Cristi et al., 1974) has also been reported. We have had no severe reactions to oily contrast material in over 700 myelograms in children.

In spite of the low incidence of the serious reactions (Harwood-Nash, 1972), it should be remembered that myelography is a procedure not to be undertaken without good reason and that as much of the oil as possible should be removed at the end of the examination.

CONGENITAL ANOMALIES
Dysraphia—general

Much has been written, but little proof given, as to the causes of dysraphia. The term itself was coined by Lichtenstein (1940), who reaffirmed Morgagni's theory of failure of fusion of the neural tube as the cause of dysraphic problems. The worst of these defects is complete nonclosure of the neural tube. Defective closure of the tube leads to other conditions, such as hydromyelia with formation of an abnormal central canal. By Lichtenstein's theory, various cellular proliferations may occur—accounting for abnormal collections and migrations of tissue. Vascular abnormalities likewise may be present, with resultant hemorrhage and destruction of normal tissue. Mesodermal and cutaneous closure abnormalities occur with the neural tube pathology, and these account for the cutaneous and bony manifestations seen in the dysraphic states.

In an excellent review and a study of dysraphic infants, Barson (1965, 1970a) mentioned practical reasons for support of Lichtenstein's (1940) theory and also the allied theory of Patten (1953) that overgrowth of neural tissue plays a part in the spinal malformations. Barson pointed out that the nerve roots are directly adjacent to their foramina until 9 weeks of gestation. Then bony growth outpaces nerve growth and there is resultant downward angulation of the nerve roots as they grow laterally. The nerve roots of the tethered cord, which are more perpendicular to the conus, or the upward-extending cervical nerve roots of the Arnold-Chiari malformation may then be explained by overgrowth of nervous tissue or decreased growth of bone.

Likewise, the kyphosis seen only in the thoracolumbar meningoceles might also be explained by neural overgrowth—and the bone would thus be shaped to the overgrowth rather than by muscle weakness. Because of the fact that the involved vertebrae are rhomboid (with the parallel sides vertical) and the clinical observation that the deformity cannot be easily corrected operatively, Barson concludes the deformity must have occurred when the bone was still in a cartilaginous state.

Oddly, Barson believes that the butterfly vertebrae and vertebral body fusions have nothing to do with dysraphia for they may occur without neural involvement.

An interesting finding in his study is that dysraphia involving T12 or L1 will always involve at least five vertebral segments, presumably because the L1-L2 area is the twenty-fifth embryological somite—which is the beginning of the tail bud. Any abnormality at that level affects the spine from there caudally.

Gardner (1959a, 1964, 1966), in a series of four articles, took an opposite view. By noting that all forms of clinical dysraphia have an enlarged bony canal he reasoned it was likely due to a dilated neural tube, in particular the central canal, which enlarges abnormally if the rhomboid roof of the fourth ventricle does not begin to perforate normally at 6 to 8 weeks of gestation. Until that time there is a physiological hydrocephalus, with dilatation of the central canal, communicating with the fourth ventricle. Later the rhomboid roof normally perforates and allows dissection of a subarachnoid space by leakage of cerebrospinal fluid with resultant absorption of the fluid as the space develops.

According to Gardner's theory, the abnormal

stretching of the central canal causes transverse sclerotome growth with resultant shortening. The neuroectoderm can become fused to the endoderm, cutaneous ectoderm, and mesoderm; the consequence can be cord tethering, diastematomyelia, or neurenteric cysts. If the rhombic roof dissects later than normal, there may be a compensatory reduction in size of the neural elements. Diastematomyelia is thought to occur as a compensatory closure of the neural tube after a complete split of both the roof and the floor plates of the tube has occurred.

The frequent association of the Arnold-Chiari malformation with spina bifida as well as with meningoceles and syringohydromyelia suggests to Gardner a neural tube distension. He also blames Dandy-Walker cysts and Chiari malformations on the identical process of obstruction of the rhombic roof and lack of fourth ventricular outlets. Whatever the weakest area then determines the defect: a Dandy-Walker cyst results when the infratentorial tissue is weaker than the supratentorial tissue; an Arnold-Chiari malformation results when the lateral ventricles are able to compress the infratentorial tissues; a meningocele results when the spinal canal is the weakest portion and dilates.

Gardner's neural tube–distension and splitting theory is an attractive thesis, but several clinical situations are difficult to explain by it. Most meningomyeloceles have the neural elements, including the central roots, at the flat skin placode area. If the tube first splits dorsally, then according to Gardner these neural elements should be at the ventral side of or all around the meningocele. If the tube has not split, the myelomeningocele should have a gigantic central canal as seen in myelocystoceles (which are uncommon). In the case of most meningoceles and myelomeningoceles, an abnormal closure of the canal represents a more likely cause.

If there has been later compensation of the distension by opening of the ventricular outlets, leaving only the dilated bony canal, why does the canal stay enlarged? Gardner theorizes a cartilaginous "set" to the sclerotomes. Bone expands in response to pressure. When pressure is removed, expansion stops—as in treatment of hydrocephalus. A logical expectation would then be for an in utero state of bone expansion to be halted if due to a passive distension. It is also difficult to explain both Arnold-Chiari and Dandy-Walker malformations on the same basis. Why is the cerebellar dysgenesis of Dandy-Walker cyst not seen in the Arnold-Chiari malformation if both simply are secondary to distension without other growth abnormality?

In other conditions, the distension theory is more attractive. Syringohydromyelia is due to dilatation of the central canal and may well be accompanied by abnormal fourth ventricular outlets. The lumbar kyphosis seen with meningoceles and supposedly due to tissue overgrowth should not be confined only to that area. Why should neural overgrowth cause a kyphosis rather than a lordosis?

Spinal dysraphia is an important congenital deformity. One third of congenital anomalies involve the central nervous system, and 90% of these are dysraphic and hydrocephalic states (Kurtzke et al., 1973). In the United States, central nervous system anomalies cause ninety-four deaths per 100,000 population before the age of 1. Age-comparable figures in the United Kingdom and Canada are 50% higher; in Ireland, 100% higher.

As confusing as how defects in embryological development occur is why the abnormalities occur. In a study of spina bifida cystica (Lawrence et al., 1968), 80% of siblings of patients with spina bifida cystica had spina bifida occulta; and a third of these showed the abnormality at more than one vertebral level. In comparison, controls had only a 44% incidence of spina bifida occulta (8% being at more than one vertebral body level). Mothers of affected children had a far higher incidence of occult spina bifida than did fathers. The findings suggest a sex-linked genetic determination of dysraphia. Renwick (1972a,b) proposed that some factor in potato blight is a likely cause of dysraphia in the United Kingdom.

Other authors (Smith et al., 1973; Spires, 1973) have disputed Renwick with equally imposing statistics. The review by Kurtzke and co-workers (1973) shows considerable racial variations, with whites having the highest incidence of dysraphia. There are large changes in the incidence rate of spina bifida over several-year periods in the same areas—and geographical differences occur in countries such as the United States, with a lowering of the rate as one proceeds from east to west. The observer can only conclude that there are multiple factors causing spinal dysraphia and probably neither of the opposing theories (abnormal dilatation versus abnormal closure) can explain all the anomalies which occur.

Widened spinal canal

We have sometimes seen a definitely widened dural sac during myelography, particularly in the lumbar area. This has occurred in 3.6% of all myelograms and often has been without any other abnormality, though most frequently seen in children being examined for suspected dysraphic lesions. We believe the finding of a widened dural sac represents the mildest form of the spectrum of spinal dysraphia. By itself, it has not been correlated with any specific symptoms.

Tethered conus

The subject of the tethered conus has had swings of popularity in the surgical literature since the 1950s. The symptoms and radiographic findings (spina bifida occulta) were noted as early as 1918 (Brickner) and the cause was then suspected. Until Gryspeerdt's (1963) report on the use of the supine myelographic technique, the diagnosis could be made only operatively.

The symptoms are often similar to those seen in diastematomyelia (in particular) and in other dysraphic states (in general). Upper motor neuron symptoms are prominent. Lower limb weakness, atrophy, and sensory loss are frequently seen. Gait disturbances are common, as are bladder or bowel weakness. Orthopedic conditions—foot deformity, scoliosis, differences in limb length—often bring the child to the attention of the physician.

More than forty cases of tethered conus have now been seen at The Hospital for Sick Children, Toronto, plus fifteen other cases with associated small meningoceles or transdural tissues (e.g., lipoma). In these groups there is a much less marked female predominance than in diastematomyelia or meningocele. It has been stated that females normally have a lower conus. We can only speculate as to the exact significance of this. The age of diagnosis of the tethered conus varies in our own series from under 1 year to 14 years. Except for being somewhat more common during growth spurts, there is no significant age pattern to the onset of symptoms.

External signs of dysraphia may include sacral dimples, hairy patches, and subcutaneous lipomas. All patients who have a tethered conus have some radiographic evidence of spina bifida, even though often only at one lumbar segment. It is not necessarily related to the actual level of the conus. More marked vertebral anomalies may exist but are uncommon in our experience.

As previously mentioned, the normal conus level has not been determined for all ages. Barson's study (1970b) is still the best work for the level of the conus at birth (Fig. 19-24). In autopsies of 252 fetuses with normal central nervous systems and varying ages from 13 to 49 weeks of gestation, he found that there is a rapid ascent of the conus between 11 and 17 weeks followed by a leveling off. The conus tip may reach the L1-L2 interspace as early as 35 weeks of gestation and normally is at that level by 48 weeks (2 months postnatal). Examining sixteen older children, he did find a 3-year-old with a conus ending at L3; and in a 12-year-old the conus was at the L2-L3 interspace. James and Lassman (1970) had similar results in their autopsies. Our myelographic experience indicates that a conus level below the L2-L3 interspace beyond age 5 years is abnormal. Empirically, we believe the conus should be at least to the mid-L2 level by age 12.

As with most conditions, we prefer oil myelography—in which case supine examination is of the utmost importance. As explained earlier, prone examination will miss the diagnosis in nearly all cases (Fig. 19-25). If the examiner depends on the level of the anterior spinal artery in the prone position as a true ending of the conus tip, he will be misled. The conus is normally suspended somewhat dorsally in the spinal canal and in abnormal cases is even more dorsally tethered by the filum. The conus may be

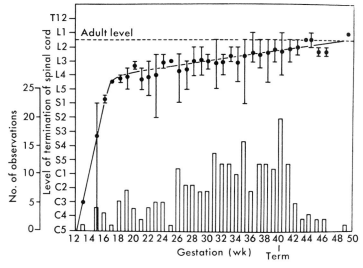

Fig. 19-24. Migration of the conus, prenatal and postnatal. (From Barson, A. J.: J. Anat. 106:489, 1970b.)

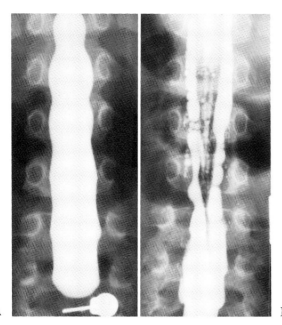

Fig. 19-25. Tethered conus. A, A prone myelogram fails to reveal the conus. B, A supine myelogram shows the conus ending at the top of the L4 vertebral body. (A 3-year-old patient.)

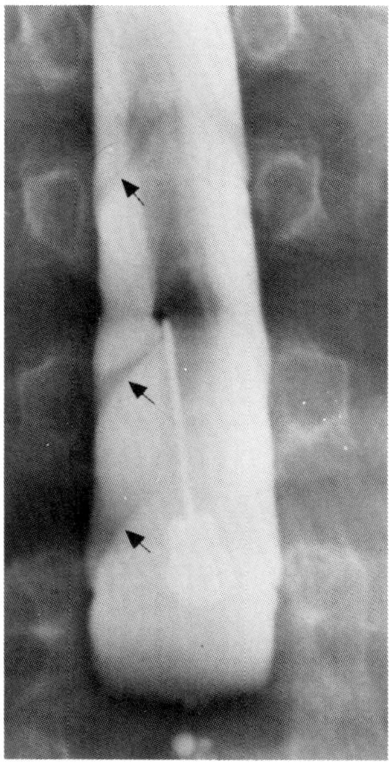

seen prone, however, if enough contrast material is used to fill the entire spinal canal to the L1 level. Then there is the risk of hiding the conus and filum in the density of the fully filled subarachnoid space. The supine position allows a surer visualization of the conus, the filum terminale, the nerve roots, and any associated masses.

In the lumbar area the subarachnoid nerve roots are normally parallel with the conus. If the conus is tethered, they will assume a more angled position—increasingly more toward the perpendicular, the lower the conus (Fig. 19-26). At times the nerve roots can even reverse their direction similar to that seen in the cervical region with an Arnold-Chiari malformation. When tethering occurs, the cord adjusts to this within five or six vertebral segments (Barry et al., 1957). The entire cord therefore is not affected by the disease and there is not a reversal of the nerve root orientation throughout the length of the cord.

The low conus may appear in a variety of shapes (Figs. 19-24 to 19-27). Usually there will be an abnormally low but normally shaped conus with a thickened filum. At times the conus will seem to have no exact termination but will gradually narrow to a very wide filum (Fig. 19-27). At operation this conus-like structure appears grossly to have normal neural elements down to its tip but actually is fibrous and without viable nervous tissue.

Fig. 19-26. Tethered conus. Lumbar nerve roots (arrows) can be seen angling off the conus at an abnormal 45° angle. The LP needle is at the L2-L3 interspace. The conus tip, not well seen on this prone film, ends at L4.

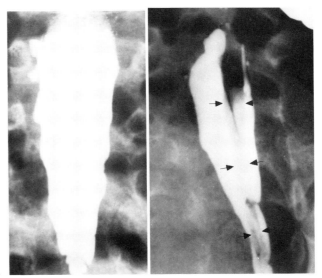

Fig. 19-27. Tethered conus. A, Prone examination shows only a widened dural sac. B, A slightly oblique supine examination shows the low conus gradually tapering (arrows) into a wide filum in the sacral region. (B from Fitz, C. R., and Harwood-Nash, D. C.: Am. J. Roentgenol. Radium Ther. Nucl. Med. **125:**515, 1975.)

Our experience indicates at myelography that a filum wider than 2 mm is suggestive of abnormality (Fig. 19-28). At times the thickness of the filum will be due in part to attached lipomatous tissue. Often lipomas, dermoids, etc. will be only subtle defects adjacent to or appearing to be part of the conus and outlined by contrast material.

As a rule—the lower the conus, the larger it tends to be and the larger is the dural sac. Then a greater than usual amount of contrast material must often be used to outline the conus adequately, even in the supine position.

An increased amount of contrast may also be useful when the conus is at a normal level in a relatively straight spine. If not, even in the supine position, the Pantopaque layers out so thinly that the conus may be quite difficult to see—the dye breaking up as it spreads along a much longer than usual segment of the subarachnoid space. Tipping the patient into an oblique supine position sometimes is helpful in these cases; the contrast material will pool in a thicker layer on one side of the conus and may outline the conus more clearly. Tipping also shows the lateral course of the nerve roots to better advantage. To demonstrate nerve root configurations in doubtful cases, a decubitus lateral position with cross-table AP filming may be a useful adjunct.

Associated lipomas and other abnormalities were

seen in fourteen of our twenty-four previously reported cases (Fitz and Harwood-Nash, 1975).

Dural bands may be seen attached to the conus or filum and possibly represent atrophic nerve roots. James and Lassman (1972) believe the tethering of the conus is not pathological but that in all cases there are intra- or extradural bands which cause traction on the cord. Additionally, these authors believe the masses sometimes associated with the low conus can be the cause of symptoms. In our own series, ten of twenty-four children had no associated masses and no bands that could be seen at operation. Differences in surgical technique might account for either the apparent presence or the apparent absence of these structures. Be that as it may, the important thing for the radiologist is that he recognize the abnormality of the conus at a low level and be aware of the technique to find the abnormality.

Although other investigators find air myelography to be quite useful in this condition, we do not think it is as reliable as oil. Air myelography does outline the conus as well as oil, especially in the lateral pro-

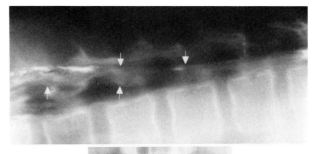

A

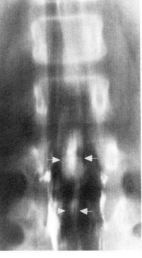

B

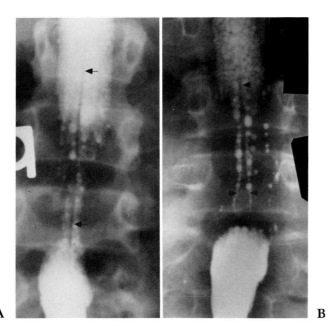

A   B

Fig. 19-28. Normal and widened filum terminale. A, Supine myelogram of a normal filum (arrows). B, Supine myelogram of an abnormal filum (single arrow), which gradually widens distally (opposed arrows) due to attached fatty tissue.

Fig. 19-29. Air myelography and a tethered conus. A, Lateral and, B, AP views outline a tethered conus (arrows). The lateral view gives best definition and also shows the dorsal location of the conus. Residual Pantopaque from a previous oil myelogram can be seen in the subarachnoid space.

jection (Fig. 19-29), but the filum and the nerve roots are not so well seen with air as with oil. There is also the theoretical possibility that at air myelography the examiner might miss a fibrous diastematomyelia because of the lesser discernability between the air and surrounding soft tissues; however, we have not encountered such a situation. Similar clinical and plain film radiographic findings occur in the two conditions, thus demonstrating the importance of myelography

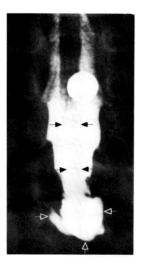

Fig. 19-30. **Tethered conus with meningocele.** A supine myelogram shows a very low conus (or an abnormally thickened filum) (solid arrows) entering the sac of a small sacral meningocele (open arrows).

to the separation of these entities. Additionally, tomography needed for good air myelography is time-consuming, particularly if the complete examination of the spinal cord is conducted (which should be done, even when only a conus lesion is suspected). If any newer water-soluble contrast agents (e.g., metrizamide) prove to be safe in large enough quantities to visualize the entire cord, they should be ideal for revealing anatomical structures without tomography or supine examination.

A Chiari malformation will occasionally be seen with diastematomyelia; but in our experience, patients having only a tethered conus have not had any evidence of a Chiari malformation. Small lumbar and sacral meningoceles, though excluded from our reported series, do also present with identical symptoms. The myelographic difference is the demonstration of the meningocele sac (Fig. 19-30). In these cases the conus and the filum may be tethered within the normal portion of the lumbosacral spinal canal or may enter the meningocele sac to form a myelomeningocele.

Once the diagnosis has been confirmed by myelography, the patient should be operated on. The technique used in our hospital is to open the dura, identify the filum, place clips across it as far distally as possible, and cut the filum. There is immediate separation of the clips, often dramatically illustrated at operation (Fig. 19-31) and verifiable by postoperative spine films (Fig. 19-32).

The results of treatment vary. At worst, progression of symptoms is halted. At best, complete recovery ensues. Exact evaluation of improvement is difficult be-

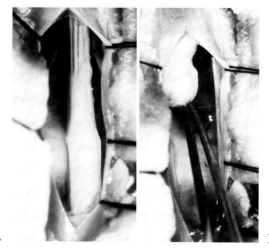

A   **B**

Fig. 19-31. **Tethered conus. A,** Exposed at operation. The thickened filum is surrounded by fat. **B,** After complete separation of the filum. The portion that was at the bottom of the operative field must now be retracted caudally to be visualized in the top of the operative field. (From Fitz, C. R., and Harwood-Nash, D. C.: Am. J. Roentgenol. Radium Ther. Nucl. Med. **125:**515, 1975.)

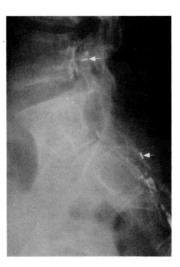

Fig. 19-32. **Tethered conus—postoperative films.** Lateral lumbosacral spine examination shows clips (arrows) that were together before sectioning of the filum now separated by almost two vertebral bodies.

cause most children have several signs and symptoms and are growing. To be completely sure that some of the improvement is not adaptation to a symptom or is simply maturation may be impossible. In our own series we believe that a significant improvement in major symptoms, such as bladder control and muscle weakness, occurred in at least half the children. Improvement was more likely to occur in children with only a tethered conus and no associated masses.

Why release of the tethering allows or causes improvement is difficult to say. Work by Hilal and Keim (1972) in patients with scoliosis suggests that stretching of the cord may cause some vascular compromise. Autopsy studies also suggest that vascular compromise may occur (Jones and Love, 1956). Perhaps there is stretching in times of rapid growth when the bony spine grows faster than the neural elements. Also with maturation and a relative decrease in neural tissue vascularity, areas having longitudinal stretching of tissues may undergo a decrease in arterial pressure relative to normal. Pressure on the nerve roots themselves might be a factor, except the roots do not appear to be under tension. Perhaps there is some pressure on the inferior surfaces of these roots at the foramina in the abnormal areas. Another theory postulates that stretching of the nerve fibers of the corticospinal tracts occurs (Yashon and Beatty, 1966).

Diastematomyelia

The true cause of diastematomyelia is obscure. According to Gardner (1964) the condition occurs when there is rupture of the central canal of the embryo both dorsally and ventrally with subsequent repair by growth of separate but incomplete neural tubes. Mesodermal tissue grows between the tubes as a result of attachment that occurs at the time of the splitting of the central canal.

Bentley and Smith (1960) suggested that the embryo may develop a partial duplication and separation of the notochord (split notochord syndrome) with the ventrally placed yolk sac or gut endoderm herniating through the canal and adhering to skin ectoderm. With further growth and repair, the defect has variable presentations. Depending on the amount of disruption, the dorsoventral placement of the remnants, and their rostrocaudal location—the theory accounts for many abnormalities, from enteric cysts, diastematomyelia and its vertebral anomalies, and central nervous system cysts and cell rests (dermoids, etc.) to posteriorly located sinuses in the skin.

Bremer (1952) suggested that the normal temporarily present neurenteric canal through Hensen's node persists for an abnormal length of time and causes diastematomyelia in various places as the newly formed neural tissues migrate cranially away from the node. This theory does not explain why diastematomyelia is so rare in the cervical area—unless the diastematomyelia is a relatively late abnormality at a time when only thoracic and lumbar tissues are being formed.

Although the incidence varies, most diastematomyelia occurs in females. The large series of Cohen and Sledge (1960), with twenty of their own cases and 112 from the literature, combined with Hilal and co-workers' thirty-four cases in 1974 show an overall incidence of 82% females and 18% males. Our own series of sixty-two cases had a 34% male incidence, a fairly marked discrepancy between relatively large series. Perhaps the greater incidence of scoliosis in females makes it more likely that they will be examined and diastematomyelia be found. Our own series is less oriented than most toward scoliosis. There is a frequent association of meningocele with diastematomyelia or diplomyelia (Emery, 1970). The incidence of Arnold-Chiari malformation with diastematomyelia is much less common than with meningocele.

Whereas diastematomyelia is usually considered as separate and distinct from diplomyelia, the latter being a complete duplication of the cord with nerve roots from both sides of both cord "halves," some authors (James and Lassman, 1972) think there is not a clear distinction; one merges with the other and there are no differences in the symptoms.

All authors point out that cutaneous signs on the back are often present, with a 50% to 75% incidence being reported (James and Lassman, 1972; Klein and Green, 1973). Hypertrichosis is the most common finding. A lipoma, hemangioma, nevus, or sinus track may also be present. The cutaneous manifestation often is directly over the diastematomyelia, but it may be several vertebrae distant from the diastematomyelia.

As mentioned, meningocele may also be present. Scoliosis is often the initial physical sign that brings a child with diastematomyelia to the physician's attention. There may also be discrepancies in leg or foot length, foot deformities, gait disturbances, muscle weakness or atrophy, and occasionally only low back pain with or without scoliosis.

Why diastematomyelia usually causes symptoms later in childhood is not clear. Since most of the migration of the conus occurs during embryonic life and early childhood, the symptoms would be expected to be prominent in infancy. Migration of the conus during childhood may not be so important. James and Lassman (1972) suggested that perhaps the increased physical activity which normal children have as they grow, combined with a lack of normal cord mobility, causes the symptoms. Barson (1970a) suggested that differentiation of the neural elements with growth decreases the possible alternative pathways for transmission of neural impulses and results in symptoms. The possible theories discussed with regard to the tethered conus may also hold for diastematomyelia.

Until the radiographic description of diastematomyelia by Neuhauser and co-workers in 1950, the diagnosis had been made almost exclusively at operation or autopsy. Neuhauser's group pointed out the important radiographic features of the disease, and little has been added since then.

Congenital bony abnormalities, usually at or near the level of the diastematomyelic spur, are *always*

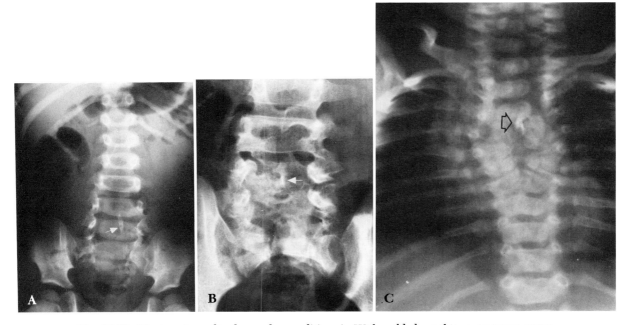

Fig. 19-33. **Diastematomyelia, bony abnormalities.** A, With mild dysraphia, a common occurrence. Note the wide interpediculate distance and the obvious bony spur in the lumbar area (arrow). **B,** More severe, with multiple areas of spina bifida and a widened interpediculate distance. Arrow denotes a lumbar bony bar. **C,** With marked dysraphia in the thoracic and cervical spine. A bony bar (arrow) is present.

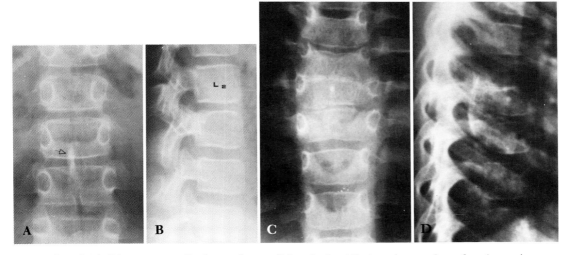

Fig. 19-34. **Diastematomyelia, bony abnormalities.** A, An AP view shows a bony bar (arrow) and a spina bifida one level below. **B,** Slight narrowing of the disk space between L2 and L3, better seen in a lateral view of the same child. **C** and **D,** More severe disk space narrowing at the level of a thoracic bony bar and adjacent levels. Note the decreased anteroposterior diameter of the midthoracic vertebral bodies in **D.**

present (Fig. 19-33). Usually both posterior elements and vertebral body abnormalities are present; but at times only one occurs. Hilal and co-workers (1974) found only three of thirty-four patients with no laminar defects and another three with no vertebral body defects. Most often there is widening of the interpediculate distance, occult spina bifida, and fused or butterfly-type vertebral bodies. Frequently there is narrowing of the anteroposterior diameter of the affected vertebral bodies and a narrowed disk space (Fig. 19-34) (Neuhauser et al., 1950).

Whereas the septum is most often bony, it can be incompletely so or even be fibrous and cartilaginous. It may occur up as far as C6, though the lumbar area is more commonly involved than the thoracic. Two spikes occasionally are seen. Hilal and co-workers (1974) pointed out that thoracic septa, on the average, are longer than lumbar septa. These authors also found that as a septum grows ventrally it may go rostrally, caudally, or straight ventrally. Associated with this is the finding of the spina bifida—being most obvious in the direction to which the spur points while going ventrally.

If scoliosis or skin abnormalities are also present, even without clinical symptoms, the neuroradiologist should be suspicious of diastematomyelia in any child with vertebral anomalies or spina bifida. To verify the diagnosis in these children, further investigation is justified. Guthkelch and co-workers (1972) followed a group of asymptomatic patients with diastematomyelia and found that nearly all later developed symptoms and required operation. The feeling of these authors was that operation is justified before symptoms occur.

Two radiological procedures are used to confirm the diagnosis of diastematomyelia.

The first, tomography, is often not necessary but does give the surgeon an excellent picture of what to expect in removal of the spur and the direction that the spur takes ventrodorsally. Lateral tomograms are especially helpful (Fig. 19-35).

Myelography is carried out in the usual manner. With scoliosis an extra large amount of contrast material may be needed. The spur and separate spinal cord segments are easily demonstrated by oil myelography. The radiologist must be sure that the defects are visible at prone myelography. In the supine position arachnoid *veils* often cause irregular splitting of the column of dye in the midline area (Di Chiro and Timins, 1974). Unless there is definite visualization of the split cord, a diastematomyelia-like defect seen only in the supine position is not an adequate basis for subjecting a child to operation.

Another function of myelography in diastematomyelia is to outline the level of the conus (Fig. 19-36). The conus is often abnormally low, particularly in lumbar diastematomyelia. The presence of a low conus means that the laminectomy should be extended or a separate laminectomy done to release the filum. Symptoms may be related to both the diastematomyelia and the conus tethering.

The septum does not always split the cord evenly. An off-center spur going obliquely to one side can rotate the cord segments into a somewhat dorsoventral

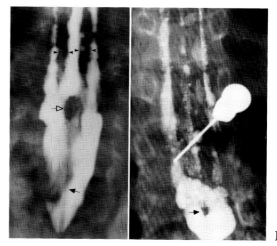

Fig. 19-36. Myelography and diastematomyelia. A, An oil myelogram shows a split spinal cord (arrowheads) extending far rostrally from a bony bar (open arrow), which causes a second defect in the dye column. The conus tip (solid arrow) is seen in the sacrum with a thick filum distal to it. B, In another patient a bony septum in the midlumbar area (arrow) can be seen with the cord ending directly at the same level. Again, separate cord halves extend far rostrally from the septum.

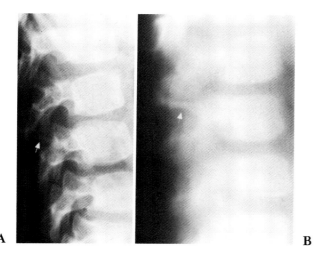

Fig. 19-35. Tomography and diastematomyelia. A bony septum (arrows) is visible on the lateral plain film (A), but its full extent is confirmed only on the tomogram (B).

orientation and make the myelographic diagnosis difficult. Tomography will more easily show the oblique spur as separate from what might otherwise be interpreted as simply an abnormal laminar process.

Air myelography in diastematomyelia was first described in 1965 (Lillequist). We do not use it frequently. Though the lateral tomographic projection may well outline both the conus and the bony spur, the situation will be less clear if the septum is cartilaginous. On occasion, the technique is useful (Fig. 19-37). As in other situations, we find oil myelography a better means of examining the entire cord and posterior fossa contents.

Syringohydromyelia

The term syringomyelia was first used by Ollivier in 1827 to describe any cavity within the spinal cord. Hydromyelia was described as a central canal dilatation communicating with the fourth ventricle by Silling in 1859. Hydromyelia is usually described as having an ependymal lining (Greenfield et al., 1958), though the cavity may break through the ependyma, and having a glial covering (Ellertsson, 1969). Syringomyelia, when differentiated from hydromyelia, is generally described as having "a cellular gliosis" (Finlayson, 1962) concentrically arranged. Greenfield and co-workers (1958) also described the lining in similar fashion. The cavity in both lesions contains CSF-like fluid.

The differentiation between dilatation of the central canal (hydromyelia) and dissection of the cord separate from the canal (syringomyelia) is at times diffi-

cult to make by radiological, clinical, or pathological methods. Excluding those cystic cavities secondary to hemorrhage and associated with tumors, we believe the combined term *syringohydromyelia* to be more appropriate. The term was first used by Gardner (1965) and avoids the confusing situation of separate names interchangeably used to describe the same type of cavity. We agree with McRae and Standen (1966) that terms such as posttraumatic or postinflammatory cavitation be used to describe the noncongenital cavities.

The theory of Gardner (1965) is the most plausible explanation for the development of syringohydromyelia. There is normally free communication between the dilated central canal and the fourth ventricle in early embryonic life until the rhombic roof begins to perforate and form the foramen of Magendie. This foramen is normally open by the fifth intrauterine month. A vestigial central canal may remain at birth; but in 70% to 80% of neonates, the canal will close. In syringohydromyelia the canal remains open due to an abnormality of the foramen of Magendie. This may in part explain the high incidence of Chiari I or other hindbrain malformations associated with syringohydromyelia, particularly in adults.

In autopsies of seventy-four patients with syringohydromyelia, Gardner found malformations, particularly Chiari type I, in all. Logue (1961) found similar abnormalities in thirty-one of thirty-five cases. In

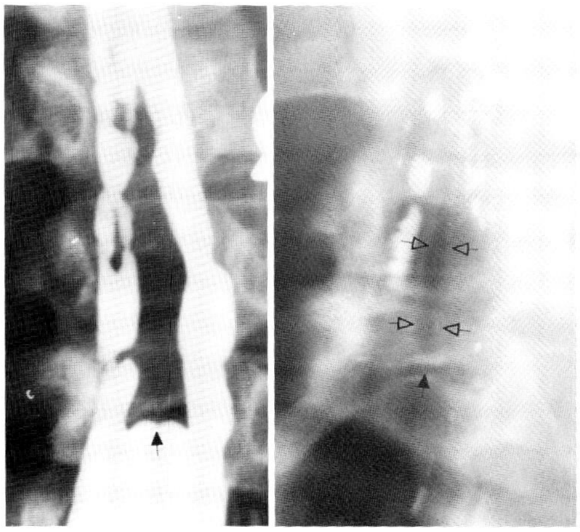

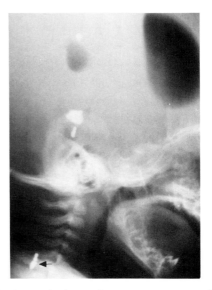

Fig. 19-37. **Air myelography and diastematomyelia. A,** An oil myelogram shows the septum (arrow) but fails to demonstrate separate cords, apparently due to adhesions of the cord against the dura. **B,** An air myelogram reveals air between the two cord halves (open arrows) over a short distance above the septum (solid arrow).

Fig. 19-38. **Syringohydromyelia.** Pantopaque can be seen in the dilated central canal (arrow) at ventriculography in an infant with adhesions of the outlets of the fourth ventricle and resultant hydrocephalus secondary to a meningitis. (From Harwood-Nash, D. C., and Fitz, C. R.: Radiology 113:661, 1974.)

children we find associations with Chiari II malformations more frequent than with Chiari I.

It is thought that arterial pulsation (Gardner, 1965) or venous pressure (Williams, 1969; Ellertsson and Greitz, 1970) keeps the canal open in abnormal cases and may cause further dissection outside the central canal. That this may occur postnatally in patients having originally a normal foramen of Magendie is suggested by our finding of a dilated central canal in a child examined for hydrocephalus after meningitis (Fig. 19-38).

In addition to association with Chiari malformations—syringohydromyelia not infrequently is also associated with spina bifida occulta, diastematomyelia, scoliosis, and occipital and C1 anomalies (Lassman et al., 1968). The most common symptoms with syringohydromyelia are decreased pain and temperature sensation (spinothalamic tracts), muscle weakness with wasting and absent reflexes (anterior horn cells), and upper motor neuron symptoms of weakness, spasticity, hyperreflexia, and abnormal plantar reflexes (pyramidal tracts) (Logue, 1971). These are related to the destruction or stretching of the central gray matter of the cord and closely adjacent structures. Because the cavity may enlarge irregularly at different levels, the symptoms may be quite varied and not at all classical.

The bony spinal canal is usually widened (Fig. 19-39), depending on the extent of the cystic cavity. The interpediculate distance is widened by the larger cavities, especially in the dorsal and lumbar areas.

Slight enlargement in the cervical area is best noted in the lateral projection. Actual interpediculate measurements are not often used by us. With experience, a subtle change from the normal contours of the bony canal is more easily seen than measured. The pedicles themselves may be flattened. The bony anomalies described give further information to suggest the diagnosis.

Myelography of syringohydromyelia is best done with a combination of oil and air techniques. Initially, Pantopaque via the lumbar subarachnoid space should be used to outline the dilated cord. The contrast material usually passes slowly around the dilated cord. The enlargement itself cannot be differentiated from any other. The length of the abnormality is greater than that of most tumors, though some neoplasms can occupy the entire cord.

In the supine position, any associated abnormal tonsillar position will be seen and will help to identify the syringohydromyelia as such. If possible, oil should be directed into the fourth ventricle, the patient should be turned prone, and an attempt made at continuing the flow of contrast into the central canal

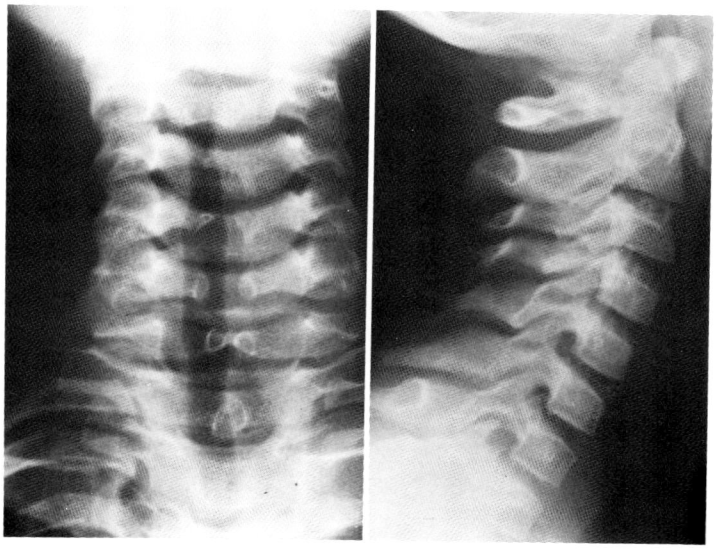

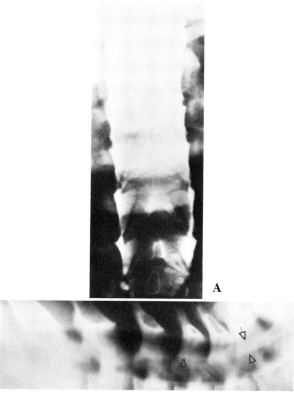

Fig. 19-39. Syringohydromyelia. AP and lateral views of the cervical spine in a child with syringohydromyelia show enlargement of the spinal canal and a spina bifida in the mid-cervical area.

Fig. 19-40. Syringohydromyelia. A, An oil myelogram demonstrates a dilated cervical cord. B, An air myelogram shows marked collapse of this widened cord (arrows). (From Harwood-Nash, D. C., and Fitz, C. R.: Radiology 113:661, 1974.)

and the dilated cavity. This will not often occur; but when it does, visualization of the abnormality is dramatic.

After oil myelography, air myelography in the upright position is performed. The cavity will either totally or partially collapse (Fig. 19-40). Such collapse of the cord was first noted by Oden (1953) and Pendergrass and co-workers (1956).

In 1963, Wickbom and Hanafee showed the change from dilatation to collapse using the combined oil and air myelographic methods. The true cause of the collapse is not certain. Heinz and co-workers (1966) suggested that the hydromyelic sac is flexible and in the upright position collapses in its uppermost portion as the lower segment expands. Conway (1967) suggested that as cerebrospinal fluid is withdrawn from the lumbar puncture site there is exchange with CSF coming down from the hemispheric convexities into the spinal subarachnoid space. This exchange allows the ventricles to expand; and the central canal, communicating with the fourth ventricle, empties into the fourth ventricle. The last theory does not explain why the collapse should occur if air goes over the hemispheres or enters the ventricles to replace the CSF and is probably incorrect.

The *collapsing cord* is a distinct myelographic sign that does not occur with solid cord enlargement or cystic tumors. We have had one case in which only a portion of the cervical cord collapsed due to noncommunication of the lower sac with the upper cervical segment (Fig. 19-41). The rostralmost portion of the cord in this case also did not collapse because of arachnoid adhesions around it, or because of lack of communication with the fourth ventricle.

In addition to showing the decreased caliber of the upright cord, *air myelography* may also demonstrate patency of the foramen of Magendie and whether or not air communicates with the subarachnoid space over the hemispheres.

Although sometimes demonstrating the displaced Chiari II fourth ventricle and what may appear to be a short dilated central canal beyond this in the cervical area, in our experience *air ventriculography* in hydrocephalic infants does not give evidence of a central canal extending below the cervical level. Since the syringohydromyelic sac is often much longer when the diagnosis of the condition is later made, the suggestion follows that either the canal continues to enlarge after birth or that possibly children with a dynamic hydrocephalus do not often have an associated syringohydromyelia.

Frequently done in a previous time period by us, *oil ventriculography* sometimes demonstrated a small central canal in hydrocephalic infants (thirty cases) (Fig. 19-42). These were not thought to be of significance when examined. We do not have a clear understanding of the circumstances that may later cause this canal to enlarge in such cases, if in fact it does.

Inadvertent sac puncture has occurred in four patients during oil myelography. In each there was a unique sausagelike appearance throughout the length of the sac (Figs. 19-43 and 19-44) suggesting the pathological descriptions of syringomyelia by Greenfield and co-workers (1958) and Finlayson (1962) of irregular circumferential glial fibers. A postmortem specimen provided by Dr. John Alcock, London, Ontario, suggested the same mechanism (Fig. 19-45). In our four cases there was not communication with the fourth ventricle, and we believed the lack of communication suggested a dissection from the central canal; however, Heinz and co-workers (1966) and James and co-workers (1971) both had similar cases which showed the identical sausage-link or stacked-coin cavities communicating with the fourth ventricle.

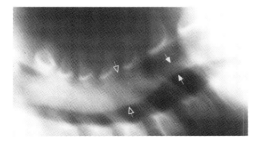

Fig. 19-41. Syringohydromyelia. On an air myelogram there is only partial collapse (solid arrows) of the large syringohydromyelic sac with return to a wide cord by the midcervical segment (open arrows).

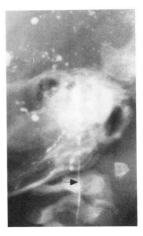

Fig. 19-42. Neonatal central canal. An oil ventriculogram in an infant with an Arnold-Chiari malformation shows a thin hydromyelic central canal (arrow) communicating with the fourth ventricle. (From Harwood-Nash, D. C., and Fitz, C. R.: Radiology 113:661, 1974.)

Indeed the contrast material in these latter cases was injected in the lumbar subarachnoid space, entered the fourth ventricle through the foramen of Magendie or Luschka, and then flowed into the central canal— demonstrating both normal and abnormal pathways to be open. The Heinz case also showed a collapse of the sac with air myelography.

Such experiences again confirm the difficulty of separating hydromyelia and syringomyelia as discrete entities. In children the condition is nearly always congenital, is frequently associated with signs of dysraphia, and even more frequently is related to Chiari type II malformations than it is in adults.

Meningocele

We use the terms meningocele, myelomeningocele, and myelocystocele as do Greenfield and co-workers (1958).

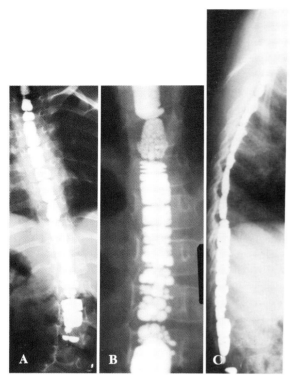

Fig. 19-43. Syringohydromyelia, injection of the sac. **A,** AP view. **B,** Enlargement of the lower thoracic area. **C,** Lateral view. Injection of contrast material into the syringohydromyelic sac shows serrated link sausagelike dilatation of the entire sac. (From Harwood-Nash, D. C., and Fitz, C. R.: Radiology 113:661, 1974.)

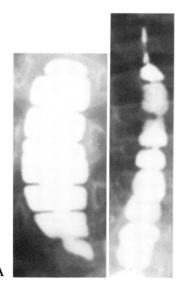

Fig. 19-44. Syringohydromyelia, injection of the sac. **A,** Lumbar and, **B,** thoracic areas of another patient with injection directly into the sac. (From Harwood-Nash, D. C., and Fitz, C. R.: Radiology 113:661, 1974.)

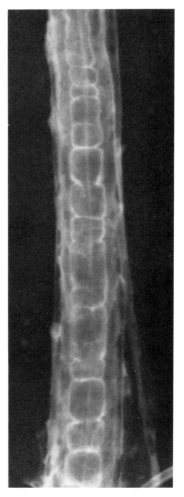

Fig. 19-45. Syringohydromyelia. Injection of a postmortem specimen shows irregular constrictions of the dilated canal similar to those seen during myelography. (Courtesy John Allcock, M.D., London, Ontario.)

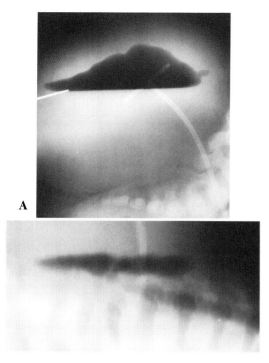

Fig. 19-46. Meningocele. An infant with a repaired lumbar meningocele and shunted hydrocephalus developed a recurrent meningocele sac. An air myelogram by direct needle puncture (**A**) shows a large thick-walled sac. A tomogram (**B**) shows a small communication with the normal subarachnoid space.

A *meningocele* is a swelling of the meninges outside the spinal canal. We include under the term meningocele intrasacral lesions that have an obviously enlarged dural canal but remain in bone. A *myelomeningocele* occurs when the cord or neural elements also pass into the bulging sac. The two may not be distinguishable by plain film radiography, except for the finding (Barson, 1965) that all dysraphic patients with a lumbar kyphosis also have a myelomeningocele. In a *myelocystocele* the central canal is grossly dilated and its dorsal part accompanies the sac posteriorly. The myelocystocele, however, is much less common than the other forms.

Subdivisions of these types of defects have been proposed (Talwalker and Dastur, 1970) and can be identified myelographically. Since the neonatal meningocele and myelomeningocele are clinically obvious, the type makes no difference as to the treatment. Myelography is not usually performed on such neonates at our institution.

Anderson and co-workers (1970) advocated pneumoencephalography in neonatal meningocele patients to determine the dynamics of any accompanying hydrocephalus. The authors emphasized that the needle puncture should not be made directly into the meningocele sac, however, since the sac usually has adhesions preventing it from communicating with the

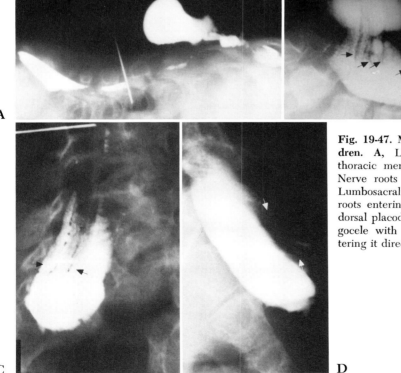

Fig. 19-47. Meningoceles in older children. **A,** Lateral view of a lower thoracic meningocele with loculations. Nerve roots do not enter the sac. **B,** Lumbosacral meningocele with nerve roots entering the sac (arrows) to the dorsal placode. **C** and **D,** Sacral meningocele with a low cord (arrows) entering it directly.

rest of the subarachnoid space. They did not give their success rate in these studies. Though examination of the meningocele may at times be useful (Fig. 19-46) and can be done via the sac, we believe ventriculography to be a more reliable procedure for these patients.

Present neurosurgical thinking is that immediate closure of the defect should be done in nearly all cases. Good reviews of the operative treatment, survival, and ethics of treatment are given in *Clinical Neurosurgery* (1973) (Chapter 8, Shillito; Chapter 9, Freeman; Chapter 10, Foltz et al.).

Operative treatment results in various survival rates, depending on the associated problems, and varied quality of survival, also related to associated defects. Overall the long-term survival is now at least 50%.

Older children presenting with skin-covered masses on their backs, especially in the lumbosacral region, are often investigated to determine the nature of the mass (which may be a meningocele) (Fig. 19-47). Lemire and co-workers (1971) reviewed thirty-one children with this situation and found twelve with meningoceles or associated defects. Several important radiographic clues were noted. Rectal displacement separated teratomas and other solid tumors from neural tube abnormalities. Dysraphia was always associated with neural tube defects but might also be seen with other abnormalities. An area of decreased density in the mass indicated a lipoma or lipomeningocele. Neurological defects were sometimes present in neural tube abnormalities. Fig. 19-48 is from their article.

Although this flow sheet is an excellent guide, myelography is still necessary. A teratoma or other tumor may have dural invasion. The tethering of the conus should be determined in any older child with a meningocele. A meningocele or associated defect

must be excluded in rarer masses that do not fit well into the dendrogram flow sheet. Examples of these are epidermoid cysts, gut duplications, and sarcomas.

Lumbar paravertebral meningoceles have also been reported (Sogani and Kalani, 1972) protruding through the absent half of a hemivertebra and extending posteriorly as an off-center mass. Their eccentric location is a confusing clinical situation also deserving myelographic confirmation.

The intraspinal meningocele, commonly located in the sacrum, usually has no signs of dysraphia externally. Neurological abnormalities involving the nerve roots are present with bladder and bowel symptoms, sacral pain, and sensory deficits. Though dura covered, such defects may be arachnoid herniations (Young and Bruwer, 1966). These herniations may not be true meningoceles yet are indistinguishable from true meningoceles by clinical or myelographic means. Even those that are dura covered are not accepted as true meningoceles by some investigators (Howieson et al., 1968) since they do not extend outside the bony canal. They may be associated with neurofibromatosis or possibly represent a forme fruste of neurofibromatosis.

Regardless of the semantics of its origin, any expansion of the bony sacral canal needs myelography to reveal its cause and contents. Some of these meningoceles communicate with the subarachnoid space. Others have an opening so small as to be invisible at initial myelography and a small portion of the contrast material must be allowed to remain in the canal. Reexamination in 24 to 48 hours may reveal contrast in the abnormal sac. If possible, the examiner should determine whether or not neural elements enter the sac (Fig. 19-49). Swedberg (1963) advocated air myelography in these cases, believing that the oil would enter the opening more slowly. Our own experience with oil ventriculography in tracking down

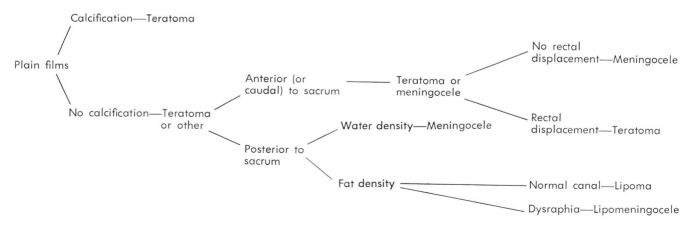

Fig. 19-48. Lumbosacral masses, dendrogram.

stenotic aqueducts suggests that oil, if anything, flows more easily than air through small-diameter openings.

The embryology of intraspinal meningocele may be somewhat different from that of other types. Palozzoli (1963) suggested the normal caudal central canal begins as two or more secondary canals which merge and then degenerate in the fifth to eleventh weeks of intrauterine life; later there is normally no sacral central canal; therefore, localized problems during this early time period must cause the sacral meningocele.

Anterior sacral meningoceles are quite uncommon. They do not present as an external mass, and they usually are noticed when mild neurological symptoms of a lesser degree than those accompanying posterior meningoceles occur. The symptoms are often related to pressure on pelvic organs. Though sometimes not

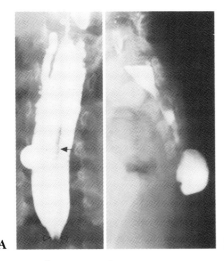

Fig. 19-49. Sacral meningocele. A, A prone view shows the conus ending at the needle tip (solid arrow) with a thickened filum (opposed open arrows) extending further distally into the meningocele sac. **B,** A lateral view shows filling of the meningocele sac at the sacrococcygeal level.

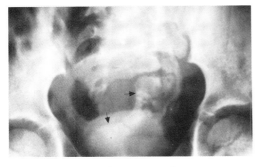

Fig. 19-50. Anterior sacral meningocele. An AP view of the lumbosacral spine shows a large defect (arrows) from the meningocele in the right half of the sacrum.

showing sacral defects, they typically are lacking a portion of the most distal sacrum (Fig. 19-50). Frequently this lack is unilateral and the remaining half has a characteristic "beak" around the meningocele (Sherman et al., 1950). Since other neoplasms (particularly teratomas) may occur as a pelvic mass with sacral destruction, myelography is of the utmost importance. Blind per rectum biopsy may cause a meningitis in a meningocele. As with the posterior meningoceles, the contrast material will fill the sac.

Lateral thoracic meningoceles are even more rare, usually presenting as a mediastinal mass and more often on the right side. Vertebral and rib anomalies are common. Neurological symptoms ordinarily are absent. The lesion is most likely to be confused with a neurenteric cyst—which, however, nearly always has a butterfly-type dysraphic vertebral body. Although asymptomatic, the lateral thoracic meningocele needs myelography to determine the character of the lesion. A large percentage of these lesions are associated with neurofibromatosis (Rubin and Stratemeier, 1952). In childhood the manifestations of neurofibromatosis may not yet be evident.

Cyst

Although quite rare, spinal extradural cysts have a high incidence in the "elderly paediatric" age group. In a review of sixty-one cases, Gortvai (1963) found one third occurring in the second decade and usually in the thoracic, especially the lower thoracic area. Typical symptoms are a spastic paraplegia and mild sensory changes. The lesions are often associated with Scheuermann's disease (Ellsberg et al., 1934). The involved areas may show evidence of an intraspinal mass with local erosion of the pedicle and an increased interpediculate distance. Myelography may show only an extradural defect or may fill the cyst.

Perineural cysts are uncommon lesions apparently representing diverticula of the arachnoid. They usually occur at the junction of the posterior root with the ganglion (Shapiro, 1975). Most often in the sacrum, they may also occur in the lumbar or thoracic areas; and they have been reported in the cervical spine (Smith, 1962). They are usually incidental findings at myelography (Fig. 19-13). Those occurring in the sacrum may be impossible to distinguish from sacral meningoceles. We believe that a midline sacral lesion with expansion of the bone is more likely to be a meningocele, though the differentiation may be academic.

Sutton (1963) indicated that perineural cysts may be quite common; he found sixteen in a review of 200 myelograms in which the oil was allowed to remain until other films were taken at a later time. We have twice noted a rapid extradural tracking of contrast, leaking around a needle puncture. Perhaps the cysts occur by a similar mechanism secondary to the rises in CSF pressure that occur with lifting, coughing, laughing, etc.

Diverticula along the septum posticum are not uncommon lesions. Though reported as an associated finding with scoliosis and said to produce symptoms by filling with CSF in the erect position (Teng and Rudner, 1960), we find them as incidental occurrences during supine myelography. They act as cups which fill in the supine position as the dye flows caudally, and they can be emptied by running the Pantopaque

cranially again. They do not empty easily in the prone position. We doubt that they cause any symptoms.

Arnold-Chiari malformation

The various aspects of the Arnold-Chiari malformation are discussed elsewhere (Chapter 16). Myelography is not usually the primary diagnostic tool in the diagnosis of Arnold-Chiari malformations but is sometimes used when an intramedullary high cervical lesion is suspected and an Arnold-Chiari is also a possibility. The primary myelographic sign of Arnold-Chiari malformation is tonsillar herniation (Fig. 19-51). Since the tonsils are usually peglike and closely adherent to the medulla, they may be difficult to see or distinguish from a medullary enlargement; however, the fairly sharp enlargement of the cord in the upper cervical area is characteristic, best seen in the lateral supine position (Fig. 19-52) but sometimes also in the prone AP position if the contrast covers the dorsal cord surface. Associated with the herniation of the tonsils is a small cisterna magna caused by the posterior dislocation of the cerebellar hemispheres, and sometimes a beaking of the medulla on the cervical spine is noted.

Even with these signs present, it is not infrequently difficult to distinguish an Arnold-Chiari malformation from a craniocervical junction mass of other cause. A helpful secondary sign to differentiate the two ab-

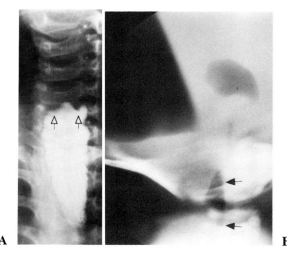

Fig. 19-51. Arnold-Chiari malformation. A, A myelogram shows complete block to flow of contrast material in the lower cervical area outlining the tonsillar pegs (arrows). **B,** A ventriculogram of the same patient shows the fourth ventricle (arrows) extending into the cervical canal, typical of a Chiari II malformation.

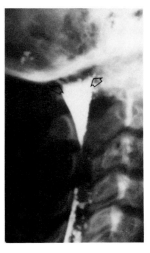

Fig. 19-52. Arnold-Chiari malformation. A lateral myelogram shows tonsillar extension (arrows) below the foramen magnum.

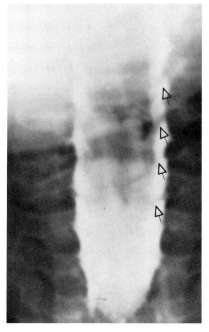

Fig. 19-53. Arnold-Chiari malformation. A cervical myelogram shows the superiorly extending nerve roots (arrows).

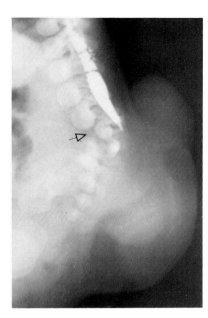

Fig. 19-54. **Prolapsed vertebral body** (arrow). This defect, just above a myelomeningocele, caused complete obstruction of contrast material in the subarachnoid space.

normalities is the upgoing cervical nerve roots present in the Arnold-Chiari malformation (Fig. 19-53). To interpret this, the neuroradiologist must be certain that the neck is not extended since neck extension will cause an apparent change in the orientation of the nerve roots at fluoroscopy in the AP position or on a spot film.

Posterior vertebral slipping

The dysraphic state not generally recognized is the posteriorly slipped vertebral body. The defect is uncommon and usually presents with a variety of other abnormalities. It may be a solitary finding in an otherwise normal spine. It may be associated with or the cause of a scoliosis.

Twice, posterior vertebral slipping was associated with a tethered conus; and once with a meningocele, in which it may represent an extreme form of the thoracolumbar kyphosis that is a concomitant of myelomeningocele (Fig. 19-54). Often there are other dysplastic vertebral bodies. The involved vertebral body is characteristically small, sometimes anteriorly beaked, and/or malformed (Fig. 19-55).

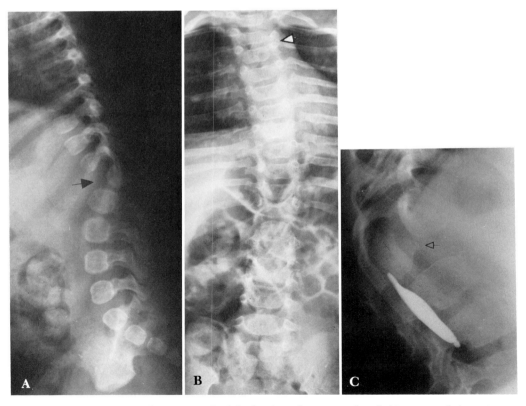

Fig. 19-55. **Posteriorly slipped vertebral body.** A and B, Lateral and AP views of the spine show slipping of the L1 vertebra (solid arrow) associated with mild scoliosis and mild vertebral abnormalities (open arrow) in the upper thoracic area. The lapsed vertebral body is small, as are the two vertebral bodies above it. C, A myelogram reveals complete obstruction to flow of contrast material by the slipped vertebral body, which has an anterior beak (arrow).

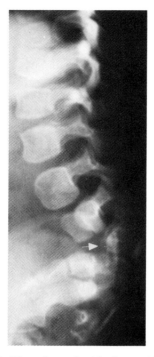

Fig. 19-56. Slipped vertebral body at L5 (arrow).

The posterior slipping usually occurs at the thoracolumbar junction but can be seen in the lower lumbar (Fig. 19-56) and even the cervicothoracic junction (Fig. 19-57) area. The cases that have come to myelography have all had some compression of the subarachnoid space as well as, in several instances, a complete block.

The condition is most likely caused by an abnormality of the anterior ossification centers of the involved vertebral body.

Spinal stenosis

Spinal stenosis is a congenital condition of unknown etiology in which the spinal canal is too small and the bony vertebral elements are large. Logically, an overgrowth of the mesoderm during embryonic life might be assumed.

The AP diameter especially, and usually the interpediculate distance as well, is narrowed. The laminae are vertically oriented, and the vertebral bodies and posterior elements have a massive appearance.

Symptoms usually do not occur until midadulthood, when degenerative processes compress the narrowed space. In a review of thirty-three cases (Roberson et al., 1973), no patient was younger than 20 years. The condition is seen rarely by us and is usually associated with low back pain and lumbar nerve root symptoms. Findings at myelography in infants resemble those in adults except the degenerative changes are not present (Fig. 19-58). There is a relatively slow flow of contrast material in a narrowed

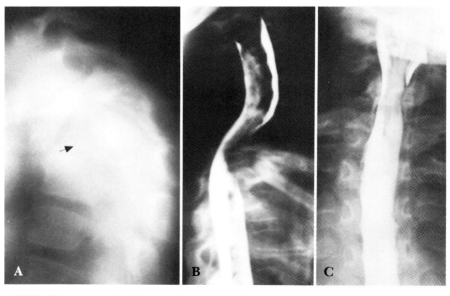

Fig. 19-57. Slipped vertebral body at T1. A lateral tomogram (A) shows a typical malformed and small vertebral body (arrow). Lateral (B) and AP (C) myelograms show compression of the subarachnoid space and cord.

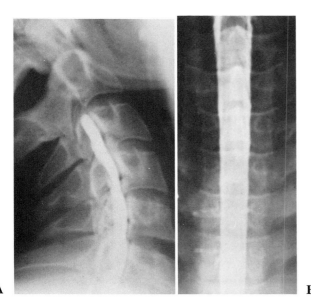

Fig. 19-58. Spinal stenoses. A, Lateral myelogram. Contrast material crowded into the ventral portion of the subarachnoid space. The diameter of the spinal canal is narrow when compared with that of the vertebral bodies. **B,** An AP view of the thoracic area in another patient shows narrowness of the subarachnoid space around the cord and a narrowed interpediculate distance.

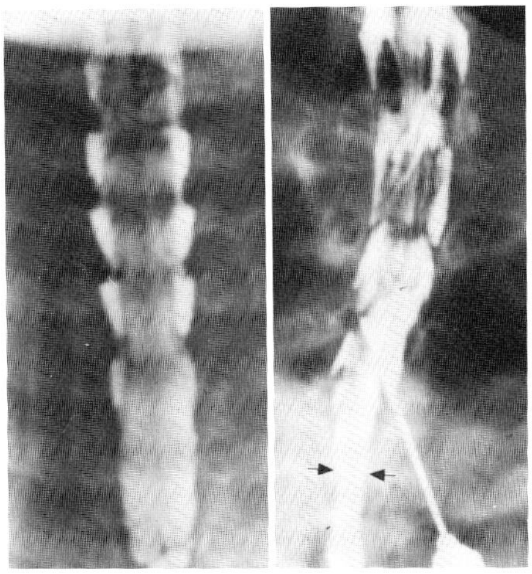

canal, and prominent intervertebral spaces cause indentations in the contrast column. Whether the prominence of the nerve roots is due partly to nerve root hypertrophy or more likely to nerve root compression in the narrowed space may be difficult to say.

Achondroplasia also causes narrowing of the lumbar spinal canal. Again symptoms usually occur during adulthood and myelographic findings are the same as those in spinal stenosis unrelated to achondroplasia, except that there is a progressively narrow canal in the lumbar region rather than the normal midlumbar enlargement (Fig. 19-59). We have also seen similar findings in a child with Maroteaux-Lamy syndrome (Fig. 19-60) due primarily to bulging of the disk, and we suspect that all the mucopolysaccharidoses would exhibit similar features at myelography.

MISCELLANEOUS DISORDERS
Dejerine-Sottas disease

Dejerine-Sottas disease or hypertrophic interstitial neuropathy is a rarely recognized slowly progressive disease often causing ataxia, sensory disturbances, muscle atrophy, and bowel and bladder dysfunction. Only forty-seven cases have been described in the English literature (Rao et al., 1974), and few of these

Fig. 19-59. Achondroplasia. A, A myelogram in the lower cervical and upper thoracic area shows crowding of the spinal cord against the narrowed subarachnoid space. **B,** A lumbar area myelogram shows that the nerve roots are prominent because of compression into a small space, which is particularly narrowed caudal to the needle (arrows).

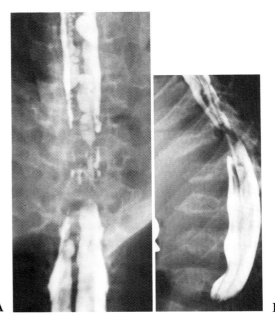

Fig. 19-60. Maroteaux-Lamy syndrome. A myelogram of a 15-year-old girl shows the relatively narrow subarachnoid space in the AP projection (**A**), particularly over the thoracolumbar kyphosis. In the lateral view (**B**), similar findings are present and there is prominence of the disk spaces.

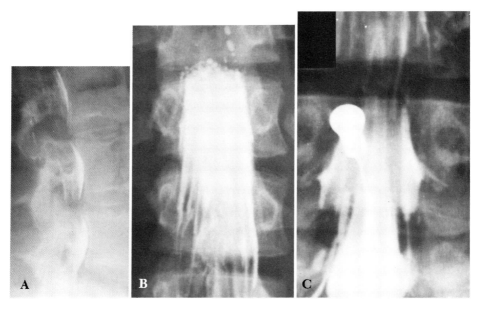

Fig. 19-61. Dejerine-Sottas disease. A, A lateral lumbar myelogram shows slight scalloping of the posterior aspect of the lumbar vertebral bodies and compression of contrast material against the bodies. **B,** An AP view of the thoracolumbar junction area shows considerable prominence of the hypertrophied nerve roots. **C,** A midlumbar view again shows the wide nerve roots. (**B** from Rao, C. V. G., et al.: Am. J. Roentgenol. Radium Ther. Nucl. Med. **122:**70, 1974.)

patients were given myelography. Though the disease often begins in childhood, it is not usually diagnosed then because of its rarity.

The plain film findings have been well described (Bellon et al., 1972). There may be scalloping of the posterior aspects of the lumbar vertebrae as seen in neurofibromatosis, a triangularly shaped pedicle due to hypertrophy of exiting nerve roots, and a widening of the spinal canal and interpediculate distance. These findings are less obvious in children because the disease has not progressed as far. Though the spinal canal is not always involved and the diagnosis may be made by peripheral nerve biopsy and hypertrophy that can be felt clinically, the myelographic findings, are quite characteristic (Fig. 19-61). The lumbar area gives the appearance of being packed with large nerve roots which are hypertrophied. The large exiting roots are outlined against the flattened pedicles. Contrast material is squeezed into the lateral gutters of the spinal canal; and transverse barlike defects—not unlike the defects seen in spondylosis—are present secondary to the enlarged nerve roots, taking up most of the available space and forcing the contrast agent into the scalloped and expanded anterior space behind the vertebral bodies.

The disk spaces do not respond to the pressure of the crowded subarachnoid space and thus narrow it relatively, causing the barlike defects. Myelography may be difficult. Typically, only a small amount of

CSF returns through the lumbar puncture needle and the injected contrast material moves very slowly as though it were subdural. The hypertrophied nerve roots may initially give a confusing appearance suggestive of arachnoid adhesions. Biopsy will confirm the diagnosis if need be. We believe the myelographic findings are characteristic enough to preclude nerve biopsy in most cases.

Isolated nerve root hypertrophy has also been reported as a myelographic finding (Gulati and Rout, 1973). Its relationship to Dejerine-Sottas disease, however, has not been established.

Disk disease

Disk disease is uncommon in childhood. It accounts for only about 2.3% of all myelograms at The Hospital for Sick Children, Toronto. Most cases seen are in teen-agers, the youngest patient being 11 years. Symptoms are well localized to a single nerve root and often follow injury or exertion. In children there are not the confusing multiple levels of disk disease and hypertrophic spurs seen in adults. The protruding disk is usually of small to moderate size and easily visualized at myelography (Figs. 19-62 and 19-63). As in adults—when performing lumbar myelography in children, the neuroradiologist must be careful not to select the involved interspace for the lumbar puncture and not to mistake a needle-related defect for a disk abnormality. Unlike adults, children never mani-

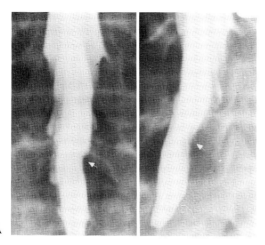

Fig. 19-62. Herniated disk. A small lateral disk compresses a lumbar nerve root (arrows) in an 11-year-old child. (**A**, AP and, **B**, oblique views.)

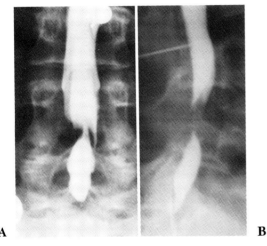

Fig. 19-63. Herniated disk. A larger anterior disk herniation also causes some narrowing of the intervertebral space. (**A**, AP and, **B**, lateral views.)

fest asymptomatic unsuspected disk disease at myelography.

Scoliosis

Scoliosis is a relatively common orthopedic problem in children. Infrequently does it come to the attention of the neuroradiologist, however. There are two occasions when myelography is needed.

The first is a *spina bifida associated with scoliosis.* Because spina bifida may signify a tethered conus, a significant percentage of which have scoliosis without neurological findings, myelography is indicated before operative treatment. With further evidence of dysraphia (e.g., hemivertebrae) or narrowed disk spaces,

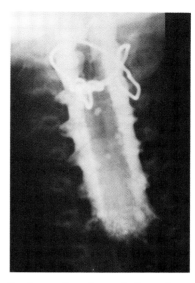

Fig. 19-64. Cord atrophy. A cervical myelogram shows the cord narrowed relative to the subarachnoid space in a quadriplegic child several months after an injury to the upper cervical spine.

the possibility of diastematomyelia should also be entertained. Operative straightening of the spine may cause neurological symptoms in tethering and diastematomyelia. A neurosurgical laminectomy is extremely difficult through a fused spine.

The second occasion when myelography is useful is a *scoliosis with progressive neurological symptoms* or a progressive scoliosis occurring at a younger age than usual. Rarely does this signify an intramedullary mass such as a tumor or syringomyelia (Curtiss and Collins, 1961).

Myelography may be difficult in scoliotic patients. A large amount of contrast material must be used and the patient often must be turned in several directions to pool the contrast in the scoliotic curves.

Spinal cord atrophy

Atrophy of the spinal cord is quite uncommon in children. It may be seen as a posttraumatic phenomenon, associated with radiation therapy for tumor, and as a part of Friedreich's ataxia. In all cases the width of the spinal cord is reduced relative to that of the subarachnoid space. This is easily seen by either air or oil myelography (Fig. 19-64). In the case of Friedreich's ataxia, it is likely to be seen in the upper cervical spine as part of a pneumoencephalographic study.

Spondylolisthesis

Spondylolisthesis is uncommon in children. We have performed myelography on only ten patients. The largest series comes from the Montreal Children's Hospital in a review of sixty-three cases of spondylolysis, fifty-two of whom had an associated spondylolisthesis (McKee et al., 1971). These investigators found that nearly all cases occurred at the L5-S1 level, with 5% at the L4-L5 level. The lesions occur equally in males and females and in most cases are not symptomatic. Though acquired, only one quarter are associated with trauma of recent origin. Five of the cases were of a congenital type in which the articular facets of the pedicles were in a sagittal rather than an oblique plane, allowing slippage of one vertebral body on another. This is the only type not associated with a spondylolysis of the posterior elements. McKee and co-workers (1971) believe that the spondylolysis is caused by either a congenital weakness which allows the pedicle to be easily fractured or a nonunion of stress fractures in any child.

Children who do present with symptoms usually have low back pain and nerve root irritation. Myelography is carried out to reveal the amount of compression of the nerve roots and subarachnoid space (Figs. 19-65 and 19-66).

There are reports of spondylolisthesis occurring in the cervical spine (Dawley, 1971). This also occurs in children and does not appear to be associated with trauma, but it may be associated with other abnormalities (Fig. 19-67).

TRAUMA
Cord edema

At myelography, cord edema resembles other intramedullary swelling such as that secondary to inflammation or intramedullary tumor. Slow flow is seen as the contrast material is made to flow over the affected area. Increased size of the cord is also noted. In the case of cord edema, the history helps differentiate this lesion from others.

Hematoma

A traumatic hematoma, either intramedullary or extramedullary, resembles other masses of the in-

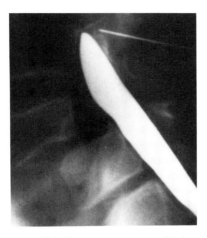

Fig. 19-65. Spondylolisthesis. A 12-year-old boy had third-degree spondylolisthesis without any compression of the subarachnoid space.

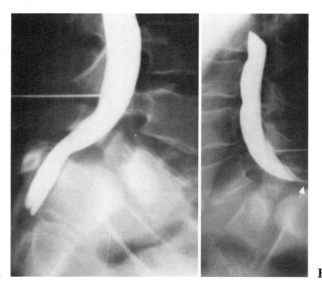

A   B

Fig. 19-66. Third-degree spondylolisthesis. In the prone position (A) there is little compression of the subarachnoid space. In the semierect position, however, there is a cutoff of the subarachnoid space at the affected level (B, arrow). (An 11-year-old boy.)

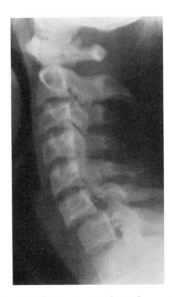

Fig. 19-67. Spondylolisthesis. A lateral cervical spine film shows mild spondylolisthesis at the C6-C7 level in an asymptomatic child with hemifacial microsomia.

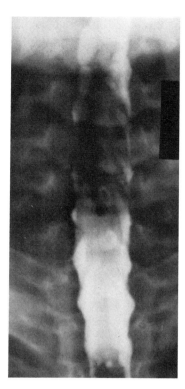

Fig. 19-68. Intramedullary hematoma. An AP cervical myelogram shows diffuse swelling of the cervical cord due to an intramedullary hematoma from fracture of the C4 vertebral body.

volved area. The intramedullary hematoma shows diffuse cord swelling (Fig. 19-68). The extramedullary hematoma, most often extradural, gives the picture of an extradural mass compressing the cord (Fig. 19-69). The history, of course, indicates the true diagnosis. Because the space dorsal to the dura is roomier, most extradural hematomas arise as posteriorly located masses.

More confusing is the spontaneous extradural hematoma. Though rare in any age, 17% of those reported have occurred below age 20 (Pear, 1972). The history may be quite variable, 2 days to several months; the myelographic picture is of an extradural mass obstructing or constricting the flow of contrast. The usually posterior and thoracic locations are clues to the correct diagnosis. Many of these spontaneous hematomas are thought to be due to bleeding of cryptic AVMs. At myelography the radiologist must look for other AVMs of the cord if the diagnosis of spontaneous epidural hematoma is suspected. Coagulation defects must also be ruled out once the diagnosis is established (Fig. 19-70).

Battered children may have both extradural hematomas and cord swelling (Swischuk, 1969). Though there is usually evidence of bony trauma on plain films, this does not have to be present. Experi-

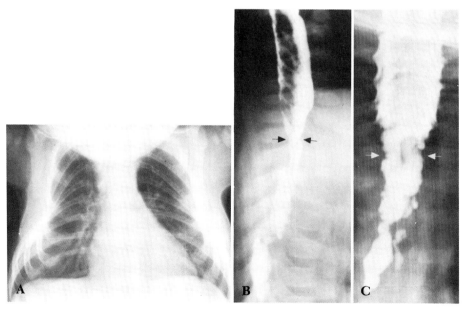

Fig. 19-69. Intradural-extradural hematoma. A 2-month-old child involved in an auto accident became quadriplegic without a vertebral fracture. **A,** A chest film shows the bell-shaped chest from loss of intercostal muscle function. **B** and **C,** Lateral and AP views of a myelogram via cisternal puncture show the cord swollen in the cervical area. The dye column and cord are compressed in all directions in the upper thoracic area (arrows). There is dorsal displacement of the dye column in the midthoracic area, with complete obstruction at T6. Operation revealed a swollen cervical cord and a thoracic subdural and extradural hematoma with a dural tear at T2.

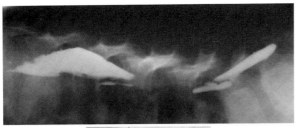

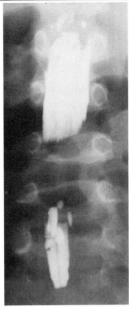

Fig. 19-70. Spontaneous extradural hematoma. This bleeding occurred in the lumbar area of a hemophiliac patient. Note the posterior location, which causes the dye column to be compressed ventrally and nearly completely blocked. (**A,** Lateral and, **B,** AP views.)

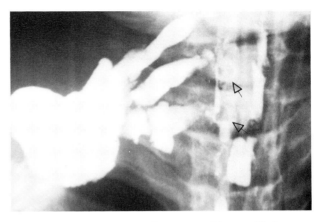

Fig. 19-71. Nerve root avulsions. A 15-year-old boy was thrown from a motorcycle and landed on his outstretched arm. Avulsion of nerve roots from C6, C7, and T1 occurred. Contrast material can be seen tracking out the nerve root sleeves into a large extradural pool. Circular rings of Pantopaque (arrows) may be areas where the nerve roots were pulled off the cord.

mental evidence in cats (Allen et al., 1974) suggests that trauma to the cord causes immediate extravasation of blood in the gray matter and loss of electrical activity in gray and white matter even without the extravasation of blood. Permanent damage probably results from direct vessel tearing within the cord rather than from ischemia secondary to an intact vessel reaction to the trauma.

Tissue disruption

Nerve root avulsions usually occur in the cervical area and are due to severe posterior extension of the arm. Often resulting from a fall on an outstretched arm in adults and children, the avulsions are also seen in infants and are the result of birth trauma. Clinically there is a paralysis of the affected limb. An Erb-Duchenneye paralysis of the shoulder and elbow indicates a C5-C7 root injury. A Klumpke's paralysis of the hand is from a C8-T1 injury. A Horner's syndrome due to T1 injury of the stellate ganglion may also be present.

The myelographic picture is unique. The term *traumatic meningocele* (Murphey et al., 1947) is a graphic description of the injury. There are pockets of extradural extravasation where the roots have been pulled from the cord (Fig. 19-71). If the dura has healed, the pockets may be small; if the avulsion is *fresh*, the contrast may flow far out into the nerve sheath. Because of the nerve root avulsion, the nerve root is not visible within the sac caused by the injury. Later healing or initial hematoma may close or obliterate the traumatic sac. The area of damage may then present as a flat arachnoid surface; but again the lucent defect of the nerve root will be absent (Lester, 1961). Less common occurrences are a smaller than normal nerve root secondary to a partial tear or displacement of the dye column by loculated CSF in a traumatic cyst (Fig. 19-72) (Davies et al., 1966).

The traumatic meningocele can be mimicked by the lateral outpouchings of the dural nerve root sacs that are sometimes associated with Scheuermann's disease. This sac is usually thoracic, however, and is rarely cervical; and it contains the root within it (Lester, 1961).

Lumbar nerve root avulsion is quite rare, though instances have been reported with severe pelvic fracture (Alker et al., 1967; Carlson and Hoffman, 1971). It has the same appearance as cervical avulsion.

In spite of studies showing spinal cord damage may be a causative factor in 10% of neonatal deaths, birth trauma is not often implicated (even by paediatric radiologists) (Towbin, 1964). Though well known as the result of breech delivery, it is rare in cephalic delivery—in which case, torsion of the cord is probably the cause (Norman and Wedderburn,

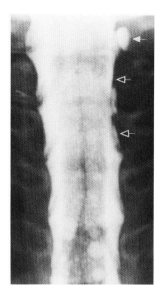

Fig. 19-72. Nerve root avulsion. An 8-year-old girl with traumatic birth and Klumpe's paralysis manifested the features of healed nerve root avulsion, including a small traumatic cyst (solid arrow) with an incomplete nerve root at that level as compared with the opposite side. Flattening of the arachnoid space two levels caudad (open arrows) was observed along with absent nerve roots at these levels.

1973). In breech delivery, traction on the cervical cord or arm is the usual causative factor.

There is often immediate clinical evidence of injury, varying from limb palsies to quadriplegia and a bell-shaped thorax due to intercostal paralysis. Myelography will confirm the diagnosis. Because of the extent of damage to the cord, decompressive surgery usually is not helpful.

The myelographic picture of birth trauma is variable. Nerve root avulsion is common (Fig. 19-73). Hematoma, both extradural and intradural, may occur. Our most traumatic case showed both plus an extradural leak of contrast material from a dural tear. At operation there was also complete transection of the cord, though no bony injury was present either radiographically or at operation. The cord may be completely transsected; but the break will not be seen at myelography, presumably because of hemorrhage and edema that accompany such extensive injury. Likewise, though it gives the diagnosis, myelography may not demonstrate all the levels of damage—especially if there is a complete block.

In birth trauma, surgery serves only as a decompressive maneuver. The severed nerve roots cannot be sewn to the cord. In accidents occurring at a later age, however, there may be clinical uncertainty as to whether the injury is at the level of the spinal cord

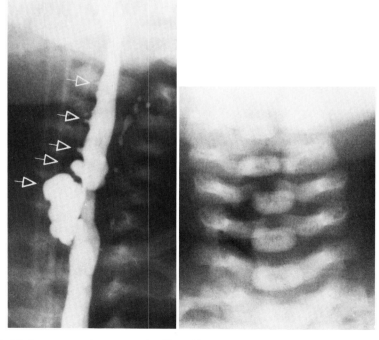

A   B

Fig. 19-73. Birth trauma. A, A 5-week-old child after traumatic forceps delivery manifested avulsion of nerve roots from C3 to C7 (arrows) and pooling of contrast in extradural sacs. (Film taken in the lateral decubitus position.) **B,** A cervical spine film shows lateral displacement of C4 on C5.

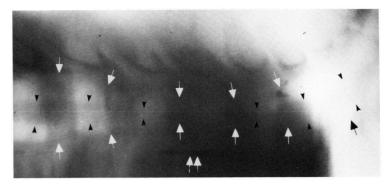

Fig. 19-74. Hypertrophic meningitis. Black and white have been reversed on this prone lateral air myelographic tomogram of the cervical spine to improve contrast. The cervical cord (opposing arrowheads) is compressed in the midcervical area by the hypertrophied meninges, which narrow the air-filled subarachnoid space (opposing arrows). A small amount of Pantopaque (double arrow) from a previous oil myelogram is caught in a pocket within the hypertrophied arachnoid.

or more peripheral. Myelography is useful in identifying the point of injury. With an extradural injury the nerve root will still be in the spinal canal. If the injury has occurred outside the bony spine, resuturing of the nerve (even several months after the injury) can result in a return of some function (Murphey and Kirkland, 1973).

INFLAMMATION

Inflammatory disease may affect the spinal cord itself or any of its covering layers.

An abscess, whether acute or chronic, usually is extradural and acts like any extradural mass. Most often abscesses are caused by local spread of a vertebral body infection or hematogenous spread from some remote infection. The history may not be suspicious for infection, and the myelographic findings may be only of a nonspecific extradural mass. Intramedullary abscesses act as any intramedullary mass and likewise cannot be myelographically separated from other intramedullary tumors. Both types of abscesses are quite uncommon, usually occurring in the thoracic and lumbar areas.

Diffuse swelling of the cord is an acute clinical phenomenon with rapidly progressing symptoms of transverse myelitis. The exact cause is often obscure, though usually it is thought to be of viral origin. The myelographic findings in these cases are also of an intramedullary mass lesion, albeit more subtle than an abscess.

At Pantopaque myelography, the radiologist first notices a subjective finding at fluoroscopy: the flow of contrast is slower than normal around the affected area of the cord. Indeed, there can be a total block of the flow of contrast. The other finding is a diffuse enlargement of the cord, which occupies more than

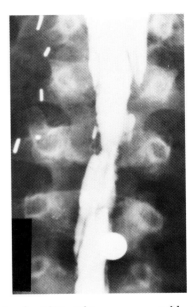

Fig. 19-75. Arachnoiditis. This was presumably secondary to irradiation in a patient from whom an intra-abdominal and extradural neuroblastoma had been removed.

the normal portion of subarachnoid space. The enlargement will most often occur over several segments without a well-defined beginning or ending to the area of involvement.

A rarer phenomenon with a similar myelographic picture is hypertrophic meningitis causing constriction of the cord (Guidetti and LaTorre, 1967; Wirth and Gado, 1973). In this case the subarachnoid space is filled by the meninges rather than by the cord (Fig. 19-74). The difference between the two situations may be difficult to distinguish at myelography, though the constricted cord size combined with the slow flow of

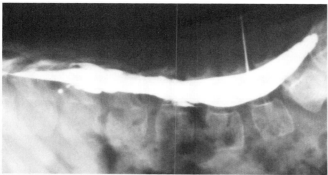
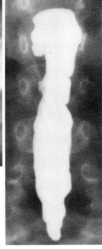

Fig. 19-76. Arachnoiditis. A, Lateral and, B, AP myelograms in a child with arachnoiditis after LP shunting. Narrowing and irregularity of the subarachnoid space occurred over several lumbar and thoracic segments.

contrast material due to the impinging meninges can be appreciated.

In children, chronic meningitis is most commonly secondary to shunts in the subarachnoid space or other operative entry into the space. We have no personal cases of meningitis occurring secondary to myelography alone. We examined one patient who had diffuse inflammatory changes in the lumbar area with a history of a single lumbar puncture and removal of CSF shortly before symptoms began. Children with chronic arachnoid inflammation often have a gradual onset of low back pain and irritation of various nerve roots. At myelography there usually is poor flow of CSF with irregular tracts of contrast material dissecting through the subarachnoid space if the dye continues to be injected (Figs. 19-75 to 19-77).

Retapping of the lumbar subarachnoid space at other levels will usually give a similar appearance. It may be very difficult to separate this picture from that of a subdural injection; subdural leakage may easily occur because of the small subarachnoid space. Due to the frequency of lumboperitoneal shunts in our institution, our experience consists mainly of cases involving the lumbar area. At times, a repeat puncture in the lower thoracic area or even a cervical puncture will be necessary to get enough flow of contrast material to be certain of not having a subdural injection.

There is a slight danger that the myelographic examination itself may cause arachnoiditis; and possibly Pantopaque in an already abnormal area will cause further inflammation. Only enough contrast material should be used therefore to confirm the diagnosis.

A meningitis may occur secondary to fluid escaping from a dermoid cyst. There are no specific myelo-

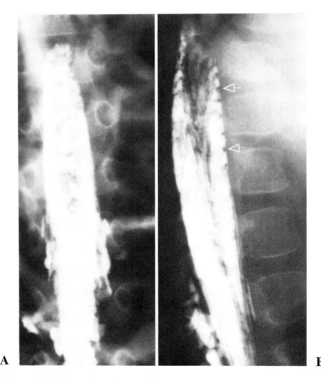

Fig. 19-77. Arachnoiditis. This is an unusual appearance of arachnoiditis, surgically confirmed, in a shunted hydrocephalic child. Small serpiginous irregularities are evident centrally in A (AP view). Ventral indentations of the dye column (B, arrows) may be dilated arteries or veins. Some extradural injection was also present.

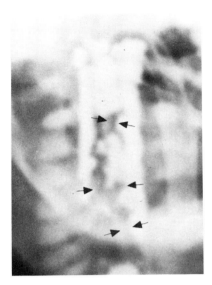

Fig. 19-78. Arteriovenous malformation. An AVM of the cord (arrows) is outlined by oil.

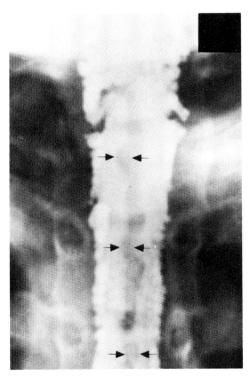

Fig. 19-79. Enlarged normal anterior spinal artery. There is severe coarctation of the aorta in an 11-year-old girl. An enlarged spinal artery (arrows) presumably acts as a collateral vessel.

graphic findings that separate this from any other arachnoid inflammation.

ARTERIOVENOUS MALFORMATION

Although arteriography, not myelography, should be the method of diagnosis of AVMs, occasionally the examiner will discover an unsuspected malformation at myelography; or he will do myelography for other reasons in a patient with a known AVM. Myelography does, in fact, fairly quickly outline the extent of external vessels on the cord surface; however, it does not show feeding arteries or abnormalities within the cord. Additionally, any contrast material left behind at myelography may interfere with visualization of the vessels at angiography.

For the neuroradiologist not accustomed to examining children, the most frequent problem is confusing the prominent anterior spinal artery of infancy and childhood with a true AVM (Fig. 19-78). Whereas the normal artery is quite large and mildly serpiginous, it will not be so large or tortuous as a true malformation.

A more difficult problem occurs when the normal artery enlarges from tumor, inflammation, or the very unusual circumstance of coarctation of the aorta (Fig. 19-79). In such cases the midline course and mild tortuosity will still help to differentiate the enlarged artery from a true AVM.

REFERENCES

Ahlgren, P.: Long term side effects after myelography with water-soluble contrast media; Conturex, Conray, Meglumin 282, and Dimer-X, Neuroradiology 6:206, 1973.

Alker, G. J., Glassauer, F. E., Zoll, J. G., et al.: Myelographic demonstration of lumbosacral nerve root avulsion, Radiology 89:101, 1967.

Allen, W. E., III, D'Angelo, C. M., and Kier, E. L.: Correlation of microangiographic and electrophysiologic changes in experimental cord trauma, Radiology 111:107, 1974.

Anderson, H., Bjurstam, N., Carlsson, C. A., and Rosengren, K.: Lumbar pneumoencephalography in newborns with myelomeningocele, Dev. Med. Child Neurol. 10(supp. 15): 17, 1968.

Barry, A., Patten, B. M., and Stewart, B. H.: Possible factors in the development of the Arnold-Chiari malformation, J. Neurosurg. 14:285, 1957.

Barson, A. J.: Radiological studies of spina bifida kyphosis, Br. J. Radiol. 38:294, 1965.

Barson, A. J.: Spina bifida; the significance of the level and extent of the defect to the morphogenesis, Dev. Med. Child Neurol. 12:129, 1970a.

Barson, A. J.: The vertebral level of termination of the spinal cord during normal and abnormal development, J. Anat. 106:489, 1970b.

Bellon, E. M., Kaufman, B., and Tucker, M. E.: Hypertrophic neuropathy; plain film and myelographic changes, Radiology 103:319, 1972.

Bentley, J. F., and Smith, J. R.: Developmental posterior enteric remnants and spinal malformations; the split notochord syndrome, Arch. Dis. Child. 35:76, 1960.

Bremer, J. L.: Dorsal intestinal fistula, accessory neurenteric canal, diastematomyelia, Arch. Pathol. 54:132, 1952.

Brickner, W. M.: Spina bifida occulta, Am. J. Med. Sci. 155:473, 1918.

Carlson, D. H., and Hoffman, H. B.: Lumbosacral traumatic meningocele, Neurology 21:174, 1971.

Cohen, J., and Sledge, C. B.: Diastematomyelia; an embryological interpretation with report of a case, Am. J. Dis. Child. 100:257, 1960.

Colquhoun, J.: The oblique approach to myelography, Radiology 108:207, 1973.

Conway, L. W.: Hydrodynamic studies in syringomyelia, J. Neurosurg. 27:501, 1967.

Crandall, P. H., and Hanafee, W. N.: Cervical spondylotic myelopathy studied by air myelography, Am. J. Roentgenol. Radium Ther. Nucl. Med. 92:1260, 1964.

Cristi, G., Scialfa, G., Di Pierro, G., and Tassoni, A.: Visual loss; a rare complication following oil myelography, Neuroradiology 7:287, 1974.

Curtiss, P. H., Jr., and Collins, W. F.: Spinal-cord tumor—a cause of progressive neurological changes in children with scoliosis; a report of 3 cases, J. Bone Joint Surg. 43-A:517, 1961.

Dandy, W. E.: Ventriculography following the injection of air into the cerebral ventricles, Ann. Surg. 68:5, 1918.

Davies, E. R., Sutton, D., and Blight, A. S.: Myelography in brachial plexus injury, Br. J. Radiol. 39:362, 1966.

Dawley, J. A.: Spondylolisthesis of the cervical spine; case report, J. Neurosurg. 34:99, 1971.

Di Chiro, G., and Timins, E. L.: Supine myelography and the septum posticum, Radiology 111:319, 1974.

Dommisse, G. F.: The blood supply of the spinal cord; a critical vascular zone in spinal surgery, J. Bone Joint Surg. 56-B:225, 1974.

Ellertsson, A. B.: Syringomyelia and other cystic spinal cord lesions, Acta Neurol. Scand. 45:403, 1969.

Ellertsson, A. B., and Greitz, T.: The distending force in the production of communicating syringomyelia, Lancet 1:1234, 1970.

Elsberg, C. A., Dyke, C. G., and Brewer, E. D.: Symptoms and diagnosis of extradural cysts, Bull. Neurol. Inst. N. Y. 3:395, 1934.

Emery, J. L.: The back lesions, lipomas, and dermoids. Presented at the American Academy of Orthopedic Surgeons Symposium on Myelomeningocele, November, 1970.

Feria, L. G., and Radberg, C.: Complete gas myelography via lumbar injection under pressure, Radiology 88:917, 1967.

Ferry, D. J., Gooding, R., Standefer, J. C., and Wiese, G. M.: Effect of Pantopaque myelography on cerebrospinal fluid fractions, J. Neurosurg. 38:167, 1973.

Finlayson, A. I.: Syringomyelia and related conditions in clinical neurology, edited by A. P. Baker, New York, 1962, Paul B. Hoeber, Inc.

Fitz, C. R., and Harwood-Nash, D. C.: The tethered conus, Am. J. Roentgenol. Radium Ther. Nucl. Med 125:515, 1975.

Foltz, E. L., Kronmal, R., and Shurtleff, D. B.: To treat or not to treat: a neurosurgeon's perspective of myelomeningocele, Clin. Neurosurg. 20:147, 1973.

Freeman, J. M.: To treat or not to treat: ethical dilemmas of treating the infant with a myelomeningocele, Clin. Neurosurg. 20:134, 1973.

Gardner, W. J.: Anatomic anomalies common to myelomeningocele of infancy and syringomyelia of adulthood suggest a common origin, Cleve. Clin. Q. 26:118, 1959a.

Gardner, W. J.: Anatomic features common to the Arnold-Chiari and the Dandy-Walker malformations suggest a common origin, Cleve. Clin. Q. 26:206, 1959b.

Gardner, W. J.: Diastematomyelia and the Klippel-Feil syndrome, Cleve. Clin. Q. 31:19, 1964.

Gardner, W. J.: Hydrodynamic mechanism of syringomyelia; its relationship to myelocele, J. Neurol. Neurosurg. Psychiatry 28:247, 1965.

Gardner, W. J.: Embryologic origin of spinal malformations, Acta Radiol. [Diagn.] 5:1013, 1966.

Gortvai, P.: Extradural cysts of the spinal canal, J. Neurol. Neurosurg. Psychiatry 26:223, 1963.

Greenfield, J. G., Blackwood, W., McMenemey, W. H., Meyer, A., and Norman, R. M.: Neuropathology, London, 1958, Edward Arnold (Publishers), Ltd.

Gryspeerdt, G. L.: Myelographic assessment of occult forms of spinal dysraphism, Acta Radiol. [Diagn.] 1:702, 1963.

Guidetti, B., and LaTorre, E.: Hypertrophic spinal pachymeningitis, J. Neurosurg. 26:496, 1967.

Gulati, D. R., and Rout, D.: Myelographic block caused by redundant lumbar nerve root; case report, J. Neurosurg. 38:504, 1973.

Guthkelch, A. N., Jones, R. A. C., and Zierski, J.: Diastematomyelia with spur; a long-term survey. Paper presented at the American Association of Neurological Surgeons, annual meeting, April 19, 1972.

Haase, J., Jepsen, B. V., Bech, H., and Langebaek, E.: Spinal fracture following radiculography using meglumine iothalamate (Conray), Neuroradiology 6:65, 1973.

Halaburt, H., and Lester, J.: Leptomeningeal changes following lumbar myelography with water-soluble contrast media (meglumine iothalamate and methiodal sodium), Neuroradiology 5:70, 1973.

Harwood-Nash, D. C.: Myelography in children, Semin. Roentgenol., vol. 7, no. 3, 1972.

Harwood-Nash, D. C., and Fitz, C. R.: Myelography and syringohydromyelia in infancy and childhood, Radiology 113:661, 1974.

Haverling, M.: Trans-sacral puncture of the arachnoidal sac; an alternative procedure to lumbar puncture, Acta Radiol. [Diagn.] 12:1, 1972.

Heinz, E. R., and Goldman, R. L.: The role of gas myelography in neuroradiologic diagnosis; comments on a new and simple technique, Radiology 102:629, 1972.

Heinz, E. R., Schlesinger, E. B., and Potts, D. G.: Radiologic signs of hydromyelia, Radiology 86:311, 1966.

Hilal, S. K., and Keim, H. A.: Selective spinal angiography in adolescent scoliosis, Radiology 102:349, 1972.

Hilal, S. K., Marton, D., and Pollack, E.: Diastematomyelia study of 34 cases, Radiology 112:609, 1974.

Howieson, J., Norrell, H. A., and Wilson, C. B.: Expansion of the subarachnoid space in the lumbosacral region, Radiology 90:488, 1968.

Howland, W. J., and Curry, J. L.: Experimental studies of Pantopaque arachnoiditis. I. Animal studies, Radiology 87:253, 1966.

James, C. C. M., and Lassman, L. P.: Diastematomyelia and the tight filum terminale, J. Neurol. Sci. 10:193, 1970.

James, C. C. M., and Lassman, L. P.: Spinal dysraphism; spina bifida occulta, London, 1972, Butterworth & Co. (Publishers), Ltd.

James, H. E., Schut, L., and Pasquariello, P. P.: Communication of hydromyelia cavity with fourth ventricle shown by combined Pantopaque and air myelography; case report, J. Neurosurg. 38:235, 1971.

Jones, P. H., and Love, J. G.: Tight filum terminale, Arch. Surg. 73:556, 1956.

Kurtzke, J. F., Goldberg, I. D., and Kurland, L. T.: The distribution of deaths from congenital malformations of the nervous system, Neurology 23:483, 1973.

Lassman, L. P., James, C. C. M., and Foster, J. B.: Hydromyelia, J. Neurol. Sci. 7:149, 1968.

Lemire, R. J., Graham, C. B., and Beckwith, J. B.: Skincovered sacrococcygeal masses in infants and children, J. Pediatr. 79:948, 1971.

Lester, J.: Pantopaque myelography in avulsion of the brachial plexus, Acta Radiol. 55:186, 1961.

Lichtenstein, B. W.: Spinal dysraphism, spina bifida, and myelodysplasia, Arch. Neurol. Psychiatry 44:792, 1940.

Lillequist, B.: Diastematomyelia; report of a case examined by gas myelography, Acta Radiol. [Diagn.] 3:497, 1965.

Logue, V.: Syringomyelia; a radiodiagnostic and radiotherapeutic saga, Clin. Radiol. 22:2, 1971.

Luyendijk, W., and van Voorthuisen, A. E.: Contrast examination of the spinal epidural space, Acta Radiol. [Diagn.] 5: 1051, 1966.

Mason, M. S., and Raaf, J.: Complications of Pantopaque myelography; case report and reviews, J. Neurosurg. 19:302, 1962.

Mayher, W. E., Daniel, E. F., Jr., and Allen, M. B., Jr.: Acute meningeal reaction following Pantopaque myelography, J. Neurosurg. 34:396, 1971.

McKee, B. W., Alexander, W. J., and Dunbar, J. D.: Spondylolysis and spondylolisthesis in children: a review, J. Can. Assoc. Radiol. 22:100, 1971.

McRae, D. L., and Standen, J.: Roentgenologic findings in syringomyelia and hydromyelia, Am. J. Roentgenol. Radium Ther. Nucl. Med. 98:695, 1966.

Murphey, F., Hartung, W., and Kirklin, J. W.: Myelographic demonstration of avulsing injury of the brachial plexus, Am. J. Roentgenol. Radium Ther. 58:102, 1947.

Murphey, F., and Kirklin, J.: Myelographic demonstration of avulsing injuries of the nerve roots of the brachial plexus—a method of determining the point of injury and the possibility of repair, Clin. Neurosurg. 20:18, 1973.

Neuhauser, E. B. D., Wittenborg, M. H., and Dehlinger, K.: Diastematomyelia; transfixation of the cord or cauda equina with congenital anomalies of the spine, Radiology 54:659, 1950.

Newton, E. J.: Syringomyelia as a manifestation of defective fourth ventricular drainage, Ann. R. Coll. Surg. Engl. 44: 194, 1969.

Norman, M. C., and Wedderburn, L. C.: Fetal spinal cord injury with cephalic delivery, Obstet. Gynecol. 42:355, 1973.

Oden, S.: Diagnosis of spinal tumors by means of gas myelography, Acta Radiol. 40:301, 1953.

Ollivier, 1827. In Logue, V., 1971.

Palozzoli, A.: Riliera clinici e patogenetici su un caso di meningocele sacrale occulto simulante un'ernia discale, Bol. Soc. Medico. Chir. 17:203, 1963.

Patten, B. M.: Embryological stages in the establishing of myeloschisis with spina bifida, Am. J. Anat. 93:365, 1953.

Pear, B. L.: Spinal epidural hematoma, Am. J. Roentgenol. Radium Ther. Nucl. Med. 115:155, 1972.

Pendergrass, E. P., Schaeffer, J. P., and Hodes, P. J.: The head and neck in roentgen diagnosis, ed. 2, Springfield, Ill., 1956, Charles C Thomas, Publisher.

Rao, C. V. G., Fitz, C. R., and Harwood-Nash, D. C.: Dejerine-Sottas syndrome in children (hypertrophic interstitial polyneuritis), Am. J. Roentgenol. Radium Ther. Nucl. Med. 122:70, 1974.

Renwick, J. H.: Hypothesis: Anencephaly and spina bifida are usually preventable by avoidance of a specific but unidentified substance present in certain potato tubers, Br. J. Prev. Soc. Med. 26:67, 1972a.

Renwick, J. H.: Potato babies, Lancet 2:336, 1972b.

Roberson, G. H., Llewellyn, H. J., and Taveras, J. M.: The narrow lumbar spinal canal syndrome, Radiology 107:89, 1973.

Roth, M.: Gas myelography by the lumbar route, Acta Radiol. [Diagn.] 1:53, 1963.

Rubin, S., and Stratemeier, E. H.: Intrathoracic meningocele; case report, Radiology 58:552, 1952.

Shapiro, R.: Myelography, ed. 3, Chicago, 1975, Year Book Medical Publishers, Inc.

Sherman, R. M., Caylor, H. D., and Long, L.: Anterior sacral meningocele, Am. J. Surg. 79:743, 1950.

Shillito, J., Jr.: Surgical approaches to spina bifida and myelomeningocele, Clin. Neurosurg. 20:114, 1973.

Silling, 1859. In Newton, T. H., 1969.

Smith, C., Watt, M., Boyd, A. E. W., and Holmes, J. C.: Anencephaly, spina bifida, and potato blight in the Edinburgh area, Lancet 1:269, 1973.

Smith, D. T.: Multiple meningeal diverticula (perineural cysts) of the cervical region disclosed by Pantopaque myelography; report of a case, J. Neurosurg. 19:599, 1962.

Sogani, K. C., and Kalani, B. P.: Paravertebral lumbar meningomyelocele; report of two cases, J. Neurosurg. 37: 746, 1972.

Spires, P. S.: Spina bifida, anencephaly, and potato blight, Lancet 1:426, 1973.

Sutton, D.: Sacral cyst, Acta Radiol. [Diagn.] 1:787, 1963.

Swedberg, M.: Meningo- and myelomeningocele studied by gas myelography, Acta Radiol. [Diagn.] 1:796, 1963.

Swischuk, L. E.: Spine and spinal cord trauma in the battered child syndrome, Radiology 92:733, 1969.

Talwaker, V. C., and Dastur, D. K.: Meningoceles and meningomyeloceles (ectopic spinal cord); clinicopathological basis of a new classification, J. Neurol. Neurosurg. Psychiatry 33:251, 1970.

Teng, P., and Rudner, N.: Multiple arachnoid diverticula, Arch. Neurol. 2:348, 1960.

Towbin, A.: Spinal cord and brain stem injury at birth, Arch. Pathol. 77:620, 1964.

Wende, S., and Beer, K.: The diagnostic value of gas myelography, Am. J. Roentgenol. Radium Ther. Nucl. Med. 104: 212, 1968.

Wickbom, I., and Hanafee, W.: Soft tissue masses immediately below the foramen magnum, Acta Radiol. [Diagn.] 1:647, 1963.

Williams, B.: The distending force in the production of "communicating syringomyelia," Lancet 2:189, 1969.

Wilson, G., Weidner, W., and Hanafee, W.: Comparison of gas and positive contrast in evaluation of cervical spondylolysis, Am. J. Roentgenol. Radium Ther. Nucl. Med. 97:648, 1966.

Wirth, F. P., Jr., and Gado, M.: Incomplete myelographic block with hypertrophic spinal pachymeningitis; case report, J. Neurosurg. 38:368, 1973.

Yashon, D., and Beatty, R. A.: Tethering of the conus medullaris within the sacrum, J. Neurol. Neurosurg. Psychiatry 29:244, 1966.

Young, I. S., and Bruwer, A. J.: The occult intrasacral meningocele, Am. J. Roentgenol. Radium Ther. Nucl. Med. 105:390, 1966.

Mass lesions of the spinal canal

Disorders of spinal cord function in children stemming from mass lesions within the canal or pressure by mass lesions without are not common. Nevertheless, the importance of clinical and neuroradiological detection of these lesions is not to be ignored. Due to the presence of cranial sutures, children may tolerate an intracranial mass lesion far better and for a longer time than they will tolerate an intraspinal mass lesion. Early clinical signs of an intraspinal mass lesion in a child may be subtle, and radiographic abnormalities of the spine will often be absent.

Comprehensive reports on the clinical characteristics of neoplasms within the spinal canal by Hamby (1935), Dodge and co-workers (1956), and Haft and co-workers (1959), Rand and Rand (1960), and Matson (1969) deal briefly with the neuroradiological aspects of these lesions. Rand and Rand (1960) describe sixty-four children with a neoplasm occupying some part of the spinal canal, and they included eight more cases of nonneoplastic mass lesions. Matson (1969), however, reports 134 children with a primary or secondary neoplasm only within the spinal canal;

but he includes neurenteric cysts as well as a chondrosarcoma and a hemangioma.

In our neuroradiological opinion, it is valid to consider mass lesions of the spinal canal in children regardless of whether the mass is neoplastic, developmental, inflammatory, traumatic, or a herniated disk.

The rationale for this statement is that often only after surgery can the histological diagnosis be known; and from a radiographic and myelographic point of view, one mass lesion may closely resemble another. We believe therefore that any spinal or paraspinal radiographic abnormality should be identified and the site and extent of the intraspinal lesion localized. Because in children a lesion may encroach on either side of the dura or within *and* without the cord itself, the specific site of the mass within the canal frequently is difficult to establish with precision by myelography. With such radiographic and myelographic evidence, however, an informed guess at the histological diagnosis can be offered.

Neoplastic and nonneoplastic mass lesions may resemble each other and may produce similar neurological deficits. The identification of the site of the lesion and its surgical treatment, and *not* necessarily the prediction of its pathology, is important. For these reasons we will consider all spinal mass lesions regardless of their pathology as they present to us from the neuroradiological point of view.

CLASSIFICATION OF INTRASPINAL MASS LESIONS

An intraspinal mass lesion in a child may be one of the following:
1. Part of a more widespread congenital abnormality of the spinal cord and vertebrae
2. A true neoplasm primary in the spinal canal or due to secondary spread to the canal
3. Due to contiguous involvement by a vertebral neoplasm
4. An acquired nonneoplastic mass

Such lesions may be within the spinal cord, within the dura but without the cord, without the dura, or within two or all of these compartments. The last combination is common in children.

Table 20-1. Classification of 200 mass lesions in the spinal canal

Mass lesion	Number	Percent
Developmental	75	38
Dermoid	24	
Teratoma	14	
Hydromyelia	14	
Lipoma	11	
Neurenteric cyst	6	
Intraspinal meningocele	6	
Primary neural neoplasm	60	30
Astrocytoma	15	
Neuroblastoma	14	
Neurofibroma	13	
Ependymoma	12	
Ganglioneuroma	6	
Cerebrospinal fluid–borne metastases	21	10
Axial neoplasm	16	8
Metastatic	12	
Vertebral	4	
Miscellaneous	28	14
Disk protrusion	7	
Hematoma	5	
Abscess	4	
Posteriorly slipped vertebra	4	
Other	8	

Table 20-2. Neoplastic mass lesions of the spinal canal

Neoplasm	Combined series (%)	Rand and Rand (1960) (%) cases	Matson (1969) (%) cases	HSC (%) cases
Developmental	24			
Dermoid	7	3	10	15
Teratoma	7	2	10	8
Lipoma	6	6	5	7
Neurenteric cyst	4	0	2	5
Primary neural	47			
Astrocytoma	15	18	18	9
Neuroblastoma	12	8	18	8
Neurofibroma	7	8	5	8
Ependymoma	8	13	5	7
Ganglioneuroma	3	2	2	4
Meningioma	2	3	2	0
CSF-borne metastases	8	9	3	13
Axial	18			
Metastatic	13	19	13	7
Vertebral	5	9	3	2
Miscellaneous	4			
Unclassified neoplastic cysts	4	1	4	6
Hamartoma	0	0	1	0
Total no. of cases	364	64	134	166

It is therefore necessary to classify mass lesions according to their pathological category and to consider the radiographic characteristics of each mass—whose pathology is determined by surgery and microscopy. The clinical characteristics and surgical management of mass lesions within the spinal canal in children are extensively detailed by Rand and Rand (1960) and Matson (1969).

The Hospital for Sick Children (HSC) series consists of 200 infants and children admitted over a twelve-year period.

Each child seen had clinical evidence of a spinal cord dysfunction alone or together with radiographic abnormalities of the vertebral column. Children in whom an intraspinal mass lesion was discovered had a lesion that was developmental in origin, a benign or malignant neoplasm, or a nonneoplastic mass (Table 20-1). Posttraumatic or myelitic swelling of the cord (Parker and Anderson, 1965), which was of a temporary nature, has been excluded.

The incidence of each group of lesions or of each type of lesion is readily obtained from Table 20-1, and the percentages of each are half the respective numbers.

Other than an associated neural or mesodermal abnormality, developmental mass lesions were the most common (38%) of all lesions presenting with a specific mass effect. The abundant fat accompanying a myelomeningocele was *not* considered to be a lipoma. Dermoids were the most common develop-

mental mass lesion (32%) and comprised 12% of all lesions discovered.

Primary neural neoplasms (30%) had no single common type. In our experience, the ratio of primary spinal neoplasms to primary cerebral neoplasms in children is 1 to 10, whereas Matson (1969) reported a ratio of 1 to 5.5.

Intra-arachnoid metastases from intracranial neoplasms (10%) are probably far more common; but the 10% figure constitutes only those detected by myelography. The actual incidence of intraspinal seeding from intracranial neoplasms therefore is much higher. Most are not clinically significant, however, and thus are not identified premortem.

Of all lesions discovered—axial neoplasms, either primary or secondary (8%), and herniated disks, extramedullary hematomas, intraspinal abscesses, and posteriorly slipped vertebrae (14%) were less common (Table 20-1).

For the sake of comparison, we have tabulated the histological type of neoplasms reported by Rand and Rand (1960) and Matson (1969) with 166 of the total 200 children in our series who had some form of *intraspinal neoplasm* (Table 20-2).

Because each series is weighted toward the particular neurosurgical activity of the center compiling it, the valid incidence of histological types within intraspinal neoplasms only is the mean of the three series. Primary neural neoplasms were the most common (47%); and of these, astrocytomas and neuroblastomas were the predominant histological types. Except that in our series dermoids were common, developmental neoplasms (24%) had no single common type. Metastatic neoplasms to the spinal column and extradural space or neoplasms of the extradural space per se comprised a significant 13% of neoplasms in the spinal canal. Neurenteric cysts have been included among developmental neoplasms since they may be considered *teratoid* lesions.

Sloof and co-workers (1964) furnish a general description of 1,322 neoplasms localized within the spinal canal in predominantly adult patients. Neurilemomas (neurofibroma group) constituted the largest group (29%), meningiomas (25.5%), gliomas (22%), sarcomas (11.9%), vascular tumors (6.2%), chordomas (4%), and others (1.4%). Intramedullary neoplasms occurred in 23% (301), and the majority of these were gliomas (91%).

Epstein (1966) describes the neuroradiological features of 187 mass lesions of the spinal canal in a predominantly adult age group and includes both neoplastic and nonneoplastic mass lesions. He presents a wide variety of histological diagnoses: primary intraspinal mass lesions (48%), metastatic vertebral tumors with intraspinal extension (26%), vertebral tumors with intraspinal extension (13%), and inflammatory and granulomatous intraspinal lesions (11%). Herniated intraspinal disks are not included, however.

Metastatic vertebral tumors, meningiomas, and neurofibromas are common in adults and rare in children, whereas developmental mass lesions are rare in adults; gliomas and developmental tumors and primary para-axial neoplasms are more common in children.

Age and sex. Mass lesions of the spinal canal in children usually present at an early age (Fig. 20-1), reflecting the higher incidence of developmental neoplastic and nonneoplastic lesions in the infant and young child. Twenty-four infants (12%) in our series were under 1 year of age, and the majority had intraspinal neuroblastomas or teratomas. Four neonates with intraspinal mass lesions were seen—two had a neuroblastoma and two a sarcomatous teratoma, all in the thoracolumbar region. Seventy-six children (38%) were seen before the age of 5 (50% in Matson's series), and again the majority had either a teratoma or a neuroblastoma. Ependymomas, dermoids, astrocytomas, and herniated disks commonly

presented after 8 years of age. Primary intraspinal neoplasms are not common in childhood; Sloof and co-workers (1964) reported that 26% of intraspinal astrocytomas, ependymomas, neurilemomas, and meningiomas occurred in patients under 19 years of age.

Mass lesions of any type occurred in as many boys (102), (51%) as girls (98), (49%). Dermoids were more common in boys; astrocytomas, ganglioneuromas, and neuroblastomas were more common in girls.

Site. The general distribution of the mass lesions

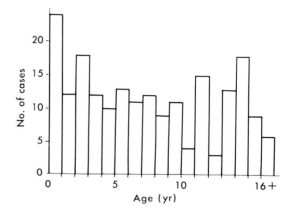

Fig. 20-1. Age and intraspinal mass lesions.

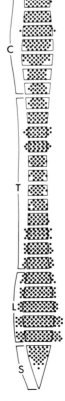

Fig. 20-2. General spinal level distribution of mass lesions.

is graphically represented by a composite diagram of the number of times each vertebral body level of the spinal canal is involved by a mass lesion (Fig. 20-2).

The majority of mass lesions occurred at more than one level and often in more than one spinal region. The cervical and the lumbar and lumbosacral regions were commonly involved whereas the midthoracic area was infrequently involved. Astrocytomas were often in the cervical region. Developmental mass lesions at the site of the embryological lumbar neuropore, ependymomas, and extradural neoplasms were more common in the lumbar region—particularly at the L4 and L5 levels, with extension into the lower thoracic or sacral segments. Midthoracic mass lesions were usually intraspinal extensions of vertebral or paravertebral neoplasms. Rasmussen and co-workers (1940) reported the locations of intraspinal neoplasms in adults to be cervical (18%), thoracic (54%), lumbar (21%), sacral (7%), and multiple (1%)—a quite different spectrum from that in children.

The locations of the mass lesions within the canal itself were *intramedullary* in 22% of patients, *intradural and extramedullary* in 44%, and *extradural* in 34%. Intramedullary lesions consisted mainly of dermoids, astrocytomas, teratomas, and ependymomas. The common intradural-extramedullary mass lesions were CSF metastases, ependymomas, dermoids, and lipomas. Extradural lesions were usually neuroblastomas and extradural extensions of axial and para-axial neoplasms, the majority of which were metastatic or para-axial malignant neoplasms such as retroperitoneal teratosarcomas and secondary rhabdomyosarcomas.

Shapiro (1968) estimates from the collected series of Rasmussen and co-workers (1940), Elsberg (1941), Woltman and co-workers (1951), and Epstein (1966) and from his own experience that in *adult patients* an intradural-extramedullary tumor occurred in 53% to 65%, an extradural tumor in 28% to 30%, and an intramedullary in 7% to 22% (average 15%). Our experience has been that the pathological identity of an intraspinal mass lesion in a child depends on the site of occurrence of the lesion. A few generalities, however, are pertinent:

1. The most common intramedullary mass lesions (in decreasing order of frequency) are astrocytoma, hydromyelia, teratoma and dermoid, and ependymoma.
2. In the intradural-extramedullary compartment the order is arachnoidal metastasis of intracranial neoplasms, dermoid, ependymoma, lipoma, and teratoma.
3. In the extradural compartment the order is neuroblastoma, extradural sarcoma and carcinoma, herniated disk, and neurofibroma.

An *intramedullary* cervical mass lesion is usually an astrocytoma or a hydromyelia; an intramedullary thoracic mass lesion is a teratoma, dermoid, or astrocytoma; an intramedullary thoracolumbar mass lesion with a dysraphic spine is either a dermoid or teratoma or a lipoma. (Without a dysraphic spine it is an ependymoma, astrocytoma, or dermoid.)

An *intradural-extramedullary* cervical lesion is likely to be a neurofibroma; an intradural-extramedullary thoracic lesion is likely to be an arachnoidal metastasis. A lesion in the cauda with dysraphia is probably a dermoid or lipoma (without dysraphia, an ependymona or arachnoid spread of a secondary neoplasm).

An *extradural* mass lesion in the cervical region may be a neurofibroma; in the upper thoracic region, an extradural neoplasm primary to that region or secondary spread to the vertebral bodies; in the lower thoracic and lumbar regions, a neuroblastoma or extradural sarcoma of infancy. Herniated disks presenting in children do so in the teen-age period and often are large.

General neuroradiology

Basic clinical features. Matson (1969) relates the clinical signs and symptoms that occur in children with intraspinal neoplasms. In our experience, the symptoms he describes are similar to those due any intraspinal mass lesion; however, they may vary in significance and prevalence depending on the age of the child and the type of lesion.

Common symptoms are weakness of the legs or a limp (in nearly half the children). In our series, back pain, torticollis, and urinary incontinence were relatively common. Abdominal pain, arm weakness, and rectal incontinence were less common. At The Hospital for Sick Children, Toronto, there has been an increasing awareness of the common association between *orthopedic* foot problems and spinal dysraphia with intraspinal developmental mass lesions (Tachdjian and Matson, 1965). Similarly, the association between *genitourinary* problems and spinal dysraphia not merely due to myelodysplasia but often associated with intraspinal developmental mass lesions or diastematomyelia has commanded interest. Furthermore, a dysraphic scoliosis may harbor an intraspinal developmental mass lesion.

We therefore believe that aggressive clinical and neuroradiological (myelographic) investigation should be directed to the identification of such mass lesions because, although their partial or total removal will not necessarily improve clinical conditions, it often prevents further deterioration.

Common signs are pathological reflexes, flaccid paralysis, diminished sensory level, and spastic paralysis. Sphincter disturbance, scoliosis (rarely kyphosis), and spinal tenderness were relatively frequent. Of all the children in our series—30% had symptoms less than 3 months prior to the definitive diagnosis of an intraspinal mass lesion, 50% had symptoms between 3 months and one year, and 20% had symptoms over one year. The majority in this last time period were children with spinal dysraphia and developmental mass lesions.

Spinal radiography. It is our custom to obtain AP and lateral radiographs of the entire spine in a child with symptoms referrable to a mass lesion of the intraspinal canal—e.g., pain, scoliosis, suspect dysraphia, paraplegia. There are, however, a few exceptions such as a clinical abnormality of the lower motor neurone lumbar root. Mass lesions may be extensive, and the clinical level of neurological abnormalities may indicate only one level of the entire mass. Furthermore, multiple spinal anomalies may be present, some at levels not related to the clinical problem.

To better visualize the intervertebral foramina, pedicles, and articular facets, *oblique* radiographs of the spine may be necessary. *Tomography* is most helpful in the accurate demonstration of subtle pediculate changes or in the elucidation of complex congenital anomalies. Both techniques must precede myelography.

Incidence of radiographic abnormalities. In our series, only 50% of patients had associated spinal abnormalities of any description—be they congenital anomalies or acquired vertebral abnormalities. Many of the acquired abnormalities are very subtle and may be easily missed.

Few mass lesions were constantly associated with spinal abnormalities (Table 20-3); and most of this group were uncommon. Teratomas and lipomas seldom had normal spinal radiographs. Conversely, 20% of astrocytomas, 28% of neuroblastomas, and 35% of dermoids had normal radiographs. Ependymomas (67%) often were associated with normal radiographs. CSF secondary neoplasms were rarely associated with bony spinal abnormalities. Matson (1969) reported an incidence of spinal abnormalities in only 66% of intraspinal neoplasms.

The 20% incidence of normal spinal radiographs with hydromyelia per se is due to the fact that positive contrast ventriculography and pneumoencephalography in infants and young children often revealed hydromyelia before the cervical cord was sufficiently enlarged to alter the spinal canal diameter (Chapters 6 and 16).

Subtle general enlargement of the spinal canal is often difficult to detect. The older the child, the more likely was the spinal abnormality to be present. Spinal abnormalities can be grouped as follows: (1)

Table 20-3. Incidence of spinal radiographic abnormalities

100%			
Ganglioneuroma			
Intraspinal meningocele			
Neurenteric cyst			
Posterior vertebral slipping			
Vertebral tumor			
50%-100%		*0%-50%*	
Teratoma	(93%)	Ependymoma	(33%)
Lipoma	(91%)	CSF secondary	
Posterior disk		neoplasms	(5%)
herniation	(86%)	Abscess	(0%)
Neurofibroma	(85%)		
Metastatic			
vertebral tumor	(83%)		
Astrocytoma	(80%)		
Hydromyelia	(75%)		
Neuroblastoma	(72%)		
Dermoid	(65%)		
Hematoma	(60%)		

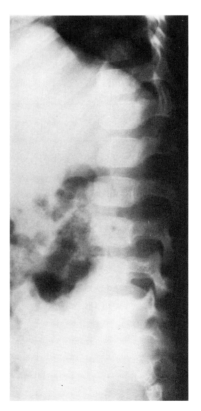

Fig. 20-3. Straight back. Once he has sat up or walked, loss of the normal lumbar lordosis in any child is a significant finding and indicates an intraspinal mass lesion, a vertebral abnormality, or a paraspinal painful lesion causing spasm.

postural abnormality, (2) paraspinal abnormality, (3) dysraphic abnormality, (4) local and general spinal canal enlargement, (5) acquired vertebral abnormality, and (6) calcification.

POSTURAL ABNORMALITY. *Loss of the normal lordosis of the lumbar spine in the absence of dysraphia* (Fig. 20-3) is the single most important radiographic sign which, if associated with signs and symptoms of spinal or neurological abnormalities, no matter how slight, demands myelography. We acknowledge that in other conditions muscle pain, renal infection, abdominal trauma, and such may produce muscle spasm and a similar lack of spinal lordosis. Astute clinical assessment, however, will obviate confusion (Richardson, 1960). Postural abnormality is valid only after infancy, once walking has commenced, for the infant's spine prior to this stage is usually flat.

Scoliosis in a nondysraphic spine is a common sign of intraspinal mass lesions (Chapter 18). It was present in 25% of our series and in 28% of Matson's (1969) series of intraspinal neoplasms. Banna and co-workers (1971), however, considered it to be quite rare. In long-standing mass lesions, kyphosis may rarely be associated with marked widening of the spinal canal. Conversely, idiopathic scoliosis may herald an otherwise latent intraspinal mass lesion, particularly an intradural neoplasm involving multiple segments of the cord, and therefore should always have careful neurological and radiographic

examinations. The idiopathic scoliosis must be a diagnosis of exclusion (Williams and Stevens, 1953). Spinal cord neurological deficit may result from a benign scoliosis (McKenzie and Dewar, 1949; Kleinberg, 1951). Due to the approximation of taut spinal dura, the scoliosis may cause a spurious appearance of pediculate thinning on the inner curved surface.

Dysraphic scoliosis (Chapter 18) caused by a simple hemivertebra, on the one hand, or by gross vertebral and arch anomalies or absences, on the other, frequently contains a lurking developmental mass lesion within the spinal curves. It is often more severe in the thoracic dysraphic states. Associated myelodysplasia or malfixed cords or diastematomyelia as well as a possible mass lesion may account for neurological abnormalities.

PARASPINAL ABNORMALITY. In addition to the pleural and aortic shadows—paraspinal mass lesions, either local and rounded or parallel and bandlike, are important indications of such lesions as neuroblastoma (Fig. 20-4), ganglioneuroma, neurofibroma, teratosarcoma, abscess, and hematoma. A predominantly extradural intraspinal location of the mass lesion is often noted. Associated rib erosion or distraction may also be observed (Fig. 20-4, A). A word of warning, however: a focal mass lesion may present in, for example, the upper thorax whereas the spinal neurological deficit and the myelographic block may be at a much lower level or vice versa.

Extradural spread occurs in these instances without

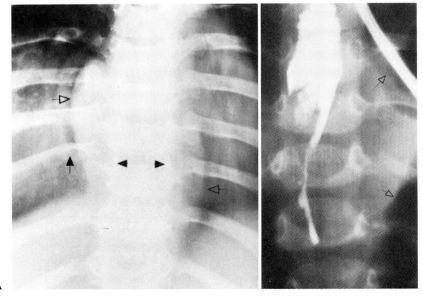

Fig. 20-4. Paraspinal neuroblastomas with intraspinal extension. A, Bilateral localized (open arrows), with destruction and upward displacement of the right ninth rib (solid arrow) and destruction of the pedicles of the ninth thoracic vertebra (arrowheads). **B,** Large paraspinal soft tissue mass (arrows) at the level of T9 to T12 extending into the extradural intraspinal space and displacing the cord to the right in another child.

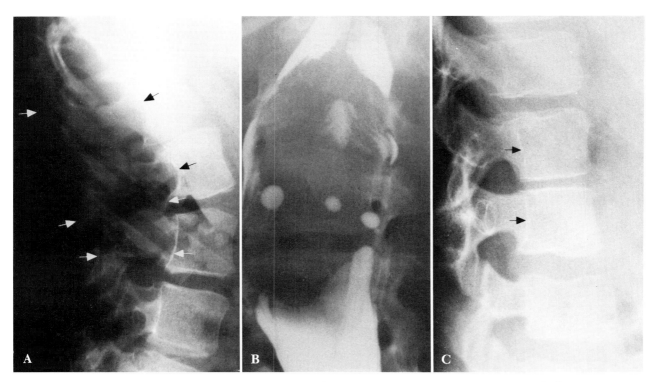

Fig. 20-5. Dysraphic abnormalities and developmental intraspinal mass lesions. A, Multiple partial block vertebrae of the lower thoracic and upper lumbar spine with scalloping of the posterior borders of the vertebral bodies (black arrows) and marked widening of the spinal canal at this level (white arrows). There is also a scoliosis. B, A myelogram demonstrates a huge intramedullary cystic teratoma with extramedullary extension. C, Minor block vertebrae formation with more subtle posterior vertebral body scalloping (arrows). A two-level intramedullary dermoid was discovered in another child.

a paraspinal mass effect and leads to greater compression of the distal spinal cord. A pelvic neoplasm may intrude within the sacral canal, as may a mediastinal teratoma into the thoracic spinal canal. The right azygous vein shadow and the phrenicopericardial ligament shadow alongside the lower thoracic vertebrae (Caffey, 1972) are normal. It is our dogmatic policy to perform myelography on any patient with a paraspinal mass lesion, even if no neurological deficit is present.

DYSRAPHIC ABNORMALITY. Spinal dysraphia and scoliosis, spinal canal widening, and anomalies of the vertebral body and arch commonly occur in the lumbar and sacral regions (Fig. 20-5, A and B) (Chapter 18). Marked scalloping of the dorsal vertebral surface suggests an underlying mass lesion (Fig. 20-5, B and C); anterior thoracic hemivertebrae may indicate the presence of a neurenteric cyst; and absent pedicles often lead to posterior slipping of the vertebral body (Fig. 20-6).

A simple discretely bifid vertebral spine may uncommonly be the only indication of an underlying developmental mass lesion (Fig. 20-7) and should

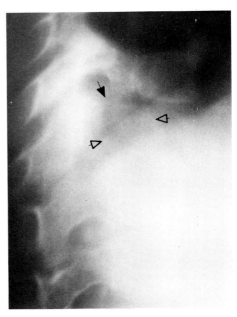

Fig. 20-6. Posterior slippage of a vertebral body with an absent pedicle. The absent pedicle (solid arrow) and the posteriorly lapsed T7 (open arrows) are seen.

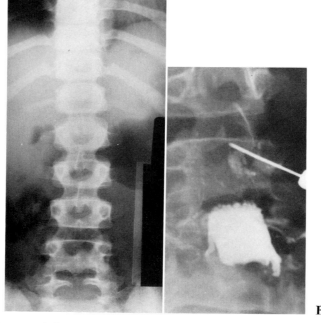

Fig. 20-7. Simple spina bifida and an underlying lipoma. A, Localized, of L5 with a mild lower thoracic scoliosis. **B,** A myelogram demonstrates a lobulated block at this level. At operation a discrete lipoma was removed.

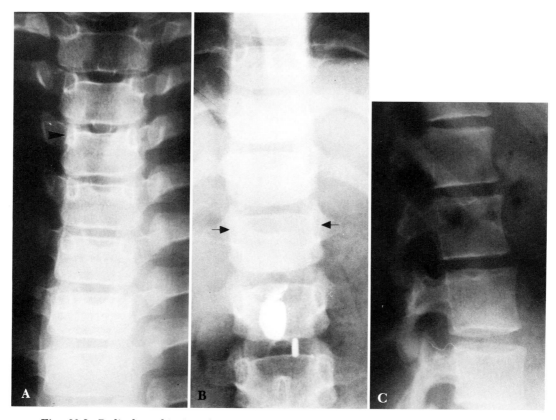

Fig. 20-8. Pediculate thinning due to intraspinal mass lesions. A, Extremely subtle, as in this child with an astrocytoma between T3 and T5. Note the thinning of the right pedicle of T4 (arrowhead). Note also the slight scoliosis. **B,** Marked, of both pedicles at L1 (arrows), and minor, of the pedicles at L2, with some inferior sharpening of the T12 pedicles both due to an intramedullary dermoid are evident. **C,** Straightening of the physiological lumbar lordosis, flattening of the normal slight concavity of each posterior vertebral body, and widening of the spinal canal in the lumbar region are due to a large ependymoma. This neoplasm, however, may also produce abnormal scalloping (Fig. 20-10, *D*).

not be confused with the cleftlike space in the midline of spinous process of young children, which is unossified cartilage. There must be some additional asymmetry between the arches.

LOCAL OR GENERAL SPINAL CANAL ENLARGEMENT. Spinal canal enlargement may be evident merely by subtle thinning of one (Fig. 20-8, *A*) or more (Fig.

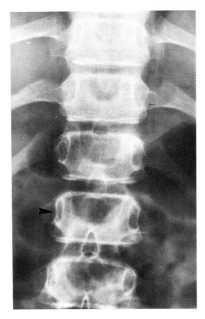

Fig. 20-9. Normal flattening of the L1 pedicle. The right L1 pedicle (arrowhead) is thinner than the left, commonly seen in normal children.

20-8, *B*) pedicles on the inner pediculate surface at the level of the enlargement; or there may be subtle flattening of the gently concave dorsal surfaces of a vertebral body (Fig. 20-8, *C*). Asymmetrical pedicles are normally common at the T12 and L1 vertebrae (Benzian et al., 1971) and may be normally slightly flattened relative to their companions on either side (Fig. 20-9).

The cervical interpediculate* distance in infants and young children is normally disproportionally wider than in older children and adults, as is the sagittal diameter of the cervical spine in the same age group. This is due partly to the immature sagittally narrow cervical vertebral bodies. Minor concavities of the dorsal vertebral bodies in the lumbar region are common in children (Fig. 20-10, *A*). Abnormal scalloping of this dorsal vertebral surface (Shealy et al., 1964; Mitchell et al., 1967) may occur in chronic progressive EVOH (Fig. 20-10, *B*), achondroplasia, Hurler's disease, Marfan's syndrome, spondyloepiphyseal dysplasia, and neurofibromatosis (Laws and Pallis, 1963) as well as in spinal dysraphia and dural ectasia (Fig. 20-10, *C*) (Heard and Payne, 1962) and in intraspinal mass lesions (Fig. 20-10, *D*). French and Peyton (1942), Simrie and Thurston (1955), and Schwartz (1956) specified the normal interpediculate distances in children; and Hinck and co-workers (1962) detailed the normal sagittal diameters. In our experience, the sagittal diameters

*Note: Interpedicular distance is the distance between one louse and another.

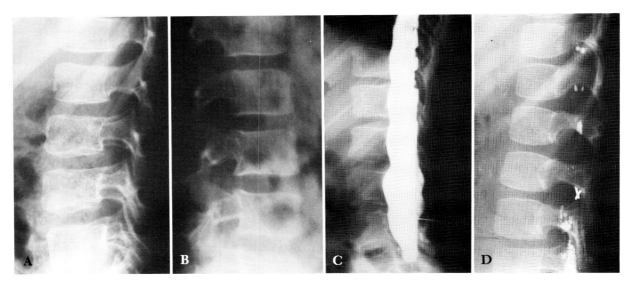

Fig. 20-10. Normal and abnormal scalloping of the vertebral bodies. A, Normal and mild, of the lower thoracic and lumbar vertebrae. **B,** More marked, of the posterior vertebral bodies, produced by a chronic EVOH. **C,** Moderate to severe, caused by spinal dysraphia with dural ectasia. **D,** Marked posterior, resulting from an extensive spinal ependymoma that extends from T12 to L5 (Fig. 20-8, *C*).

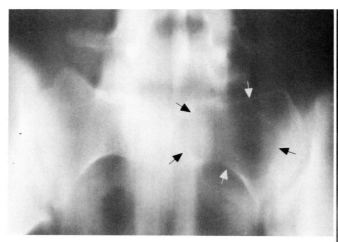

A

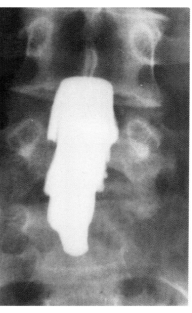

B

Fig. 20-11. Aneurysmal bone cyst of the sacrum. A huge cyst of the left sacrum (arrows) has destroyed the pedicle of S1 and caused an extradural compression of the distal spinal subarachnoid space (B).

of the C4 to C7 levels are virtually the same and any sagittal diameter of the spinal canal greater than one and a half times the sagittal width of the related vertebral body at the same level should be examined with great suspicion. Measurements do provide some assistance to the neophyte and may serve to confirm a suspicious widening, but they should not supercede in significance evaluation by the educated eye.

Banna and co-workers (1971) offer a useful rule of thumb in the assessment of interpediculate distances: the allowable difference in the interpediculate distance between adjacent levels from T2 to T10 is 2 mm; at T1 and T2 and from T10 to L1, 3 mm; from L1 to L4, 2 mm; and from L5 to S3, 3 to 4 mm. These figures apply only to the nondysraphic spine.

Anteroposterior and lateral tomography is invaluable for delineating some subtle changes in the pediculate configuration and spinal canal diameters. Extensive spinal canal enlargement throughout many spinal regions may occur with an astrocytoma, hydromyelia, or teratoma and may even extend from the upper cervical to the midlumbar region. Flattening of the pedicles may be more on one side than the other, indicating an asymmetrical lesion. Local or extensive spinal canal expansion indicates a chronic process and may be quite extensive at the time of clinically provoked spinal radiographs.

ACQUIRED VERTEBRAL ABNORMALITY. As in adults, disk space narrowing in infants and children is related to disk herniation. It may also be related to infections such as spondylarthritis. Bony destruction (Chapter 18), often with vertebral collapse, may be due to primary lesions such as chordoma, aneurysmal bone cyst (Fig. 20-11), osteoblastoma, or hemangioma, to secondary neoplasms such as leukemia, rhabdomyosarcoma, or ill-defined sarcoma, or to direct invasion by neuroblastoma or a paravertebral sarcoma. Enlargement of the intervertebral foramina occurs with neurofibroma, paraspinal ganglioneuroma, and teratoma. Inflammatory destruction will include the disk; neoplastic destruction will not.

CALCIFICATION. Paraspinal calcification may occur in a neuroblastoma or a teratoma. Intraspinal calcification rarely occurs in a teratoma (Fig. 20-12). One cervical intramedullary astrocytoma contained radiographically detectable calcium (Fig. 20-13).

Myelography. Our general principles of myelography and intraspinal mass lesions (Harwood-Nash, 1972b) are given in Chapter 19. We recommend positive contrast myelography for the investigation of intraspinal mass lesions in children. We reserve air myelography for the investigation of a tethered distal cord or filum or a cervical hydromyelia.

Myelography should be performed on children with even the *slightest suspicion clinically or radiologically of an intraspinal mass lesion,* and it should be performed within 24 hours of such a suspicion. It should never be delayed because of negative spinal radiographs. In this way many emergent mass lesions are detected and possible neurological deterioration can be avoided.

Regardless of the absence of neurological symptoms or radiological evidence of an intraspinal mass lesion, myelography should be performed on any child with a *paraspinal mass* (Kirks et al., 1976). Prone, supine, and decubitus lateral views at the level of the extra-axial mass will detect possible intrusion into the

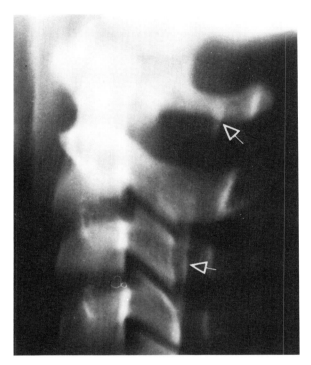

Fig. 20-12. Calcification and a cervical teratoma. An extensive intramedullary cervical teratoma contains a thin line of calcification (arrows) seen best at tomography.

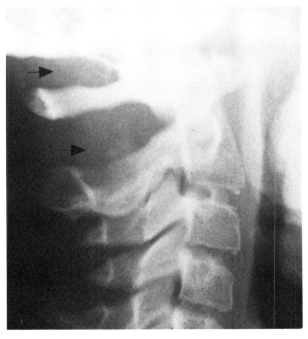

Fig. 20-13. Calcification and a cervical astrocytoma. A high cervical intramedullary astrocytoma has widened the spinal canal at C1, C2, and C3. This neoplasm contained faint floccular-type calcification (arrows).

spinal canal. A laminectomy at this level should *always* precede planned thoracotomy or laparotomy. If not, removal of the mass via these routes may often cause severe bleeding from a possible intraspinal extension and thus constitute a neurosurgical emergency. Renal tumors (e.g., Wilms') do not commonly act in such a manner.

A developmental *intraspinal mass lesion* may exist at a dysraphic site and should be detected or excluded by myelography prior to orthopedic spinal correction procedures, as should diastematomyelia or a low-fixed conus or filum terminale (Chapters 18 and 19).

Certain technical refinements are often required. An intraspinal mass lesion may extend beyond standard radiographic or clinical estimation of its level; and if it is in the lumbar region, the needle may enter it and cause possible bleeding—as may occur with an extensive intraspinal neuroblastoma or leakage of the contents of a cyst like a dermoid, both necessitating an emergency laminectomy.

A lumbar puncture will very rarely cause a more craniad intraspinal mass lesion to cone within the

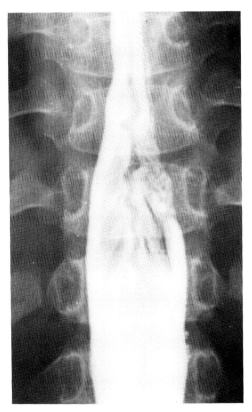

Fig. 20-14. Accentuation of the anterior spinal artery and an intraspinal mass lesion. A diffuse astrocytoma of the conus led to an accentuation of the size and tortuosity of the anterior spinal artery. This does not necessarily indicate increased blood supply to the neoplasm, however.

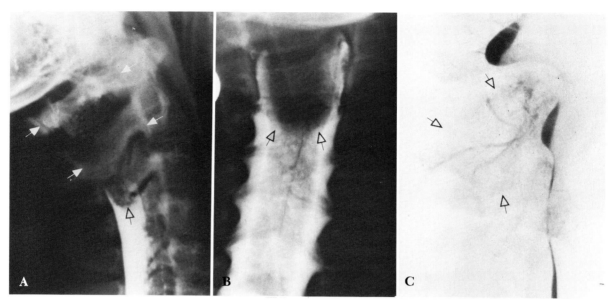

Fig. 20-15. Angiography and spinal cord tumors. A and **B,** A large intramedullary astrocytoma with extramedullary extension in the upper cervical region has expanded the upper cervical spinal canal (solid arrows) and created a characteristic extramedullary myelographic defect (open arrows). **C,** A vertebral angiogram in the lateral projection shows some layering of contrast at the back of the vertebral artery plus marked vascularity in the region of the neoplasm (arrows).

spinal canal. We have seen only one child who deteriorated after a myelogram due to this phenomenon. A totally craniad spinal subarachnoid block may prevent reflux of CSF up the needle. Experience will dictate whether an arbitrary insertion of contrast medium should be performed. Cerebrospinal fluid protein may be so high as to clot within the needle. Supine, prone, decubitus, and cross-table lateral views are necessary at the site of a partial or complete block of the spinal subarachnoid space.

Our practice is to scratch the skin overlying the level of the lesion and to leave 2 ml of contrast behind in the subarachnoid space to facilitate a limited postoperative reexamination if necessary. In instances of a complete subarachnoid space block, we do not insert contrast via the cisternal route unless we fail to insert it via the lumbar route or the neurosurgeon specifically requests additional information. On select occasions we have performed a thoracic subarachnoid puncture using our short-bevel needle.

Determination of whether a mass lesion is truly intramedullary, intradural-extramedullary, extradural, or a combination of these is often difficult—though in most cases an educated guess will be correct. Some intramedullary mass lesions (e.g., a dermoid) will create a straight block of contrast material similar to that produced by an extradural mass effect. Intradural-extramedullary lesions or extradural mass

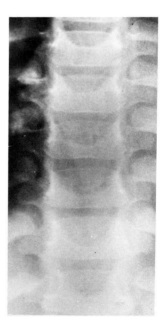

Fig. 20-16. Spinal arteriovenous malformation with large varices. A spinal AVM with huge venous varices widens the interpediculate distance in the lower thoracic spine.

lesions may compress and widen the cord to simulate an intramedullary mass (Traub, 1972). An intramedullary mass may have a small rounded extension into the intradural-extramedullary space to simulate a mass in this compartment.

Specious widening of the cord may occur in the prone position when the spinal canal is posteriorly convex and the amount of contrast material around the cord varies over the involved segment (Shapiro, 1968). The classical myelographic signs of a lesion exclusively within each compartment are often not present. Shapiro (1968) details the myelographic appearances of mass lesions in the different compartments of the spinal canal.

A mass lesion near the conus region often results in an accentuation of the anterior spinal artery to the conus (Fig. 20-14) (Harwood-Nash, 1972b).

Angiography. Vertebral angiography will outline the cervical cord by opacification of its pial coverings (Harwood-Nash, 1972a) and may reveal the vascularity of some neoplasms—especially ependymomas and astrocytomas (Fig. 20-15). Large venous varices of a spinal cord angioma may create an intraspinal mass effect (Fig. 20-16) and are visualized by selective spinal artery angiography.

DEVELOPMENTAL MASS LESIONS
Dermoid

Epidermoids, derived from epithelium alone, and dermoids, derived from epithelium and dermis, including accessory organs such as hair follicles and sebaceous and sweat glands, are lesions that can be differentiated only by histology. They are identical from a neuroradiological point of view. The history of their identification and details of their embryogenesis and occurrence have been discussed by Rand and Rand (1960) and Sloof and co-workers (1964).

Both epidermoids and dermoids have a benign and progressively expanding course that is due to a deranged closure of the neural tube, occurring during the third to fifth week of fetal life. Such sequestered inclusions of epithelium alone or with dermis may be isolated within the cord, within the dura outside the cord, in the extradural space, or in a combination of two or three of these sites. A persistence of a tube of epithelium and dermis may occur from the surface to the mass itself or merely end at the dura, a *dermal sinus.* These are commonly in the lumbosacral region and are rare elsewhere.

Dermoids are seen slightly more often than epidermoids (Sachs and Horrax, 1949; Rand and Rand, 1960). Epidermoids occur within the thoracolumbar spine and are more likely to be intradural; a quarter of them are intramedullary (Rand and Rand, 1960). Dermoids occur intradurally. Dermal sinuses asso-

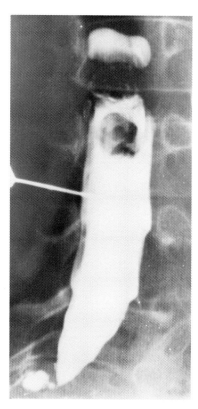

Fig. 20-17. **Implantation dermoids.** Two discrete masses were discovered in a patient who had had repeated lumbar punctures with a nonstyletted lumbar puncture needle for the treatment of meningitis.

ciated with a mass are usually associated with dermoids (Sachs and Horrax, 1949); but in our experience, dermal sinuses are uncommon.

Wright (1971) collected ninety-seven patients from the literature with a spinal dermal sinus. Of these patients, forty-two had associated congenital tumors and all the tumors were intradural. Most sinuses passed through an area of spinal dysraphia; 78% presented because of meningitis or an intraspinal abscess. Thirty-five of forty patients with meningitis had a bacterial meningitis. These episodes of meningitis may occur either in a pyogenic form with intra-arachnoid infection via the sinus or in an aseptic form due to rupture of the dermoid cyst and the resultant arachnoid irritation from the contained fatty acids (Craig, 1943).

Implantation dermoids have been caused by use of an open lumbar puncture needle without a stylet (Manno et al., 1962; Boyd, 1966; Pear, 1969) and have resulted from multiple lumbar punctures (Fig. 20-17), especially during the treatment of tuberculous meningitis (Choremis et al., 1956).

In our series, there were twenty-four children (12%) with an intraspinal dermoid cyst, the most

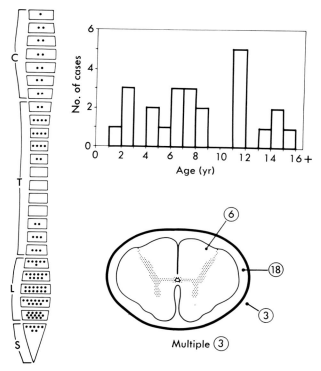

Fig. 20-18. **Age and site of dermoids.** Seven boys and seventeen girls were included in this survey.

common single group of mass lesions in children that were primary to the spinal canal. Dermoids constituted a third of developmental mass lesions. A dermal sinus was present in six children, and purulent meningitis occurred in four of these; two children had a chemical meningitis due to rupture of the dermoid.

Age and sex. No child seen was under the age of 1 year, and most were between 2 and 8 years of age (Fig. 20-18). There was a preponderance of girls (seventeen) to boys (seven). Rand and Rand (1960) reported a series of thirty-eight children collected from the literature between 1893 and 1957 in which only three were infants less than 1 year of age; a similar presentation was found between 2 and 8 years of age, in which twenty-four were boys and only fourteen were girls.

Site. The lumbar region was most common (Fig. 20-18). Dermoids generally extended over more than one vertebral segment. The upper thoracic region was also involved but less often; the cervical region was not often involved. A dermoid within the cauda was a frequent finding, but some of these extended by a continuous mass out from the conus and were considered to be intramedullary lesions.

The intradural-extramedullary compartment was involved most frequently (Fig. 20-18) (eighteen); the intramedullary less frequently (six); and the extramedullary uncommonly (three). In three children the dermoid involved the intramedullary and the intradural-extramedullary compartments as lobulated masses.

Neuroradiology of dermoids

Spinal radiography. Abnormal vertebrae were associated with 65% of dermoids—i.e., 35% of patients had normal radiographs. Of the children with abnormal vertebrae, half manifested dysraphic changes (Fig. 20-19, A and B) that were often mild such as a single vertebral anomaly. Gross vertebral anomalies were not common. In nondysraphic spines, gentle widening of the canal occurred with pediculate thinning (Fig. 20-19, C), and often dorsal scalloping over numerous contiguous vertebral bodies. In some cauda equinal dermoids, a subtle inner erosion of one or two pedicles was present. Scoliosis and a dermoid were not commonly associated (Fig. 20-20). Intraspinal dermoid calcification was not seen. The upper sacral canal was infrequently involved.

Myelography. If no spinal abnormalities are present, our practice is to insert the needle at the L4-L5 interspace. If an abnormality does exist and is nondysraphic, the needle is inserted below or rarely above the abnormality. If spinal dysraphia is present, a similar insertion is performed—unless the dysraphia is extensive, in which case we insert the needle into the general area. Our experience indicates that the dural sac is often wide enough to enclose the mass and maintain a generous subarachnoid space. We have on three occasions inadvertently entered the cystic dermoid itself (Fig. 20-21). This latter event prompts immediate surgery due to the danger of a chemical meningitis. Great care must be taken to avoid this.

The mass is usually lobulated, often continuous with or part of the conus (Fig. 20-22). Less commonly it consists of bilobed (Fig. 20-23, A) or multiple nodules. The dermoid often intertwines itself within the cauda equina, and a complete subarachnoid block by large dermoid may occur (Fig. 20-23, B). Cervical dermoids are rare and may involve the intradural-extramedullary and the intramedullary spaces (Fig. 20-24).

A smaller dermoid may have a smooth surface and present as a focal well-defined subarachnoid defect (Fig. 20-23, A). Recurrent growth after incomplete removal is common, and seeded nodules in the lower lumbar sac may occur. One bilobed dermoid was definitely related to numerous lumbar punctures three years prior to diagnosis of bacterial meningitis (Fig. 20-17). No dermal sinus was present.

From the myelographic point of view, a *large dermoid* and an *intradural teratoma* or *lipoma* are

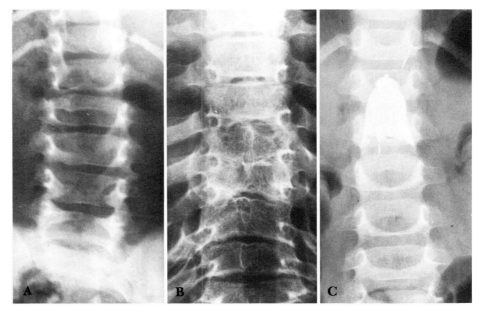

Fig. 20-19. Bony spinal changes and dermoids. A, Widening of the lumbar spinal canal with spina bifida of L3, L4, and L5. A large lumbar dermoid extended up into the lower thoracic canal. **B,** Segmentation defects with block vertebrae involving the midthoracic spine from T5 to T10. Again a large intramedullary dermoid was found. **C,** A nondysraphic spine and a large dermoid of the conus with a markedly irregular upper edge were shown at myelography. Note the thinning of the pedicles at L3 and the slight widening of the lower lumbar canal without marked pediculate thinning.

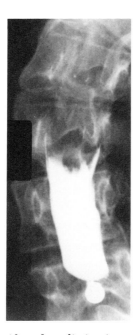

Fig. 20-20. Dermoid and scoliosis. An uncommon scoliosis presented in this child with a large lumbar cord dermoid. Again note the irregular tumor margin.

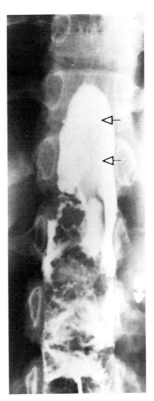

Fig. 20-21. Dermoid cyst puncture at myelography. Inadvertent puncture of a dermoid cyst shows contrast medium in the interstices of the cheesy contents of the large cyst. The spinal cord shadow (arrows) merges with the cyst.

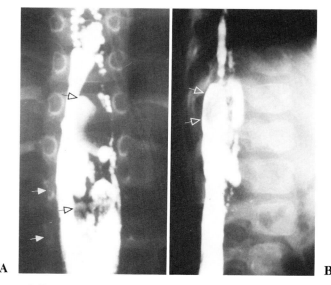

Fig. 20-22. **Intramedullary and extramedullary dermoid. A,** Large and lobulated, of the conus and lower thoracic cord (open arrows). Note the thinning of the pedicles at L1 and L2 (solid arrows). **B,** A supine lateral myelogram clearly demonstrates the upper large lobule of the dermoid (arrows) presenting as an extramedullary mass.

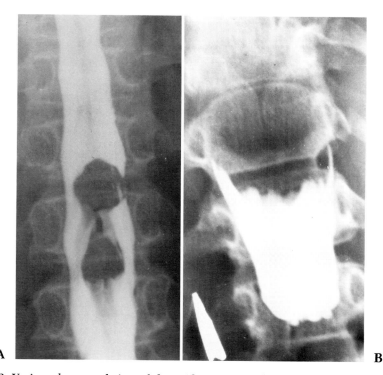

Fig. 20-23. **Various shapes and sizes of dermoids. A,** Discretely binodular, in the lower lumbar cord and extramedullary space. Note the distortion of the nerve roots around the lower dermoid. **B,** Huge intramedullary, in the lower thoracic area.

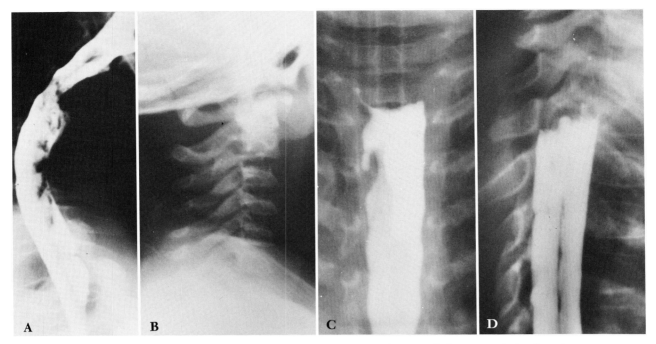

Fig. 20-24. Cervical dermoid. A, An extensive intradural-extramedullary irregularly shaped mass in the posterior cervical canal markedly compresses the cord. It was associated with a posterior midline dermal sinus track. **B to D,** A large intramedullary and extramedullary dermoid extends from T1 to C1 with marked widening of the sagittal diameter of the cervical canal (**B**), producing a complete block to contrast on a prone myelogram (**C**) and in the lateral projection (**D**). Note the mildly irregular block.

indistinguishable. The latter lesion is more commonly associated with marked dysraphic spinal change.

Teratoma

Teratomas contain derivatives from the epithelial, dermal, and endothelial germ layers. Willis (1953) defined teratomas as true tumors comprised of multiple tissues foreign to the part in which they arise. Early embryonic sequestration of tissues results in these lesions, and Rand and Rand (1960) summarized the various theories of morphogenesis and pathological characteristics. Though confusing, the term *teratoid* (Hosoi, 1931) is a pathological description of a lesion very much like a teratoma but lacking endothelial elements. Most teratoids are cystic, as are true teratomas, and may uncommonly become malignant. Sacrococcygeal teratomas of infancy are not considered to be masses of the spinal canal (Chapter 18).

Fourteen children (7%) in our series had a teratoma within the spinal canal; ten lesions were cystic, and five of these were classified as teratoid cysts. Most were extensive. Two were malignant and involved the extradural space, extending from the retroperitoneal tissue.

Age and sex. Contrary to dermoids, teratomas presented at a younger age—seven children under 2

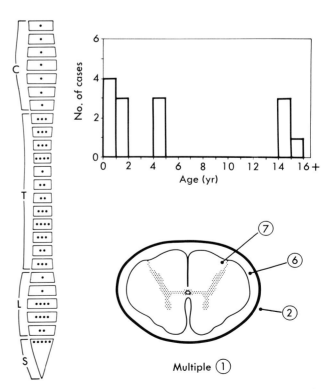

Fig. 20-25. Age and site of teratomas. Eight boys and six girls were studied.

years (50%) and four under 1 year (Fig. 20-25). The older children all had teratoid cysts, indicating that these lesions are a little different from true teratomas of the spinal canal. Boys (eight) were more common than girls (six), again contrary to the situation of children with dermoids.

Rand and Rand (1960) reviewed twenty-one children with a teratoma reported between 1905 and 1955. Ten neoplasms were teratoid tumors, and eleven were teratomas. Seven were cystic, and one was malignant. Boys and girls were equally represented, and 50% were younger than 2 years of age.

Site. Many of the lesions in our series were extensive, involving as many as fifteen vertebral segments (far greater involvement than with dermoids). Lesions were found in the thoracic, lumbar, and sacral regions and were relatively evenly distributed. One cystic teratoma occurred in the cervical cord. Half the lesions were within the cord, six were in the intradural-extramedullary compartment, and two in the extradural compartment. One teratoma involved the intramedullary and the intradural-extramedullary compartments, with discrete globulated masses in both these sites. A teratoma occurred only in the cauda, and another only in the conus.

Neuroradiology of teratomas

Spinal radiography. The majority of teratomas (93%) were associated with spinal abnormalities. Dysraphic changes (Fig. 20-26) were more common in teratomas than in dermoids; but other lesions, especially teratoid cysts, were associated with either dysraphia or simple intraspinal expansile abnormalities including thinning of the pedicles (Fig. 20-27, *A* and *B*), widening of the canal, and scalloping of the dorsal aspects of the vertebrae (Fig. 20-27, *C*). Most extradural teratomas eroded and infiltrated adjacent vertebrae with destruction. Linear calcification was present in the wall of a cervical cystic teratoma (Fig. 20-12).

Myelography. A lobulated large mass is commonly present in the conus or cauda equina (Fig. 20-27) and is indistinguishable from a dermoid or lipoma. An extradural teratoma is malignant and extensive, and a general extradural compression of the subarachnoid space is present. Angiography assists in detecting the vascular lesion within the extradural space and its involvement of vertebrae, often with interposed normal vertebrae (Fig. 20-28).

The cystic teratoma of the intramedullary compartment appears as a smooth diffuse extensive en-

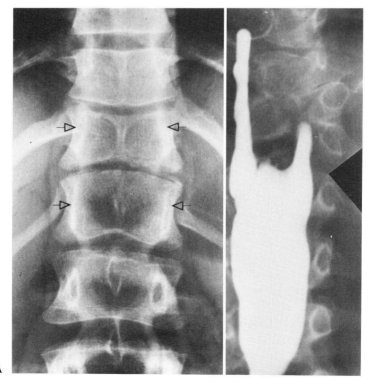

A **B**

Fig. 20-26. Teratomas and spinal dysraphia. A, There is pediculate thinning with interpediculate widening, especially at T11 and T12 (arrows). **B,** An upper intramedullary thoracic teratoma in another child causes partial block to contrast and is associated with marked segmentation anomalies, vertebral body fusions, and butterfly vertebrae.

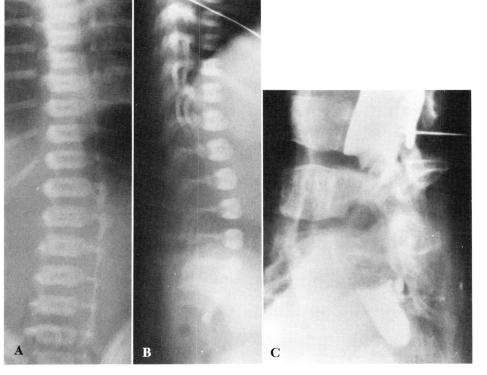

Fig. 20-27. Intraspinal teratomas. A and B, An extensive neoplasm of the lower thoracic and lumbar cord in a neonate extends into the cauda equina, widening the spinal canal in both lateral and sagittal directions with marked thinning and elongation of the pedicles. C, A large local teratoma in the cauda equina of another child has widened the sagittal diameter of the canal and scalloped the posterior borders of the lower lumbar vertebrae.

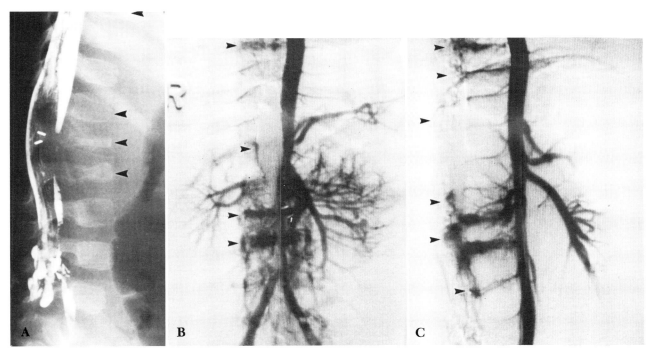

Fig. 20-28. Malignant extradural teratoma and vertebral body destruction. A, A myelogram shows a large neoplasm that has displaced the cord posteriorly and has destroyed numerous vertebrae (arrowheads), which are partially or completely collapsed. B and C, Anteroposterior and lateral aortograms demonstrate the vascular teratoma within the vertebral bodies, its vascular supply, and its extradural spreading (arrowheads).

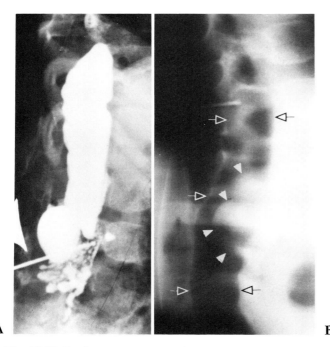

A   B

Fig. 20-29. Inadvertent puncture of cystic teratomas. A, Puncture of the lower aspect of an extensive thoracolumbar neoplasm has filled the cyst itself with contrast medium. B, Lumbar puncture entered another extensive cystic teratoma. The injected air outlines the cyst in the lateral view extending down into the sacral canal (arrows). A large tumor nodule within the cyst is clearly seen (arrowheads).

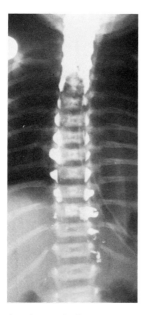

Fig. 20-30. Extensive intraspinal teratoma. An intramedullary neoplasm in an infant extends from the upper thoracic to the lumbar region with arachnoid pockets between the pedicles and the thoracic vertebrae.

largement of the cord, commonly extending over many cord segments or maybe located in the cauda equina. Inadvertent needle puncture during myelography will provide an outline of the cyst and possible intracystic tumor nodules (Fig. 20-29). A complete subarachnoid block may occur, or a slow passage of contrast will be seen through the thinned subarachnoid space. Thus an intramedullary or an intradural-extramedullary mass lesion, often extensive and associated with vertebral anomalies and dysraphia, that presents in a child under the age of 2 is likely to be an intraspinal teratoma (Fig. 20-30). Small vascular nevi of the back frequently overlie the site of a teratoma. A cervical intramedullary teratoma is indistinguishable from an astrocytoma or hydromyelia. Air myelography is necessary to differentiate the former two from the latter.

Syringohydromyelia

A benign cyst within the spinal cord may occur as a dilated central canal or within the substance of the cord. Acquired causes of cysts within the substance of the spinal cord are spinal cord trauma (Barnett et al., 1966, 1973), associated spinal cord tumors (Poser, 1956), or arterial insufficiency to the cord (Blackwood et al., 1963; Feigin et al., 1971).

Dilatation of the central canal per se or cysts within the substance of the cord that are associated with dilatation of the central canal may be concomitants of congenital anomalies of the neural and spinal axis, in particular the dysraphic states (Gardner, 1965; Conway, 1967). They may be associated with myeloceles (Gardner, 1965), with a Chiari malformation (type II in children) (Cameron, 1957; Gardner et al., 1957), with the Dandy-Walker syndrome (Gardner et al., 1957; Baker and Rydell, 1971), and with occipital and cervical spinal abnormalities such as basilar impression (Gardner, 1973). These cysts may also be associated with the Klippel-Feil syndrome, spinal segmentation defects, and cervical dysraphia (Spillane et al., 1957; McIlroy and Richardson, 1965; McRae and Standen, 1966). Additionally, basal arachnoiditis has been implicated (McLaurin et al., 1954; Appleby et al., 1969; Barnett et al., 1973).

Syringomyelia, well described by Ollivier in 1827, is the name given a cavity that is considered to be a diverticulum of the central canal due to rupture of the canal and dissection of the cerebrospinal fluid within the cord (Blackwood et al., 1963; Conway, 1967). The wall of the canal is not lined by ependyma.

Hydromyelia is a term given the dilatation of the persistent central canal that communicates or has communicated with the fourth ventricle at its obex. The wall of this canal is lined by ependyma. Obstruction of the outlet of the fourth ventricle, either in embryonic life (Gardner, 1965) or postnatally due to adhesions and some form of mild tonsillar ectopia (Barnett et al., 1973), suggests a hydrodynamic development of hydromyelia—the driving force being an arterial pulse (Gardner, 1965) or a venous pressure wave (Williams, 1969, 1970; Bertrand, 1973). Gardner's triad is cord cavitation, defective ventricular drainage, and a patent central canal.

Williams (1969, 1970) prefers the term "communicating syringomyelia," applying to both syringomyelia and hydromyelia as just described. The noncommunicating form related to cysts is associated with tumors, trauma, or degenerative conditions. Barnett and coworkers (1973) provide an extensive review of the subject of syringomyelia and consider every aspect of the abnormality, from history to treatment. These cysts, however, are only a clinical expression of a variety of causes. A cyst of the central canal and a cyst of the cord both have the same myelographic appearance. It seems valid to us therefore to avoid confusion by using the term *syringohydromyelia* (Harwood-Nash and Fitz, 1974) which, though perhaps cumbersome, is comprehensive.

Neuroradiology of syringohydromyelia

Fourteen children (7%) of our series had a syringohydromyelia sufficiently large to create a space-oc-cupying effect in the spinal canal. Serendipitously discovered filling of a slitlike central canal by positive contrast ventriculography occurred during the examination of three infants with Arnold-Chiari malformation (Chapter 15) (Tjaden et al., 1969; Harwood-Nash and Fitz, 1974). These children were under 2 years of age and, though the cord was widened, the spinal canal was normal. The ages of the remaining eleven, all of whom had a widened spinal canal, ranged from 6 to 16 years. There were nine girls and five boys. The cervical cord was involved in every case. In three children the cyst extended into the thoracic cord only, and in five children the cyst extended all the way into the lumbar cord.

Spinal radiography. Widening of the cervical bony canal in both the sagittal (Fig. 20-31, *A*) and the coronal planes occurred in eleven of the fourteen children (70%). Thoracic spinal cord widening occurred in two of the children, with extension of the cyst into the thoracic cord (Fig. 20-31, *B*); thoracolumbar canal widening occurred in all five children with lumbar cord extensions. The widening of the spinal canal was regular and symmetrical, leading to thinning of the pedicles (which was often marked). Scalloping of the dorsal aspects of the vertebrae was uncommon and, if present, occurred in older children.

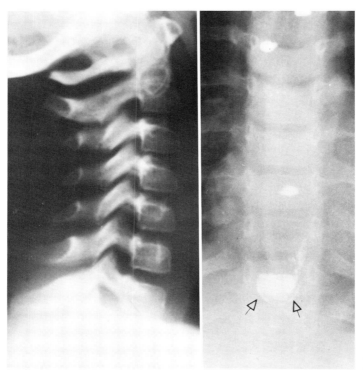

A   **B**

Fig. 20-31. **Syringohydromyelia and spinal cord widening. A,** Moderate generalized widening of the sagittal diameter of the entire cervical canal. **B,** Interpediculate widening and pediculate thinning of the cervical and thoracic spinal canal in an extensive syringohydromyelia. The dilated central canal is demonstrated by positive contrast ventriculography, with the Pantopaque entering the sac itself (arrows).

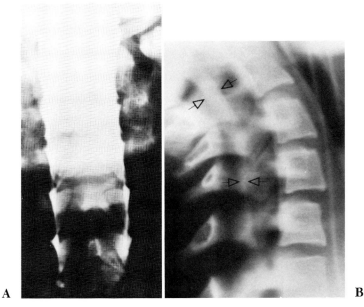

A   **B**

Fig. 20-32. **Myelography and syringohydromyelia.** A Pantopaque myelogram (**A**) demonstrates an extensively dilated cervical cord. A subsequent air myelogram (**B**) reveals collapsing of the cord (arrows), especially at the C4 level (lower arrows).

Scoliosis was present in seven children, four of whom had an associated spinal dysraphia. This dysraphia was present in a total of seven children—five in the lumbar region and two in the cervical spine (one in a child with a vertebral spinal dysraphia and one in a child with a Klippel-Feil syndrome). Another child had occipitalization of the arch of C1.

Myelography. A Chiari malformation (type II), demonstrated by ventriculography was present in six of the children.

The three forms of myelography—positive contrast, air, and myelocystography (direct instillation of oil into the cyst)—will reveal the smooth enlargement of the cord by Pantopaque (Fig. 20-32, *A*), the collapsing cervical cord by air (Fig. 20-32, *B*), and the strange serrated outline of the cyst cavity itself by oil (Fig. 20-33) (Heinz et al., 1966; Harwood-Nash and Fitz, 1974). This serrated appearance, not usually seen with the Chiari malformation but with scoliosis, may represent a syringomyelia rather than a hydromyelia (which usually has a smooth central canal).

A syringomyelocele was present in two children, in one child in the lumbar region and in the other in the cervical region (Fig. 20-34). The cyst within the cord communicates with the meningocele. Air ventriculography demonstrated a large dilated central canal in another child with a Chiari type III and an occipital encephalocele (Fig. 20-35).

The *differential diagnosis* between syringohydromyelia and intramedullary lesions such as an astrocytoma or teratoma is not possible without air myelography or myelocystography.

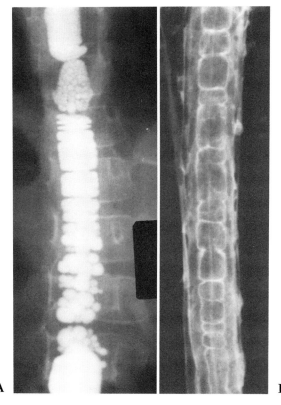

A   **B**

Fig. 20-33. **Myelocystography and syringohydromyelia. A,** Injection of Pantopaque into an extensive syringohydromyelic sac demonstrates a strange serrated appearance throughout the sac. **B,** Postmortem contrast injection in a similar case shows the lobulations and serrations. (**B** courtesy J. Allcock, M.D., London, Ontario.)

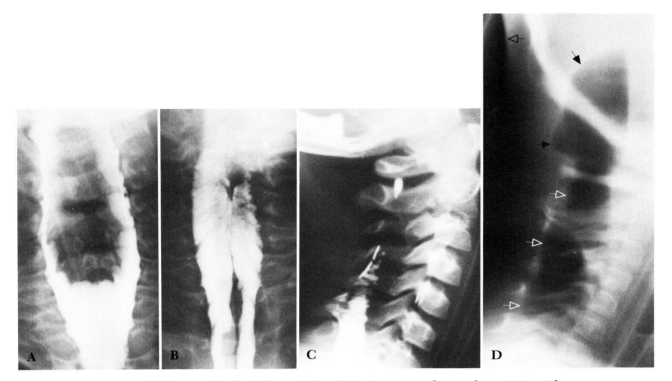

Fig. 20-34. Syringomyelocele of the cervical cord. A, A prone myelogram demonstrates widening of the lower cervical cord. A local spina bifida of C5, C6, and C7 is also seen. Supine myelograms in the anteroposterior (**B**) and lateral (**C**) projections show the cord and nerves puckered through the spinal dysraphia into a small meningocele. At operation this patient had a cystic dilatation of the central canal connecting directly with the meningocele. **D, Chiari type III and hydromyelia.** A child with an occipitoencephalocele (open arrows) had a large low fourth ventricle (solid arrows) and a hydromyelic sac extending the entire length of the cervical canal (white arrows). Note the widening of the sagittal diameter of the cervical canal. These abnormalities were demonstrated by air ventriculography.

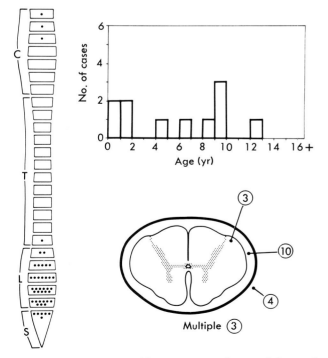

Fig. 20-35. Age and site of lipomas. Seven boys and four girls were studied.

Lipoma

Fatty tissue in the spinal canal, spinal muscles, and extradural layers is commonly associated with spinal dysraphia. Fatty tissue may also extend into the dural space and involve the cord and filum terminale. We excluded from our series, however, the majority of these cases with spinal dysraphia with or without meningoceles which had a preponderance of fatty tissue. We consider a lipoma to be a discrete localized mass lesion in the spinal canal that is causing specific neurological symptoms identical to those of other developmental mass lesions. We do not consider the mere presence of fat to be a lipoma. The majority of lipomas were of localized lesions often with extensive lobulations containing fibrous tissue and intermingled adult fatty tissue.

Metaplasia of spinal connective tissue, the existence of embryonic rests, and the proliferation of fatty cells usually within the pia are a few of the various theories that have been advanced to explain the embryogenesis of these lipomas (Sperling and Alpers, 1936; Ehni and Love, 1945). Rand and Rand (1960) provide a full review of the literature. This embryo-

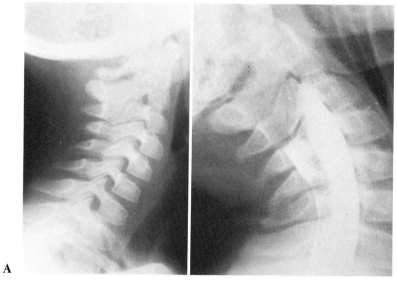

Fig. 20-36. Spine and cervical lipoma. The upper cervical canal is widened (**A**) due to an intramedullary cervical lipoma (**B**). A spina bifida of C2 and C3 was present, and a subcutaneous fatty lipoma with a connecting stalk was also discovered.

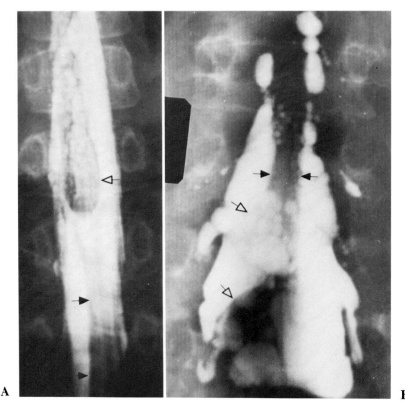

Fig. 20-37. Sites of lipomas. A, In the upper lumbar region posterior to the cord in the extramedullary space (open arrow). A low conus is also present (solid arrows) extending to L5. **B,** In the distal lumbar cord (solid arrow), which is low fixed. Open arrows indicate an extensive lipoma. Note the markedly dysplastic dura and wide subarachnoid space.

genesis associated with spinal dysraphia leading to a compact contained *mass lesion* accounts for most lipomas in infancy and childhood.

Lipomas occurred in eleven children (5%) in our series—a subcutaneous lipoma together with an associated intramuscular lipoma in eight children, and a skin dimple (similar to that associated with dermoids) over the site of the lipoma in three. A fibrofatty stalk may connect the subcutaneous lipoma with the intraspinal component.

Caram and co-workers (1957) reviewed fifty-one cases of intraspinal lipoma occurring at all ages. Rand and Rand (1960) summarized the literature and added five cases of their own to the seventeen thus obtained. Lassman and James (1967) reported fifteen children with an intraspinal lipoma. Gold and co-workers (1969) described the myelographic evaluation of four children with invasion of the spinal canal by a lipoma.

Age and sex. Four of the children in our series were under 2 years of age, and three were aged 9; but a scattered distribution was the order (Fig. 20-35). Boys (seven) were commoner than girls (four). In Rand and Rand's (1960) collected series, eight of the twenty-two children were under 1 year of age and seven were 10 years or older; girls slightly outnumbered boys.

Site. Virtually all lipomas in children of our series occurred in the lower spinal canal, particularly the lower lumbar and upper sacral region. One extended up into the lower thoracic region, and one was localized to the cervical segments (Fig. 20-36). Lassman and James (1967) reported that all of their fifteen children had a lipoma of the lumbar region. Caram and co-workers (1957), however, reported a preponderance of cervicothoracic (22%) and thoracic (35%) lipomas; these occurred mainly in adults and were less commonly associated with spinal dysraphia.

Lipomas presenting as an intraspinal mass lesion in a child are associated with lumbar spinal dysraphia. Lipomas without dysraphia and at other sites will usually present in adulthood. Caram and co-workers (1957), furthermore, described five cases in which the entire cord was involved by lipomatous tissue.

Lipomas commonly involve the intradural-extramedullary space (ten of the eleven in our series) (Fig. 20-37, *A*)—three incorporated into the cord (Fig. 20-37, *B*), four in the extradural space, and three involving the three compartments. Those occurring in the lower lumbar sac generally incorporated the lumbar roots within lipomatous tissue.

Neuroradiology of lipomas

Spinal radiography. Nine of our eleven children had a spinal dysraphia and commonly a moderate degree of segmentation abnormalities. Widening of the interpediculate distances occurred as part of the dysraphia (Fig. 20-38, *A* and *B*); but in most cases, some thinning of the pedicles could be ascribed to the mass. Dorsal vertebral scalloping again was common (Fig. 20-38, *C*). Partial sacral agenesis was prevalent among lipomas of the sacral canal (Fig.

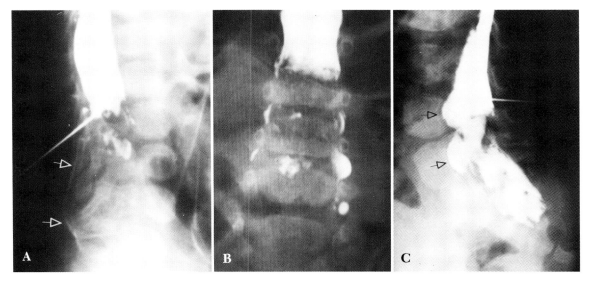

Fig. 20-38. Lipoma with spinal dysraphia and spinal abnormalities. A and B, Marked spina bifida (arrows) with posterior arch deformity (A) and widening of the interpediculate distance (B) due in part to the dysraphia and in part to a large lipoma of the lower lumbar spinal canal which created a complete block to the downward passage of contrast. C, A large lower lumbosacral lipoma with pronounced scalloping of the posterior vertebral body margins (arrows). Pantopaque shows the lobulated appearance of the lipoma.

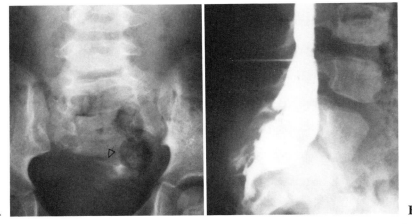

Fig. 20-39. Lipoma and partial agenesis of the sacrum. A, Widened upper canal and partial agenesis of the lower sacrum (arrow). **B,** A myelogram in the same child demonstrates a large intrasacral lipoma with numerous posterior arachnoid herniations.

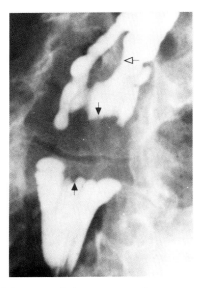

Fig. 20-40. Lipoma and diastematomyelia. Open arrow designates the diastematomyelia; solid arrows, a large inferiorly placed lipoma.

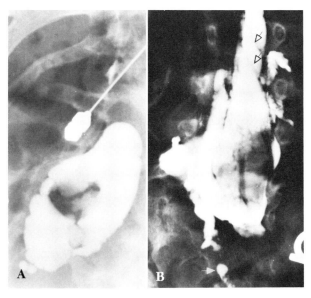

Fig. 20-41. Small and large lipomas. A, Discrete bilobed upper lumbar, associated with a major spinal dysraphia. **B,** Huge lumbosacral, with intertwined roots (open arrows). There is also dysplasia of the dura with enlargement of the subarachnoid space. Note the inferior sinus track (solid arrow).

20-39), a finding that suggests the possible association of a lipoma with an anterior meningocele. Two patients had a high lumbar diastematomyelia (Fig. 20-40). We have not detected the lucency of a lipoma on spinal radiographs, probably because of the associated fibrous content.

Myelography. A low lumbar puncture is recommended unless marked sacral anomalies are present, in which case a high lumbar puncture is effected. Since dorsally situated lipomas are common, supine myelography should be performed. A large irregular-bordered dural sac in the subarachnoid space is commonly associated with a lipoma and represents dural dysplasia (Fig. 20-37, *B*).

The mass lesion may incorporate an enlarged filum and be associated with a low conus (Fig. 20-37, *B*). It may be relatively small and lobular (Fig. 20-41, *A*) or large and lobular through which the lumbar sacral nerve roots intertwine and conus involvement occurs (Fig. 20-41, *B*). In some instances the lipoma may be impossible to separate from the cord and such a distinction can be made only at operation. The myelographic differential diagnosis between lipomas and other developmental mass lesions, particularly dermoids, is often very difficult.

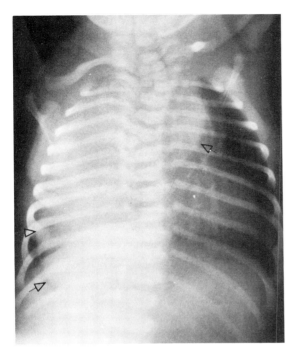

Fig. 20-42. Neurenteric cyst. A neonate had a sagittal cleft vertebra at C6, a left hemivertebra at C7, a maloriented sagittal cleft vertebra at T1, and a right hemivertebra at T5. An enormous right-sided thoracic mass (arrows), extending to the left through the superior mediastinum, was a neurenteric cyst which connected with the spinal canal at the level of C7 and T1. This case is not included in our statistical series.

Neurenteric cyst

Neurenteric cysts within the spinal canal are quite rare (Knight et al., 1955, one case; Matson, 1969, two cases). We have had six infants and children with what was described pathologically as a neurenteric cyst. To most pathologists, whether such an intraspinal cyst is teratomatous or neurenteric is a moot point. We make the differentiation by considering as neurentric cysts only those with *endothelial elements and anterior vertebral dysraphia*.

Neurenteric cysts occur subsequent to persistence of a transient open passage at the third embryonic week between the yolk sac and the notochordal canal, the neurenteric canal (of Kovalevsky) connecting the primitive gut and the dorsal surface of the embryo (Bremer, 1952; Fallon, 1954; Bentley and Smith, 1960). This persistence of the canal of Kovalevsky causes the notochord to split around the canal; and therefore the normal interposition of mesodermal notochord, and hence the vertebra between ectoderm and endoderm, fails to materialize (Elliott et al., 1970). Depending on the completeness of closure in these primitive structures—the result is a wide variety of cysts, cords, and fistulas. Posterior mediastinal masses, cord anomalies, vertebral body anomalies,

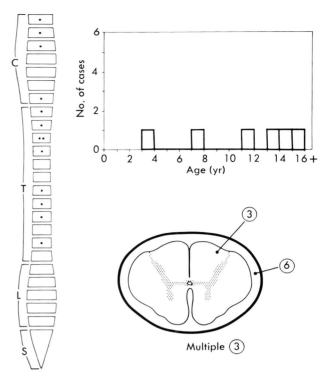

Fig. 20-43. Age and site of neurenteric cysts. Four boys and two girls comprised this group.

diastematomyelia, and enteric duplications either alone or in various combinations may occur (Klump, 1971; Madewell et al., 1973). The vertebral anomalies, which must be of the body at least, are usually complex; but they may be quite subtle and missed if tomography is not performed (Veeneklaas, 1952; Fallon et al., 1954; Wilson, 1969).

Neuhauser and co-workers (1958) describe in detail the radiographic characteristics of neurenteric cysts. The cysts within the spinal canal may occur in the intramedullary, extramedullary, or extradural spaces (Matson, 1969). Neurenteric cysts must have associated spinal abnormalities, and most occur in the lower cervical and upper thoracic area. The intrathoracic paraspinal mass may be quite large (Fig. 20-42).

The six children in our series (4%) presented at a relatively older age (Fig. 20-43). Four were boys and two were girls.

Site. One cyst occurred in the upper cervical spine, and five within the thoracic spine (Fig. 20-43); one of the latter extended into the lower cervical spine. All had an intradural-extramedullary location, and three were also within the cord itself.

Neuroradiology of neurenteric cysts

Spinal radiography. The bodies of the vertebrae at the level of the cyst were dysraphic (Fig. 20-44)

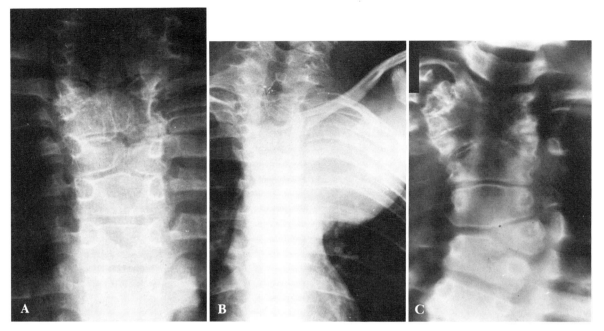

Fig. 20-44. Spinal vertebral anomalies. A, Fusion of the bodies of C7 and T1, hypoplastic hemivertebra at T2, unilateral hemivertebra at T3, and sagittal cleft vertebra at T4. B, These defects were associated with a large left apical paraspinal mass, a large neurenteric cyst. C, Gross vertebral body fusion of T2 through T5 with a hemivertebra at T8 in another child. No thoracic mass was present in this child, who also had a neurenteric cyst.

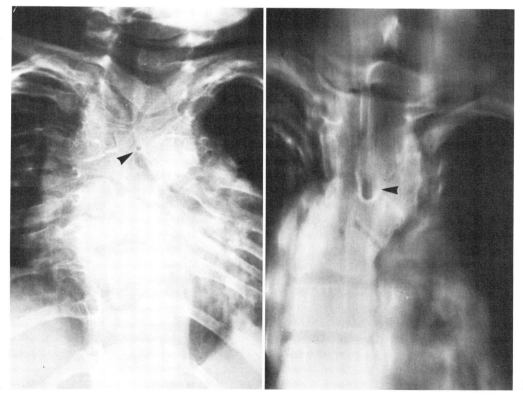

Fig. 20-45. Canal of Kovalevsky. A, Marked anterior spinal dysraphic anomalies with absent ribs in the left upper thorax and a well-defined canal (arrowhead). B, A tomogram in another child demonstrates a large well-corticated canal (arrowhead).

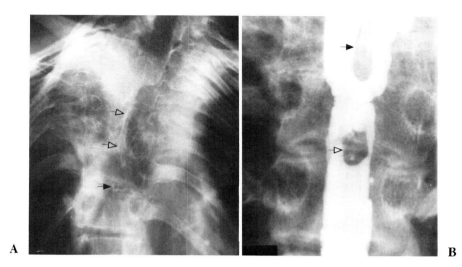

Fig. 20-46. Neurenteric cyst, diastematomyelia, and canal of Kovalevsky. A, The gross spinal dysraphia, diastematomyelic spur (open arrows), and canal (solid arrow) are clearly seen on this standard radiograph. **B,** A myelogram shows the intradural-extramedullary neurenteric cyst (open arrow) and the diastematomyelic spur (solid arrow).

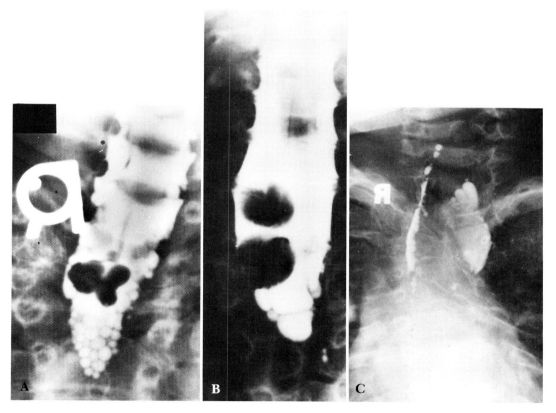

Fig. 20-47. Myelography and neurenteric cysts. A and **B,** Multiple grapelike appearance of the intradural-extramedullary component in two children. The cord is also involved. **C,** A large intradural-extramedullary cyst associated with marked spinal dysraphia widens the canal itself.

and varied from hemivertebrae to vertebral body fusion; all were associated with dysraphia and disorganization of the pedicles and spinous processes. There was a clearly defined canal of Kovalevsky in three cases (Fig. 20-45), and the neurenteric connection passed through this canal. In three children a paraspinal mass was found (Fig. 20-44, A and B). Widening of the spinal canal occurred as part of the dysraphia, but in two children the cysts were large enough to cause expansion of the canal itself. A diastematomyelia and a canal of Kovalevsky were noted in one child (Fig. 20-46).

Myelography. The characteristic myelographic fea-

ture of neurenteric cysts was multiple grapelike clusters. The intramedullary portions produced a nonspecific widening of the cord (Fig. 20-47, A and B); and if the clusters were large, they also widened the spinal canal (Fig. 20-47, C). Contrast did not egress through the canal.

The *differential diagnosis* of posterior mediastinal paravertebral masses includes neurofibroma, ganglioneuroma, ganglioneuroblastoma, neuroblastoma, enteric cyst, bronchogenic cyst, arachnoid cyst, and rarely teratoma; but these lesions do not have anterior dysraphic abnormalities.

Intraspinal and intramedullary cysts that occur and

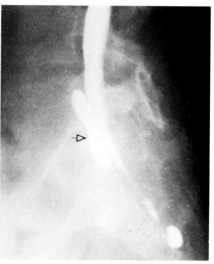

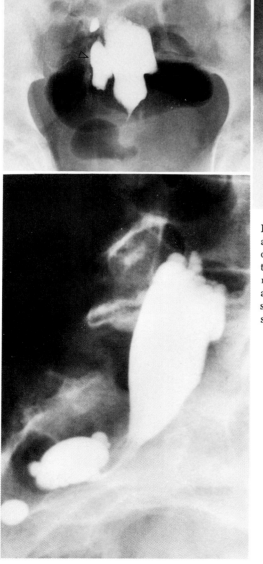

Fig. 20-48. Intraspinal meningoceles. A and B, Sacral, herniating through the dura (arrows) and presenting as an extradural mass which compresses the sacral roots. C, Herniating through the dura in another child, but contained within the sacral canal and again compressing the sacral roots.

may simulate neurenteric cysts are teratomatous, ependymal, and extramedullary arachnoid and extra-dural arachnoid cysts as well as any teratomatous cyst that may be associated with a dysraphic spine.

Intraspinal meningocele

In our opinion, intraspinal meningocele is a valid term for a space-occupying lesion within the spinal canal that is due to herniation of the meninges through the dural coverings but still contained within the spinal canal. Though spinal dysraphia is always associated with this condition, the intraspinal meningo-cele differs from the ordinary meningocele insofar as it expands and hence compresses the cord and root structures like an extradural mass lesion within the canal. A sacral meningocele, however, is contained within the sacral canal and is either an expansion of the meninges *within* the dura (Chapter 18) or a meningeal herniation through a spinal defect *outside* the spinal canal (Chapter 18), often occurring an-teriorly in the sacral region. An arachnoid cyst of the spinal canal is a cystic compartment of the sub-arachnoid space within the dura.

Intraspinal meningoceles are rare lesions and oc-curred in six children (3%) of our series. All were associated with minor forms of spinal dysraphia; and all presented with cauda equinal symptoms necessi-tating surgical intervention, for they were indeed intraspinal masses of consequence. One child was an infant of 6 months; the others were 2, 3, 7, 8, and 13 years of age. Sites were the lower lumbar and upper sacral regions exclusively. Myelography dem-onstrated a small connection between the meningocele and the spinal canal alongside a patent subarachnoid space (Fig. 20-48).

The *differential diagnosis* of an intraspinal arach-noid cyst is difficult; but the intraspinal cyst is usually not associated with dysraphia and, though rare in children, is more common in the thoracic region. It is usually acquired (due to arachnoiditis), or it oc-curs in association with neurofibromatosis. In the latter instance, such a cyst may indeed herniate through dura into the paravertebral space.

PRIMARY NEURAL NEOPLASMS

Neoplasms of neural origin that are within or encroach on the spinal canal constitute 30% of mass lesions of the canal. The majority are slow growing, and 75% produce erosive defects on the spine. Our practice is to perform myelography on an emergency basis at the slightest clinical and/or spinal radio-graphic evidence of an intraspinal mass lesion. This aggressive approach is necessary since severe com-promise of spinal cord function may occur within days.

Astrocytoma

Astrocytomas are the most common glioma of the cord in children and the commonest neoplasm of neural origin in patients of all ages (Sloof et al., 1964; Shapiro, 1968). They constituted 8% of mass lesions of the spinal canal in our series, and they comprise 9% of neoplastic mass lesions of the spinal canal. Both Rand and Rand (1960) and Matson (1969) report a higher incidence (14% and 18%) of mass lesions in their respective series, but the two series contained far fewer developmental neoplasms.

Age and sex. Boys (eleven) far outnumbered girls (four). The sexes are equally represented in adults, however (Sloof et al., 1964). Children were commonly seen after 8 years of age (Fig. 20-49). Astrocytomas were rarely found in the very young. Those that were tended to be of a more malignant character.

Site. The cervical cord was commonly involved, followed in incidence by the lower thoracic cord. The lumbar cord was involved by downward exten-sion of a lower thoracic astrocytoma in only two children. In adults, however, though some associated cervical cord extension may be observed, the thoracic area is by far the commonest site of occurrence (Sloof et al., 1964).

In four children a cervical cord astrocytoma was contiguous with a brain stem astrocytoma (Fig.

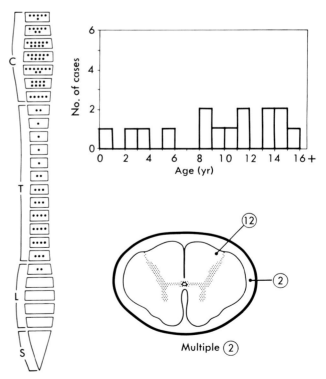

Fig. 20-49. **Age and sites of astrocytomas.** Eleven boys and four girls comprised this study.

20-50). In one child an astrocytoma of the vermis significantly extended down into the upper cervical canal (Fig. 20-51). All astrocytomas commonly involved more than two or three vertebral segments, usually five to ten segments, which also is common in adults (Sloof et al., 1964). In one child an astro-

cytoma extended from the cervicomedullary junction to the L1 level.

Involvement may be equal at all levels or may taper gently superiorly and inferiorly. The tumors were cystic in four of our children, in two of nine in Rand and Rand's (1960) series, and in twenty-one

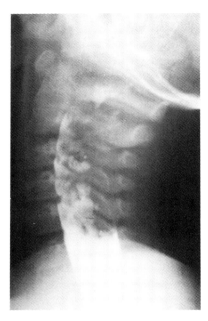

Fig. 20-50. Cervical cord astrocytoma continuous with a brain stem glioma. Note the widening of the upper cervical canal. This extensive neoplasm of the upper cord was malignant and nodulated into the subarachnoid space. It is continuous with a brain stem component.

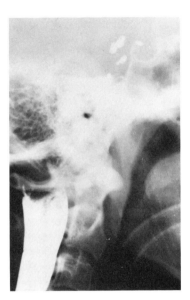

Fig. 20-51. Astrocytoma of the vermis extending down the cervical canal. This neoplasm presented as an upper cervical cord lesion rather than an intracranial lesion.

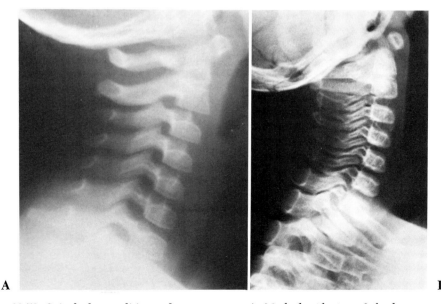

Fig. 20-52. Spinal abnormalities and astrocytomas. A, Marked widening of the lower cervical sagittal diameter in an infant. B, Widening of the sagittal diameter of the upper cervical canal in an older child. This astrocytoma continued into the brain stem.

of eighty-six patients of all ages in the series of Sloof and co-workers (1964). The cysts were mainly astrocytomas of low-grade malignancy. A syringomyelia was associated with an astrocytoma.

The majority of our astrocytomas were intramedullary; however, two appeared to be extramedullary but intradural at myelography. These were found to involve the cord. Cooper and Kernohan (1951) presumed that astrocytomas may form from heterotopic glial rests outside the cord.

Neuroradiology of astrocytomas

Spinal radiography. A spinal abnormality was present in 80% of children with an astrocytoma. The telltale loss of lumbar lordosis was almost invariable. Widening of the spinal canal in the cervical region was more pronounced in the sagittal diameter and often extended over many vertebral segments (Fig. 20-52). Interpediculate widening of the thoracic spine over many segments was a frequent finding (Fig. 20-53, A). On occasion, however, only one or two pedicles were thinned (Fig. 20-53, B) and the thinning was subtle. At least 50% of the children had no erosive changes of the spine whatsoever (Fig. 20-53, C); rather a scoliosis and loss of lumbar or cervical lordosis were observed (Fig. 20-52, A). Unless the astrocytoma was confined to two or three levels, posterior vertebral body scalloping was usually not marked. Scoliosis was not common in the astrocytomas that occurred in the cervical region; and if present, it was not severe. It was generally associated with extensive neoplasms and those occurring in the thoracic region.

Myelography. The widening of the spinal cord by the neoplasm was either gentle (Fig. 20-53, A), in which case the contrast often passed slowly along the widened cord (Fig. 20-54), or quite abrupt, in which case total block was common (Fig. 20-53, B).

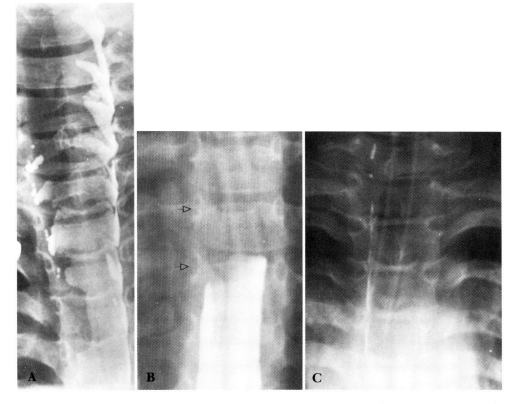

Fig. 20-53. The spine and astrocytomas. A, Huge astrocytoma involving the entire spinal cord. The interpediculate distances were widened throughout the cervical, thoracic, and upper lumbar spine—as seen here in the cervical and upper thoracic spine. The pedicles were not markedly thinned, however. This neoplasm contained a large cervical upper thoracic cyst. **B,** Localized intramedullary astrocytoma in another child. Note the subtle thinning of the pedicles (arrows) on the right side of the seventh and eighth thoracic vertebrae. The myelographic block appeared to have been caused by an extramedullary mass, but at surgery an intramedullary location was observed. **C,** An extensive cervical and upper thoracic astrocytoma with no pediculate changes or spinal canal widening. At biopsy, this astrocytoma had ganglioglioma elements.

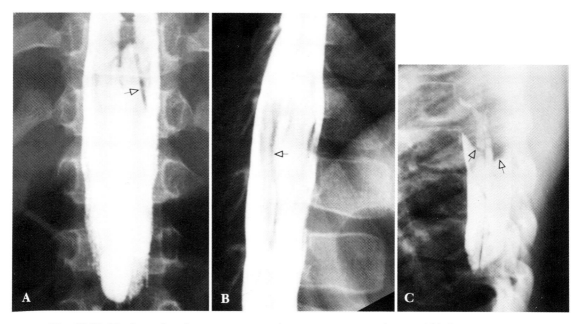

Fig. 20-54. Myelography of an astrocytoma. A prone position myelogram (**A**) demonstrates an intramedullary neoplasm over which passes a large nerve root (arrow). With the patient on his left side, a lateral view (**B**) shows free passage of contrast around the mass. Again a nerve root is clearly seen (arrow). A similar position but with the right side down (**C**) shows a large nodule (arrows) extending into the subarachnoid space.

Although not frequently encountered, an irregular edge of the neoplasm may give a myelographic block similar in appearance to that caused by an extradural mass. Furthermore, an eccentric nodular extension of the astrocytoma may also give the appearance of an intradural-extramedullary mass (Fig. 20-53, *B*). Careful attention to prone, supine, and lateral myelographic views will obviate confusion (Fig. 20-54). Air myelography will detect intradural-extramedullary nodules (Fig. 20-55), and the cord will not collapse as in hydromyelia (Fig. 20-56).

It is not possible to detect a cyst within the astrocytoma, though local eccentricity may occur with a cyst or a fusiform nodule of solid neoplasm may extend into the subarachnoid space. Prominent spinal vessels will often be shown to course over the neoplasm, but this does not indicate neoplastic vascularity (Fig. 20-56).

Mass lesions that closely simulate an astrocytoma neuroradiologically are intramedullary ependymoma, intramedullary teratoma, syringohydromyelia, and dermoid. The former three conditions all may be quite extensive and produce generalized irregular widening of the spinal canal and cord. Air myelography of the cervical cord must be performed to differentiate between a solid intramedullary neoplasm (e.g., an astrocytoma) and a possible syringohydromyelia (Fig. 20-56) (Westberg, 1966; Harwood-Nash and Fitz, 1974).

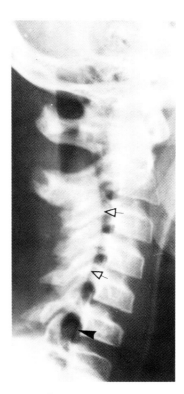

Fig. 20-55. Intramedullary and extramedullary astrocytoma. A large intramedullary astrocytoma of the cervical cord (arrows) is shown by air myelography to have a discrete extramedullary nodule (arrowhead).

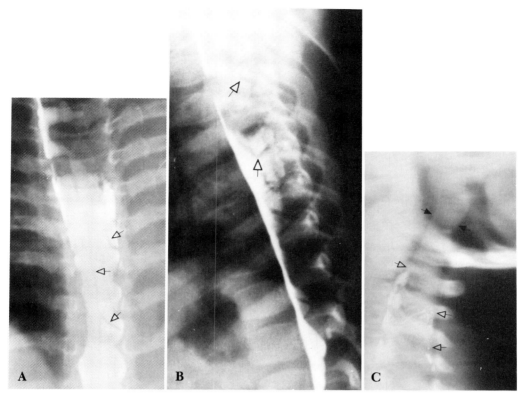

Fig. 20-56. Positive contrast and air myelography in astrocytoma. A and **B,** Prone and lateral positive contrast myelograms demonstrate an extensive neoplasm from the cervical into the lumbar region with marked narrowing of the subarachnoid space and enlargement of the radiculomedullary and anterior spinal vessels (arrows). Notwithstanding the compressive effect of the neoplasm, however, the prominent vessels do not indicate a neoplastic tumor but apparently are secondarily dilated. **C,** An air myelogram in the same patient shows the neoplasm extending into the cervical cord to the level of C1 (open arrows). The medulla (solid arrow) is clearly seen and is normal.

Neuroblastoma

Neuroblastoma is a relatively common thoracic and abdominal neoplasm in infants and young children. It is a neoplasm of the adrenal glands and sympathetic chain extending from the base of the skull to the pelvis; and it arises mainly from primary ganglia, less commonly from the secondary ganglia. Common sites are the adrenal glands, the thoracolumbar region, and the superior and posterior mediastinum. Willis (1953) simplified the terminology to include exotic names like sympathicoblastoma, gangliosympathicoblastoma, neurocytoma, and ganglioneuroma under the name neuroblastoma. Because they present in a different fashion for neuroradiological investigation, we have elected to separate ganglioneuromas, a more benign differentiated neoplasm, from the more malignant neuroblastoma. We acknowledge that some neuroblastomas contain ganglioneuroma elements, and vice versa, and that a neuroblastoma may mature into a ganglioneuroma; but the dominant cell type is what we considered for our classification.

The usual presentation of these tumors was a mass in the abdomen and weakness of the legs (if the child was old enough to walk). Less usual presentations were scoliosis or vertebral pain and neurological bladder symptoms. If a clear-cut level of neurological deficit was present, it was often some distance from the paravertebral mass. Clinical evidence of widespread skeletal or soft tissue involvement by the neuroblastoma was uncommon at the time of the appearance of symptoms referrable to the spinal canal and occurred in only one of our fourteen cases.

The bone marrow, however, was frequently involved at the time of presentation; and, furthermore, radionuclide bone scans revealed bony involvement when radiography did not. One child presented with a cerebellar ataxia, which may be associated with generalized neuroblastoma. In our experience, Wilms' tumor rarely involved the spinal canal. Rand and Rand (1960) provide excellent discussion of neuroblastomas within the spinal canal and report on the clinical features of six additional cases.

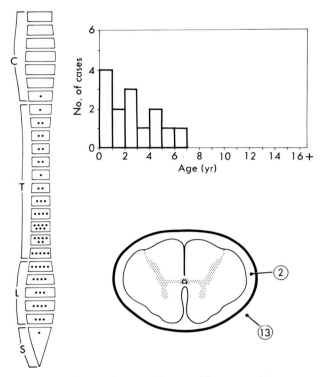

Fig. 20-57. **Age and site of neuroblastomas.** There were fourteen patients in this study, ten boys and four girls.

Intraspinal involvement by neuroblastoma occurred in fourteen children (7%)—8% of neoplasms within the spinal canal. Eighteen percent in Matson's (1969) series of intraspinal neoplasms and 8% of Rand and Rand's (1960) series were neuroblastomas.

Age and sex. Spinal canal involvement by neuroblastoma occurs in infancy and early childhood, the youngest in our series being 19 days old (Fig. 20-57); the other three infants less than 1 year of age were 5 months, 7 months, and 11 months old. The oldest patient was 6 years. Males (ten) outnumbered females (four). All ganglioneuromas in our series, however, were in girls.

Site. Although a *paraspinal* mass lesion was common, the neuroblastoma often created an extradural defect or block some distance from the main mass due to spread of sheets of tissue within the extradural space (Fig. 20-58). The common *intraspinal* sites were the lower thoracic and upper lumbar regions (Fig. 20-57).

In only one child did the lesion extend into the lower cervical region, and that was from a superior mediastinal neuroblastoma. In another child a neuroblastoma was confined to the intradural-extramedullary space (Fig. 20-59). A third child had both intradural-extramedullary and extradural involvement, however. The intradural site occurs rarely (Fig. 20-57).

Grant and Austin (1956) reported one intradural-extramedullary neuroblastoma. Dargeon (1962) reported one child in a series of 236 with a neuroblastoma in the extradural space. Fortner and co-workers (1968) reported a child in a series of 133

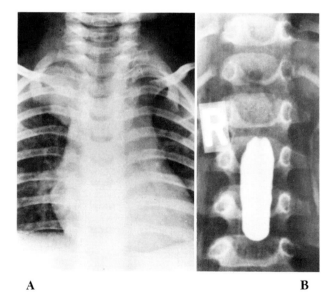

A   B

Fig. 20-58. **Paravertebral neuroblastoma with distant intraspinal block.** A large right apical paravertebral neoplasm apparently caused no bony vertebral changes. The myelogram, however, shows complete block due to extradural spread at the L1-L2 level (**B**).

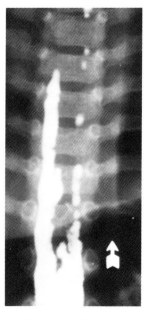

Fig. 20-59. **Intradural-extramedullary neuroblastoma.** An irregular virtually total subarachnoid block.

who had an intradural neuroblastoma. Thus the dura does seem to present a successful barrier in the majority of extradural neuroblastomas.

The rarity of intraspinal involvement by neuroblastoma in the foregoing reports reflects, we think, the unfortunate lack of myelographic investigation of paraspinal mass lesions in children—in whom a surprisingly high number extend into the spinal canal (Kirks et al., 1976). The remaining twelve children in our series all had an extradural neuroblastoma.

Neuroradiology of neuroblastomas

Spinal radiography. In ten children (72%) an abnormality of the spine was detected, whereas in four no abnormality was found. In one infant no vertebral, paravertebral, or intravenous pyelographic abnormality was present. An extradural neuroblastoma was discovered at myelography performed to investigate the onset of bilateral leg flaccidity. A rib erosion or rib separation and pediculate and vertebral destruction of varying degrees were common at the site of the paraspinal mass lesion (Fig. 20-60, A). The myelographic block was often at a distance, however.

Generalized skeletal involvement occurred in only one child, and in another a single sclerotic lumbar vertebra was present. Unilateral pediculate erosions may be confined to one or two levels and may consist merely of subtle thinning. Scoliosis was uncommon and when present was only slight (Fig. 20-60, B). The spinal canal was not enlarged from within except in one case (Fig. 20-60, A). Two of the adrenal neuroblastomas were calcified.

Myelography. We customarily urge that myelography be performed on a child with a paraspinal mass lesion prior to treatment *even if the vertebral radiograph and neurological examination are normal.* To prevent inadvertent intraspinal bleeding and/or cord compromise during the procedures, any intraspinal extension must be removed by laminectomy before intrathoracic or intra-abdominal removal or radiotherapy is contemplated.

In two instances the myelographic lumbar puncture was frankly bloody. Being sure of an intradural placement of the needle, we proceeded to inject 2 ml of contrast—notwithstanding the fact that a laminectomy was to be performed in any case. In both, an irregular lumbar subarachnoid block was present due to diffuse intradural neuroblastoma.

In eight children there was either a gradual tapered (Fig. 20-61, A and B) or a sudden (Fig. 20-61, C to E) extradural block; in the remaining four a partial block due to either a unilateral intraspinal mass lesion or a circumferential dural involvement (Fig. 20-61, C) occurred. We commonly identified an extradural neuroblastoma some distance from the paraspinal mass or vertebral erosions without evidence of either abnormality at these distant sites

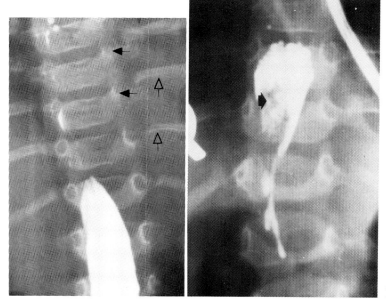

A   B

Fig. 20-60. **Vertebral abnormalities and neuroblastomas.** A, Left lower thoracic soft tissue mass thinning the ribs (open arrows) and the adjacent pedicles (solid arrows). B, Low thoracic paraspinal mass with extradural extension and a scoliosis away from the mass. Note the prominent tortuous anterior spinal artery (arrow), which is of no significance. (**B** from Harwood-Nash, D. C.: Semin. Roentgenol. 7:297, 1972.)

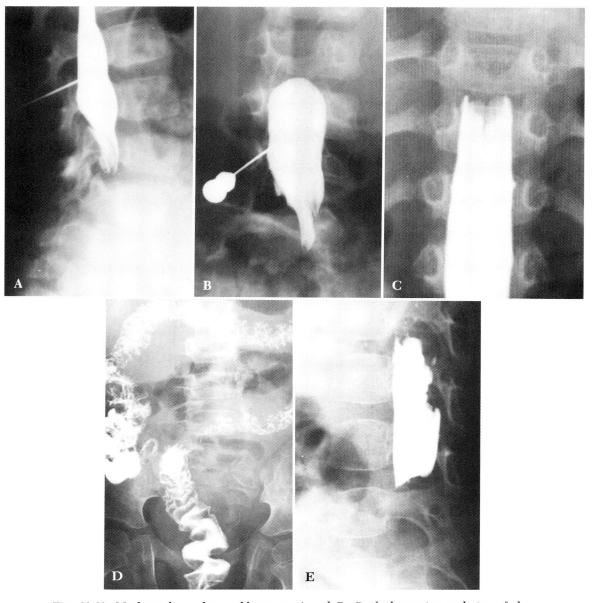

Fig. 20-61. Myelography and neuroblastomas. A and **B,** Gradual tapering occlusion of the lumbar sac by this lumbosacral extradural neoplasm. **C,** Abrupt irregular extradural block by a circumferential neuroblastoma. Note the normal spine. **D** and **E,** A large intrapelvic neuroblastoma caused marked displacement of the sigmoid colon upward and to the right (**D**). The intraspinal extension (**E**) created a complete extradural block at L4. Intradural-extramedullary spread also occurred, as seen by the upper irregular defects in the contrast column.

(Fig. 20-58). If there is a total block and the surgeon wishes to know the upper limit of the intraspinal mass, a cisternal puncture myelogram may be obtained.

Neurofibroma

Tumors arising from the nerve sheath, probably from the cells of Schwann, are blessed with many names—common among which are neurolemmoma, schwannoma, and neurofibroma. Acknowledging the

various pathological nuances that may be present, and with some neuroradiological license, we prefer the term neurofibroma. We have, furthermore, grouped together solitary neurofibromas and multiple neurofibromas as part of von Recklinghausen's disease (Chapter 16) and malignant degeneration of neurofibromas as neurofibrosarcoma.

There were thirteen children (7%) with such a rare intraspinal neoplasm in our series. According to the Mayo series, however, 29% of all intraspinal

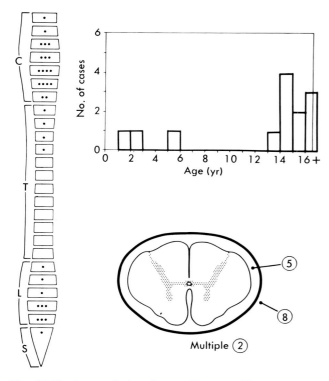

Fig. 20-62. Age and site of neurofibromas. Thirteen patients comprised this study, five boys and eight girls.

neoplasms are neurofibromas (Sloof et al., 1964). Four of the thirteen children had generalized neurofibromatosis. There were four neurofibrosarcomas— and these neoplasms generally were large and infiltrated the paraspinal muscles and facial planes, often destroying bone. Two of the four neurofibrosarcoma patients had neurofibromatosis. Herrman (1950) reported four cases of sarcoma in neurofibromatosis, and Cuneo (1957) reported spinal cord compression by a neurofibrosarcoma. The other two children with neurofibromatosis had multiple intraspinal neurofibromas existing in both the extradural and the intradural-extraspinal areas. The remaining nine children had neurofibromas that were focally located in the spinal canal and were usually large. Rand and Rand (1960) provide an extensive discussion of the literature and clinical features of neurofibroma in children.

Age and sex. The majority of children presented in the early or middle teen-age period; two children under 3 years of age had a neurofibrosarcoma (Fig. 20-62). Ingraham (1938) reported one child aged 13 months. In a review of 115 cases of spinal neurofibromas, Gautier-Smith (1967) reported only one child below 10 years of age; but ten children in his study were between 10 and 20 years of age. There is no particular difference in incidence between boys and girls.

Site. The most common site was the cervical region (Fig. 20-62)—contrary to the experience of Sloof and co-workers (1964), who found that 43% of neurofibromas occurring at all ages were located in the thoracic region. In our series, the thoracic region was spared but the lumbar region was commonly involved. Sacral canal extension of the neurofibroma occurred in one child. Multiple neurofibromas occurred only in the two children with neurofibromatosis. Most of the single lesions were moderately large, and three were very large plexiform neoplasms involving many tissue planes. In three children the neurofibroma was primarily in the intradural-extramedullary compartment, two were intradural and extradural, and the remainder were extradural.

In the Mayo series, however, Sloof and co-workers (1964) reported 62% of neurofibromas in the intradural, 32% in the extradural, and 6% in both areas. An intramedullary neurofibroma is extremely rare and usually presents in adulthood (McCormick, 1964; Mason and Keigher, 1968). All the extradural neurofibromas in our series extended, either slightly or greatly, through one or more intervertebral foramina to create the so-called dumbbell tumor (Fagan and Swischuk, 1974). Apparently neurofibromas that present in children do so because they are unusually large early in life and thus there is early accompanying pain with compression of the nerve and cord.

Neuroradiology of neurofibromas

Spinal radiography. Multiple and plexiform neurofibromas and neurofibrosarcomas present with the bizarre spinal dysplasia (Fig. 20-63) of neurofibromatosis, kyphoscoliosis, or scoliosis per se and dysplasia of the related ribs in the thoracic region (Fig. 20-64). If the neurofibroma is of the dumbbell type—it may itself enlarge the intervertebral foramina (Fig. 20-65) or indeed may enlarge the spinal canal, in addition to the intrinsic spinal canal enlargement that is part of the dysplasia of neurofibromatosis (Chapter 16). Such changes may occur without a neurofibroma, however, and lateral herniations of arachnoid may themselves enlarge intervertebral foramina; but this is uncommon in children. Furthermore, a wide spinal canal and dural sac with scalloping of the posterior borders of the vertebrae are relatively common in neurofibromatosis (Chapter 16). Solitary neurofibromas without neurofibromatosis are not associated with vertebral dysplasias as just described.

Extradural and extraspinal neurofibromas of the dumbbell type will smoothly enlarge intervertebral foramina (Fig. 20-65) and thin or destroy pedicles. The intraspinal component of the lesion will often widen the interpediculate distance or erode one or

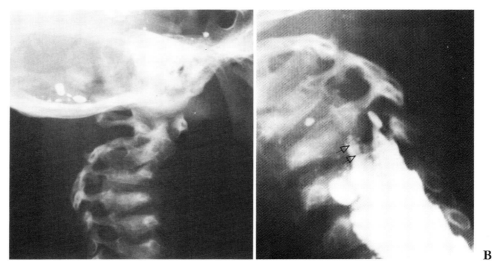

Fig. 20-63. Spinal dysplasia and neurofibromatosis. A, Marked kyphoscoliosis with distorted and thinned upper cervical vertebrae caused by a large neurofibroma. **B,** A myelogram demonstrates complete block to contrast medium at C4 with displacement of the cervical cord (arrows).

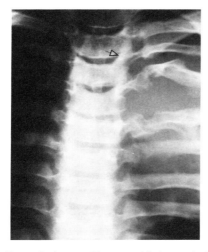

Fig. 20-64. Paraspinal neurofibroma with intraspinal extension. A large left thoracic paraspinal neurofibroma in neurofibromatosis caused marked dysplasia, distraction, and thinning of the ribs. There is thinning of the left T3 pedicle (arrow) with widening of the distance between it and its companions at T4 and T5. The intraspinal component of the neoplasm passed between these pedicles.

more pedicles from within the canal. Congenital abscence of the pedicles (Steinbach et al., 1952) must not be mistaken for an erosive enlargement of the intervertebral foramina. Adjacent ribs may be thinned as a result of direct compression or as part of the dysplasia of neurofibromatosis, and a large paraspinal mass may be seen (Fig. 20-63).

The neurofibrosarcomas in our series were all large; vertebral destruction occurred in the region of the mass lesion itself in three of the patients (Chapter 16).

Abnormal spinal films were present in 85% of all children with neurofibromas. Two of the three patients with an intradural neurofibroma alone had a single lesion with no vertebral abnormalities (Fig. 20-66). The third child had generalized neurofibromatosis and multiple intradural neurofibromas without extradural components. Another child with neurofibromatosis had both extradural and intradural neurofibromatoses. A fifth child, with an intradural and an extradural component, had a single neurofibroma.

Myelography. The classical intradural-extramedullary mass lesion effect at myelography is produced by a neurofibroma (Figs. 20-65 and 20-66). This effect is an inferiorly convex edge identified outside the cord and displacing the cord to the other side. The block may be partial or complete. The neurofibroma may be lobulated or smooth. Extradural masses usually produce an abrupt obstruction to the contrast with flattening of the cord if the mass is anterior or posterior (Fig. 20-67). The result is a pseudoexpansion of the cord. Multiple small neurofibromas may be seen arising from many roots of the spinal cord and cauda equina (Fig. 20-68). These multiple small lesions occur in neurofibromatosis. The associated dural ectasia with sacculations in neurofibromatosis may also be seen and are usually associated with considerable vertebral dysplasia (Chapter 16).

An intradural meningioma may produce a picture similar to that of a single intradural-extramedullary neurofibroma; but these intradural lesions occur pre-

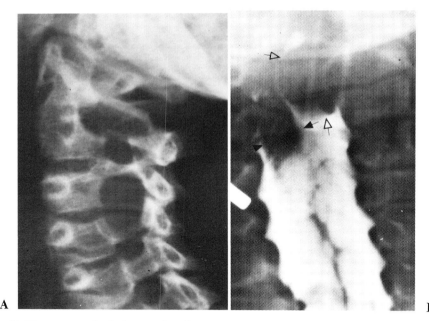

Fig. 20-65. Intervertebral foraminal enlargement and neurofibroma. A, A large dumbbell-shaped neoplasm enlarges the intervertebral foramen between C3 and C4 on the left. **B,** A myelogram shows the classical appearance of the intradural-extramedullary neurofibroma (open arrows) displacing the cord to the right (solid arrow).

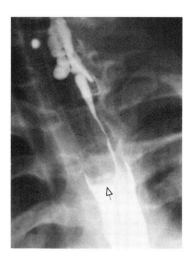

Fig. 20-66. Intradural-extramedullary neurofibroma. A large tubular neoplasm in the intradural-extramedullary space produced a classical inferiorly convex edge (arrow). Note the total lack of vertebral changes.

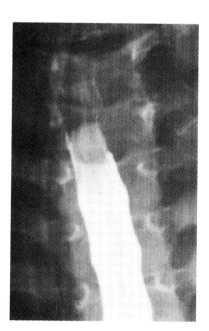

Fig. 20-67. Extradural neurofibrosarcoma. There is marked flattening of the cord with an abrupt block to the contrast column and displacement of the entire sac to the right. Note the slight interpediculate widening and thinning of the upper pedicles.

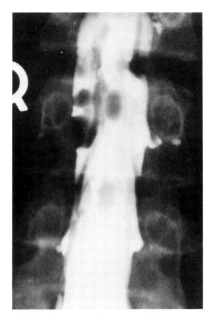

Fig. 20-68. **Multiple neurofibromas.** These were associated with lumbar nerve roots in a patient with neurofibromatosis.

dominantly in adults (Haft et al., 1959). We have not had experience with this neoplasm in the spinal canal of children.

Ependymoma

Ependymomas constituted 6% (twelve cases) of spinal canal mass lesions in our series—or 7% of intraspinal neoplasms. Rand and Rand (1960) report an incidence of 13%, and Matson (1969) an incidence of 5%. Rand and Rand (1960) and Sloof and co-workers (1964) discuss at length the pathological and clinical features of intramedullary ependymomas and intraspinal ependymomas in children and adults respectively.

Ependymomas arise from ependymal cells within the cord or filum terminale. We have excluded those that have seeded downward from a cranial ependymoma and have classified them as CSF-borne metastases. Cooper and co-workers (1951) cite nine ependymomas of the spinal canal which were thought to be primary extramedullary neoplasms. These authors theorize that the neoplasms arose from heterotopic glial tissue within the spinal subarachnoid space. Spontaneous subarachnoid hemorrhage may rarely originate from a spinal ependymoma (Fincher, 1951; Tarlov and Keener, 1953).

Age and sex. The majority of the twelve children in our series were older than 9 years, the youngest being 7 (Fig. 20-69). Girls and boys were equally common. Rand and Rand (1960) report eight children with an ependymoma, two of whom were 4 years old; and boys were predominant.

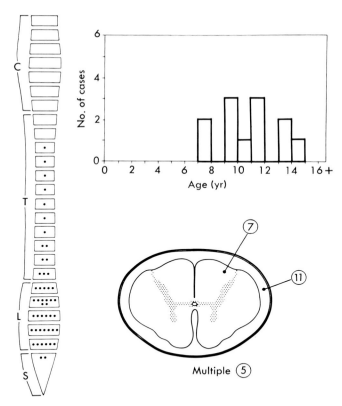

Fig. 20-69. **Age and site in ependymomas.** Six boys and six girls comprised this study.

Site. The lumbar region was the most commonly involved, and three ependymomas extended up into the thoracic area. Cervical involvement was extremely rare. Half the eight lesions reported by Rand and Rand (1960) were in the thoracic region, however; and thoracic and thoracolumbar distribution was common in the mainly adult series of Sloof and co-workers (1964).

From a myelographic point of view, we have considered an ependymoma of the filum alone to be extramedullary. Thus seven were intramedullary, usually at the conus—but one extended from the conus to T3, a truly remarkable neoplasm. Horrax and Henderson (1939) described an ependymoma extending from the medulla of the brain to the conus of the cord. Eleven neoplasms were intradural and extramedullary. There were six ependymomas in five children arising from the filum terminale, one child having two discrete lesions. Five of the seven intramedullary ependymomas had significant mass extensions outside the conus and spinal cord. Sloof and co-workers (1964) report 37% located in the cord and 63% in the filum in patients of all ages. A filum ependymoma may rarely be mobile (Wotzman and Botterell, 1963). None of our series extended extradurally, but one seeded up into the quadrigeminal cistern of the brain (Fig. 20-70).

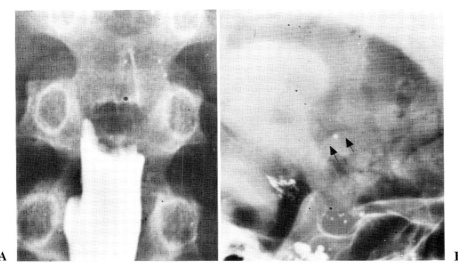

Fig. 20-70. Ependymoma of the spinal canal seeding up to the cranial cavity. A, Of the filum terminale. B, Of the anterior third ventricle (in the same child), indenting the ventricle (arrows). Upward seeding of the ependymoma into the cranial subarachnoid space caused this indentation.

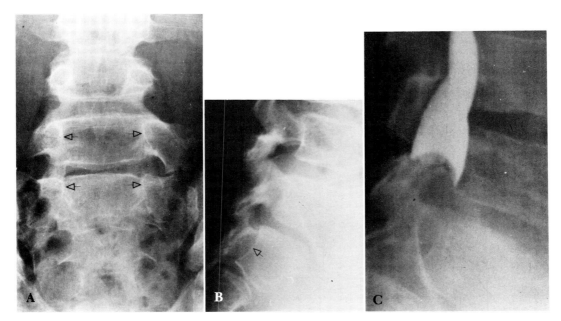

Fig. 20-71. Spinal abnormalities and ependymomas. A, Subtle widening of the L5 and S1 interpediculate distances (arrows). B, Minor scalloping of the L5 vertebra (arrow). C, A myelogram demonstrates the characteristic superiorly convex defect due to an ependymoma of the filum terminale in the same patient.

Neuroradiology of ependymomas

Spinal radiography. Vertebral abnormalities were uncommon (in only 33%). Subtle interpediculate widening and thinning of lumbar pedicles, minor posterior vertebral scalloping (Fig. 20-71), and a generalized widening of the interpediculate distances (Fig. 20-72) were abnormalities that did occur.

Scoliosis was not common, but a straightened lumbar spine was seen in seven of the twelve children.

Myelography. An ependymoma appears as a discrete moderately large smooth-surfaced (Figs. 20-70 and 20-71) or mildly lobulated mass lesion surrounded by nerve roots and all within the conus and cord. The spinal cord itself and conus are widened, but

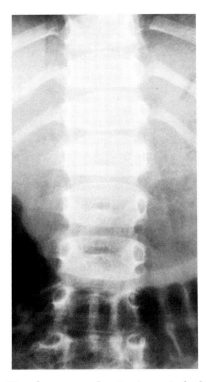

Fig. 20-72. Ependymoma and extensive spinal abnormalities. A neoplasm of the proximal filum terminale and conus extends up into the lower thoracic spine with marked thinning of the pedicles and widening of the interpediculate distances at many levels.

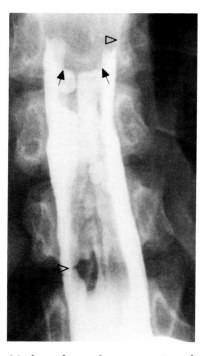

Fig. 20-73. Myelography and an extensive thoracolumbar ependymoma. A large mass in the cauda (open arrow) extends superiorly into the extramedullary space (solid arrows). Note the relative lack of spinal abnormalities except for thinning of the left pedicle at T10 (arrowhead).

the extramedullary extension may be abrupt and lead to the erroneous conclusion that a primary extramedullary mass lesion with compression of the spinal cord is present (Fig. 20-73). The contrast material may slowly pass up a progressively narrowed subarachnoid space to reach a complete block in the thoracic region (Fig. 20-74); or there may be a complete block in the lumbar region. As in all mass lesions of the spinal canal, it is essential to obtain films in multiple positions, particularly supine views, since the ependymoma will often spread posteriorly.

The absence of spinal dysraphia obviates the diagnosis of a teratoma or lipoma, but a dermoid of the conus or cauda or an astrocytoma of the cord itself may be quite similar to an ependymoma at myelography. An extensive ependymoma may also simulate an extensive hydromyelia, and air myelography should be performed to differentiate the two.

Ganglioneuroma

Although a sympathetic chain neoplasm, commonly a neuroblastoma in infants and children, a ganglioneuroma is considered separately from neuroblastomas. It is different, first, in character—being localized, firm, and fibrous and containing mature ganglion cells (Willis, 1953)—and, second, in clinical presentation and neuroradiological characteristics.

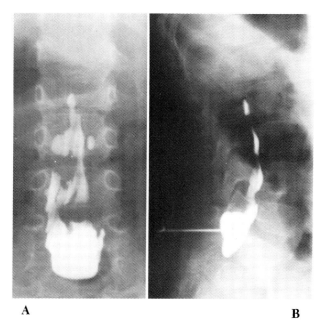

A **B**

Fig. 20-74. Myelography and an extensive lobulated ependymoma. Supine and lateral myelograms demonstrate an ependymoma of the filum terminale which has wrapped the lumbar roots. **A,** The neoplasm extends to T10 and considerably widens the upper lumbar interpediculate distances. **B,** Contrast medium slowly passes anteriorly within the scalloping of the posterior vertebral bodies. Note also the marked sagittal widening of the spinal canal.

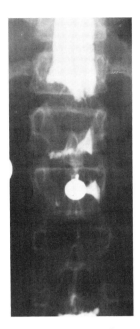

Fig. 20-82. Subarachnoid seeding of a chromophobe carcinoma. Large secondary deposits in the lumbar area are due to seeding from a primary chromophobe carcinoma. There is a virtually complete block to the contrast medium.

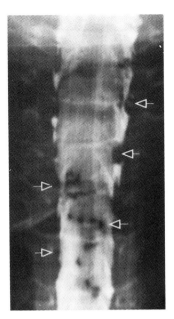

Fig. 20-83. Extensive subarachnoid seeding of a medulloblastoma. Sheets of neoplastic cells clothe the cervical spine and create several small nodular defects (arrows). The resultant effect is an apparent marked widening of the cord.

noid space, a parasitic disease such as cysticercosis, or multiple hydatid cysts may vaguely simulate these multiple deposits.

AXIAL NEOPLASMS

Vertebral neoplasms, either primary or secondary or part of a generalized disease, are by far more common in adults (Epstein, 1969).

Primary vertebral neoplasm

Primary vertebral neoplasms are rare in children, and even more rarely do they compress the spinal cord. In our series, four such lesions (occurring between the ages of 10 and 14 years, and all benign) were large enough to compress the cord. One was an osteoblastoma in the cervical region (Lichtenstein, 1956; Crabbe and Wardill, 1963), and two were aneurysmal bone cysts (Winter and Firtel, 1961; Matson, 1969). Both were large lesions, one occurring in the lower cervical region and the other in the upper lumbar region. The cord in the latter patient had partial vertebral collapse (Fig. 20-84). The clinical and pathological details of this cyst in the spine of children are considered in detail by Rand and Rand (1960).

Wisniewski and co-workers (1973) describe a rare benign chondroblastoma of the spine in a 17-year-old boy which did not compromise the cord. Hereditary multiple exostosis involving the vertebrae may com-

press the cord in children (Vinstein and Franken, 1971). A rare isolated osteochondroma compressed the cord in another child (Fig. 20-85). A primary osteogenic sarcoma or Ewing's tumor (Epstein, 1966, 1969) is rare at any age—and more especially in a child —as is a chordoma in a site other than the sacrum, a fibrosarcoma, chondrosarcoma, and small cell sarcoma of the vertebrae. Each may compress the cord.

Metastatic vertebral neoplasm

Vertebral neoplasms due to metastases from extra-axial origins, due to direct contiguous spread from the paraspinal mass (e.g., a retroperitoneal sarcoma, teratoma, neuroblastoma), or due to distant neoplasms are rare in children. We have included leukemia in this group. Twelve (6%) children had such lesions.

The primary neoplasms for such metastases were four rhabdomyosarcomas (two in the nasopharynx, one in the thigh, one in the uterus), two malignant teratomas of the pelvis and abdomen (Fig. 20-86), a Ewing's tumor of the femur (Fig. 20-87), a hypernephroma, a malignant teratoma of the mediastinum, a Wilms' tumor (Fig. 20-88), an extradural mass produced by vertebral leukemic deposits, and a reticulum cell sarcoma spread to the extradural space.

There was an even distribution in ages from 6 months to 14 years (Fig. 20-89). The sites were predominantly thoracic; but no vertebra was exempt from involvement alone or in concert with others (except for the third to the sixth cervical vertebrae). One rhabdomyosarcoma in the nasopharynx extended into the intradural space; however, the remainder were all extradural masses.

Although we did not commonly encounter children with a significant mass of extradural leukemic cells (one child), Wilhydre and co-workers (1963) report twenty children under the age of 16 years with such a lesion. The best description of extradural leukemia exists in the writings of Critchley and Greenfield (1930) and Hamby (1944). Intraspinal extradural bleeding may complicate leukemia (D'Angio et al., 1959).

Epidural lymphomas of any type are rare in children. Bharati and Kalyanaraman (1973) described a malignant lymphoma in the extradural space in a 1½-year-old boy; and in our series, a 6-year-old girl had a reticulum cell sarcoma in the thoracic extradural space spread by contiguity from a mediastinal lesion. Other possible neoplasms of the verte-

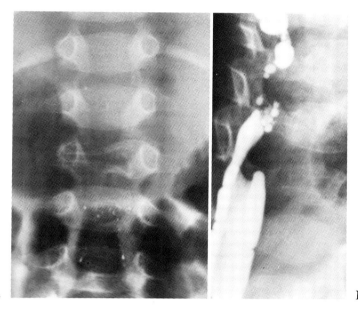

Fig. 20-84. Collapsed aneurysmal bone cyst and cord compression. An aneurysmal bone cyst of the right side of L2 has collapsed (A). The cyst mass itself produced a large extradural block (B).

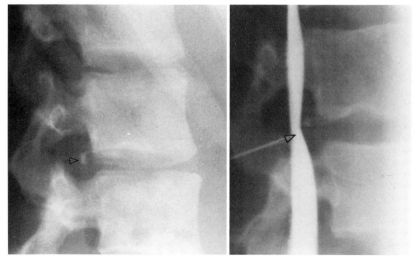

Fig. 20-85. Isolated osteochondroma and root compression. A small isolated neoplasm at the inferior border of L2 (A, arrow) compressed the dural sac (arrow) at the L3 nerve root (B).

brae and extradural space, or extradural space alone, are undifferentiated small cell sarcoma tissue originating from a paraspinal lesion with a similar histology. Dodge and co-workers (1956) report a secondary extradural osteogenic sarcoma.

MISCELLANEOUS SPINAL AND INTRASPINAL LESIONS

A gamut of other lesions of the spine and spinal canal rarely occur in infants and children. Some are common in adults but rare in children; others with exotic pathology are rare at any age.

Disk protrusion

Herniated disks are rare in children (Webb et al., 1954; Rand and Rand, 1960; Matson, 1969) but may present clinically as a classical nerve compression syndrome or if large as a cauda equinal lesion mimicking an ependymoma of the filum terminale.

Seven herniated disks (4%) occurred in our series.

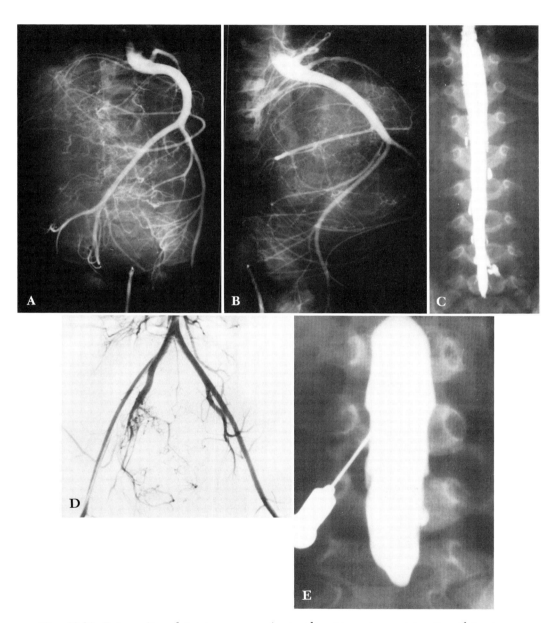

Fig. 20-86. Retroperitoneal teratosarcomas. A vascular sarcomatous retroperitoneal teratoma in a neonate (**A** and **B**) has spread into the extradural space, wrapping and compressing the subarachnoid space (**C**). A retroperitoneal teratoma of the ovary (**D**) is quite vascular and has spread into the lower lumbar region, producing an extradural compression at L5 and S1 with L5 and S1 root compression (**E**). Vertebral body infiltration by each neoplasm was found at autopsy and operation respectively.

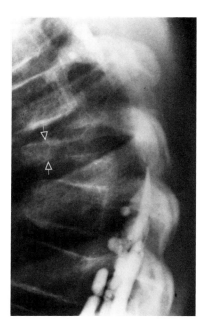

Fig. 20-87. Secondary Ewing's tumor. This neoplasm in the femur has spread to T8 (arrows), causing collapse and a complete extradural block to contrast medium.

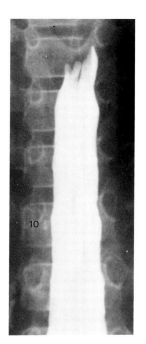

Fig. 20-88. Wilms' tumor and extradural spread. This right-sided mass spread to the extradural space at T7 and produced a complete block.

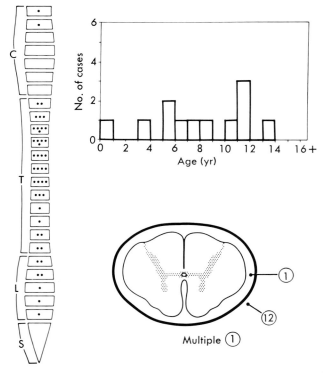

Fig. 20-89. Neoplasms of the spinal canal due to extra-axial origins. Seven boys and five girls made up this study.

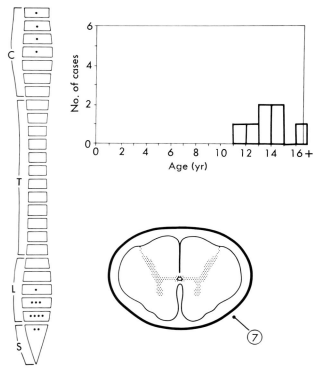

Fig. 20-90. Age and site of disk protrusions. Five boys and two girls were in this survey.

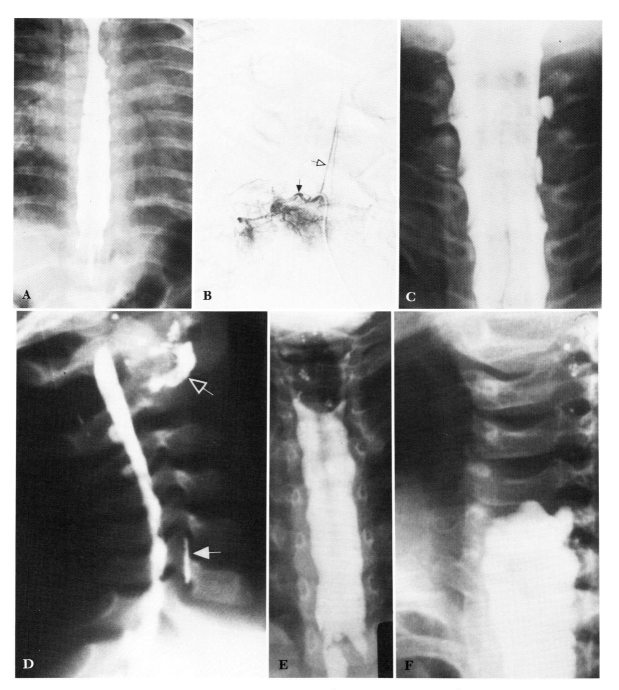

Fig. 20-100. Miscellaneous intraspinal lesions. A, A hemangiopericytoma in the T10, T11, T12 region creates a total extradural block to contrast inserted by the cisternal route. B, A selective spinal angiogram demonstrates the extent of this vascular tumor at T12. The artery of Adamkievicz (open arrow), which is a radiculomedullary artery to the anterior spinal artery, arises from the intercostal artery of T12 (solid arrow). C, An extradural cyst containing clear fluid unlike CSF is present on the left side between C6 and T2 and produces an extradural compressive defect. Small subarachnoid pouches are also seen. D, An extensive traumatic arachnoid cyst of the cervical and thoracic cord or canal displaces the subarachnoid space posteriorly. Note the upper branchial plexus avulsion with extravasation of contrast (open arrow). The contrast has leaked into the cyst itself (solid arrow). E and F, In the Chiari malformation, myelograms in the cervical canal will show prolapsed tonsils as smooth (E) or irregular (F) defects. The tonsils can herniate down to C5 or C6 in some Chiari malformations.

kyphosis may be mild or severe, and treatment is removal of the offending vertebra and spinal fusion.

Tomography is an essential addition to vertebral radiographs, and myelography reveals the marked extradural compression defect (which is very focal) (Fig. 20-99). The presence of a low-fixed cord in two children further complicated the picture.

Other intraspinal lesions

There were eight other lesions of our series in the spinal canal: an intra-arachnoid melanoma (Kiel et al., 1961), a hemangioblastoma (Kendall and Russel, 1966), a paraspinal hemangiopericytoma with extradural extension (Fig. 20-100, *A* and *B*) (Kriss et al., 1968), a large venous varix of a spinal AVM producing widening of the canal, and three extradural cysts (Fig. 20-100, *C* and *D*) (Nugent et al., 1959; Banna and Gryspeerdt, 1971), one of which was traumatic in origin (Fig. 20-100, *D*) (Shahinfar and Schechter, 1966). All occurred in the thoracic spine.

Two cysts had normal spinal radiographs, one with some pediculate thinning and scoliosis. Two were connected with the subarachnoid space at myelography. Two were anteriorly, and one was posteriorly, placed. A congenital dural defect may account for the herniation of arachnoid; these differ from intraspinal meningoceles insofar as no associated spinal dysraphia is present. There was one additional cyst which was an intradural space-occupying mass rather than merely a loculation of the subarachnoid space (Palmer, 1974).

Care must be taken not to misdiagnose prolapsed tonsils in the Chiari malformation as a neoplastic mass lesion in the cervical spinal canal at myelography (Fig. 20-100, *E*).

Other rare lesions with which we have not had experience are intramedullary and intradural-extramedullary tuberculomas (Lin, 1960; Jakoby and Koos, 1961), cryptococcosis (Skultety, 1961), schistosomiasis granuloma (Bird, 1964), intraspinal mass lesions of spinal cord compression due to extramedullary hematopoiesis (Sorsdahl et al., 1964), lymphangioma (Epstein, 1966), and hemangioendothelioma.

REFERENCES

Allen, J. P., Myers, G. G., and Condon, V. R.: Laceration of the spinal cord related to breech delivery, J.A.M.A. 208: 1019, 1969.

Appleby, A., Bradley, W. G., Foster, J. B., Hankinson, J., and Hudgson, P.: Syringomyelia due to chronic arachnoiditis at the foramen magnum, J. Neurol. Sci. 8:451, 1969.

Baker, G. S., and Rydell, R. E.: Dandy-Walker malformation: association with syringomyelia, Minn. Med. 54:889, 1971.

Banna, M., and Gryspeerdt, G. L.: Intraspinal tumours in children (excluding dysraphism), Clin. Radiol. 22:17, 1971.

Banna, M., Pearce, G. W., and Uldall, R.: Scoliosis; a rare manifestation of intrinsic tumours of the spinal cord in children, J. Neurol. Neurosurg. Psychiatry 34:637, 1971.

Barnett, H. J. M., Botterell, E. H., Jousse, A. T., and Wynn-Jones, M.: Progressive myelography as a sequel to traumatic paraplegia, Brain 89:159, 1966.

Barnett, H. J. M., Foster, J. B., and Hudgson, P.: Syringomyelia; major problems in neurology, vol. 1, Philadelphia, 1973, W. B. Saunders Co.

Bentley, J. F. R., and Smith, J. R.: Developmental posterior enteric remnants and spinal malformations, Arch. Dis. Child. 35:76, 1960.

Benzian, S. R., Mainzer, F., and Gooding, C. A.: Pediculate thinning; a normal variant at the thoracolumbar junction, Br. J. Radiol. 44:936, 1971.

Bertrand, G.: Dynamic factors in the evolution of syringomyelia and syringobulbia, Clin. Neurosurg. 20:322, 1973.

Bharati, R. S., and Kalyanaraman, S.: Epidural spinal lymphoma in an infant, J. Neurosurg. 39:412, 1973.

Bird, A. V.: Acute spinal schistosomiasis, Neurology 14:647, 1964.

Black, S. P. W., and Keats, T. E.: Generalized osteosclerosis secondary to metastatic medulloblastoma of the cerebellum, Radiology 82:395, 1964.

Blackwood, W., McMenemey, W. H., Meyer, A., Norman, R. M., and Russell, D. S., editors: Greenfield's neuropathology, ed. 2, London, 1963, Edward Arnold (Publishers), Ltd.

Boyd, H. R.: Iatrogenic intraspinal epidermoid, J. Neurosurg. 24:105, 1966.

Bremer, J. L.: Dorsal intestinal fistula; accessory neurenteric canal; diastematomyelia, Arch. Pathol. 54:132, 1952.

Caffey, J.: Pediatric x-ray diagnosis, vol. 1, ed. 6, Chicago, 1972, Year Book Medical Publishers, Inc.

Cairns, H., and Russell, D. S.: Intracranial and spinal metastases in gliomas of the brain, Brain 54:377, 1931.

Cameron, A. H.: The Arnold-Chiari and other neuroanatomical malformations associated with spina bifida, J. Pathol. Bacteriol. 73:195, 1957.

Caram, P. C., Scarcella, G., and Carton, C. A.: Intradural lipomas of the spinal cord, with particular emphasis on the "intramedullary" lipomas, J. Neurosurg. 14:28, 1957.

Choremis, C., Economos, D., Papadatos, C., and Gargoulas, A.: Intraspinal epidermoid tumours (cholesteatomas) in patients treated for tuberculous meningitis, Lancet 271:439, 1956.

Conway, L. W.: Hydrodynamic studies in syringomyelia, J. Neurosurg. 27:501, 1967.

Cooper, I. S., Craig, W. M., and Kernohan, J. W.: Tumors of the spinal cord, Surg. Gynecol. Obstet. 92:183, 1951.

Cooper, I. S., and Kernohan, J. W.: Heterotopic glial nests in the subarachnoid space. Histopathologic characteristics, mode of origin and relation to meningeal gliomas, J. Neuropathol. Exp. Neurol. 10:16, 1951.

Crabbe, W. A., and Wardill, J. C.: Benign osteoblastoma of the spine, Br. J. Surg. 50:571, 1963.

Craig, R. L.: Epidermoid tumor of the spinal cord, Surgery 13:354, 1943.

Critchley, M., and Greenfield, J. G.: Spinal symptoms in chloroma and leukemia, Brain 53:11, 1930.

Cuneo, H. M.: Invasion of the spinal cord by malignant schwannoma, J. Neurosurg. 14:242, 1957.

D'Angio, G. J., Evans, A. E., and Mitus, A.: Roentgen therapy of certain complications of acute leukemia in childhood, Am. J. Roentgenol. Radium Ther. Nucl. Med. 82:541, 1959.

Dargeon, H. W.: Neuroblastoma, J. Pediatr. 61:456, 1962.

Dodge, H. W. Jr., Keith, H. M., and Campagna, M. J.: Intraspinal tumors in infants and children, J. Int. Coll. Surg. 26: 199, 1956.

Ehni, G., and Love, J. G.: Intraspinal lipomas: Report of

Index